We are pleased to provide you with the **Healthwise® for Life** handbook that offers guidelines on how to recognize and cope with more than 200 of the most common health problems.

In addition to this handbook, our program consists of several new tools that are designed to inform you of the best care for you and your family, **all offered to you at no charge**.

SCAN OnCall

A free health information hotline answered by our registered nurses who can assist you in making the right decisions about your health. Available 24 hours a day, 365 days a year, SCAN OnCall is just a phone call away. Call today: **(800) 793-1717**.

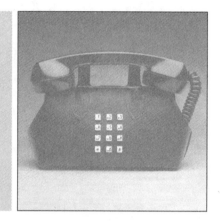

Healthwise® Knowledgebase

Your best online resource for locating comprehensive health information. You and your family can search thousands of health topics to make important lifestyle and treatment decisions.

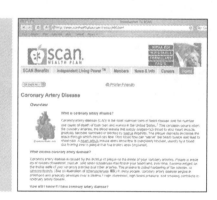

We are continuously striving to better meet all aspects of your health care needs. If you have any questions, please call your SCAN Member Services Department at (800) 559-3500 from 7 a.m. to 6 p.m., Monday through Friday. For the hearing impaired, we offer TDD service at (800) 735-2929.

Thank you for your membership and the opportunity to serve you.

Healthwise® for Life

A Handbook for Healthy Aging

Molly Mettler, MSW, and Donald W. Kemper, MPH

Katy E. Magee, Editor

Steven L. Schneider, MD, and A. Patrice Burgess, MD, Medical Editors

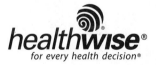
healthwise®
for every health decision®

Healthwise, Incorporated
P.O. Box 1989, Boise, Idaho 83701

Illustrations by Nucleus Communications

Copyright© 1992, 1996, 1998, 2000, 2003, 2004 by Healthwise, Incorporated,
P.O. Box 1989, Boise, Idaho 83701

First Edition, 1992
Fifth Edition, 2003

5th HWFL/SCAN-1st/3-04
ISBN: 1-932921-02-8

Printed in the United States of America.

Table of Contents

Chapter 7: Chest, Lung, and Respiratory Problems 131

Chapter 8: Heart and Circulation Problems 157

About This Book

No book can replace the need for doctors—and no doctor can replace the need for people to care for themselves. This new edition of *Healthwise® for Life* contains the latest medical information to help you make the best decisions about prevention, home treatment, and when to call a doctor for over 200 common health problems specific to adults over 50. This book will also help you and your doctors work together to manage your health problems.

The guidelines in this book come from evidence-based medical information and the input of doctors, nurses, and other health professionals. We have made every effort to present the information in a way that is unbiased, easy to read, and easy to use.

We recommend that you review pages 1 and 2 right away. Page 1, the Healthwise Self-Care Checklist, is a process you can follow every time a health problem arises. Page 2, the Ask-the-Doctor Checklist, will help you get the most out of every doctor visit. You may also wish to read Chapters 1 and 2 before using the rest of the book. Chapter 1, Making Wise Health Decisions, presents a process to make a health decision, ways to develop a partnership with your doctor, and information to reduce your health care costs. Chapter 2, Aging With Vitality, presents information on staying healthy and detecting health problems early. The rest of the book is designed to be used on a topic-by-topic basis whenever a problem or interest develops.

 But this is not just a book. This icon is your link to more in-depth information on the Internet. Simply go to the Web site address listed on the back cover and "search" for the underlined text next to the icon. This will link you to more information about the topic.

If you receive professional advice in conflict with this book, please follow your doctor's advice. Because your doctor is able to take your specific history and needs into consideration, his or her recommendations may prove to be the best. Likewise, if any self-care advice fails to provide positive results within a reasonable period, you should consult a health professional.

This book is as good as we can make it, but we cannot guarantee that it will work for you in every case. Nor will the authors or publishers accept responsibility for any problems that may develop from following its guidelines. This book is only a guide; your common sense and good judgment are also needed.

We wish you the best of health!

Molly Mettler and Donald W. Kemper

About Healthwise

Healthwise is a nonprofit organization whose mission is to help people make better health decisions. We create consumer health information that is based on the most current and reliable medical studies available. Expert writers and editors put medical evidence into user-friendly terms, and a team of nationally recognized medical specialists from key centers of excellence reviews every word.

Healthwise information reaches more than 22 million families worldwide each year through our self-care handbooks, online content, and nurse call center resources. Health plans, employers, hospitals, physician groups, community organizations, government agencies, and e-health care companies trust Healthwise to support successful self-care, shared decision making, and Information Therapy™ programs. Healthwise products and consulting services have been shown to improve health and satisfaction while reducing unnecessary costs.

We publish the *Healthwise® Handbook* (a medical self-care guide for families), *La salud en casa: Guía práctica de Healthwise®* (a Spanish translation of the *Healthwise Handbook*), and *Healthwise® for Life* (a medical self-care guide for adults over 50).

The online content of the Healthwise® Knowledgebase is recognized by many as the most comprehensive and reliable source of consumer health information on the Web. The "More Info" icons in this handbook link the basic self-care information in the handbook to in-depth medical information in the Healthwise Knowledgebase. People trust the Healthwise Knowledgebase for evidence-based, commercially unbiased, and referenced information on thousands of health problems, surgeries, medical tests, treatments, medications, and support groups.

Our readers often provide the best ideas for improving this book. If you have a suggestion that will make this book better, please write to us at *Healthwise Handbook* Suggestions, c/o Healthwise, Incorporated, P.O. Box 1989, Boise, ID 83701, or e-mail us at moreinfo@healthwise.org. To learn more about our health information programs, products, and services, visit our Web site at www.healthwise.org.

Acknowledgements

The 5th edition of *Healthwise for Life* was edited by Katy E. Magee, A. Patrice Burgess, MD, and Steven L. Schneider, MD. We greatly appreciate Jo-Ann Kachigian and Marilyn Allen for their proofreading and editing assistance; Terrie Britton and John Kubisiak for their layout and design work; and Andrea Blum for her production management. Special thanks go to the Healthwise Health Information Team for their invaluable assistance.

We are grateful to the following health professionals who reviewed this edition and shared their wisdom to make it better:

Steven N. Blair, PED
Randall D. Burr, MD
Arden G. Christen, DDS
Lisa Cooper, MD, MPH
Alan C. Dalkin, MD
Seymour Diamond, MD
Terry J. Golden, DO
William M. Green, MD
Carla Herman, MD
Barrie Hurwitz, MD
Peter J. Kahrilas, MD

Robert B. Keller, MD
Robert A. Kloner, MD
Steven T. Kmucha, MD
Joy Melnikow, MD, MPH
Scott H. Pressman, MD
Ruth Schneider, RD, MPH
Avery L. Seifert, MD
Peter Shalit, MD, PhD
Brent T. Shoji, MD
R. Steven Tharratt, MD, FACP, FCCP
Lisa Weinstock, MD

We also wish to thank the hundreds of physicians and other health professionals who have reviewed and helped to improve *Healthwise for Life* over the years.

The Healthwise® Self-Care Checklist

Step 1. Observe the problem.

- When did it start? What are the symptoms? _____
  _____
  _____

- Where is the pain? Dull ache or stabbing pain? _____
  _____

- Measure your vital signs:

  Temperature: _____   Blood pressure:_____/_____

  Pulse: _____/ minute   Breaths:_____/ minute

- Think back:

  Have you had this problem before?   Yes _____   No _____

  What did you do for it? _____
  _____

  Any changes in your life (stress, medications, food, exercise, etc.)?
  _____
  _____

  Does anyone else at home or work have these symptoms?_____
  _____
  _____

Step 2. Learn more about it.

- *Healthwise® for Life* (note page number): _____
- Other books or articles: _____
- Advice from others (lay or professional):_____
- Information on the Internet: _____

Step 3. Make an action plan.

- What do you think is wrong?_____
- What is your home care plan? _____
  _____

- When will you call your doctor? _____

Step 4. Evaluate your progress.

- Are you getting better or worse? _____
  _____
  _____

Ask-the-Doctor Checklist

Before the visit:

- Complete the Healthwise Self-Care Checklist on page 1 and take it with you.
- Take a list of medications you are currently taking. If you have seen a doctor before for similar problems, take the record from the last visit with you.
- Write down the two or three questions you most want answered.

During the visit:

- State your main problem first.
- Describe your symptoms (use page 1).
- Describe past experiences with the same problem.

Write down:

- Temperature: _____   Blood pressure: _____ / _____
- The diagnosis (what is wrong): _____
- The prognosis (what might happen next): _____
- Your self-care plan (what you can do at home): _____

  _____

  _____

For drugs, tests, and treatments, ask:

- What is its name? _____
- Why do I need it? _____
- What are the costs and risks? _____
- Are there alternatives? _____
- What if I do nothing? _____
- (For drugs) How do I take this? _____
- (For tests) How do I prepare? _____

At the end of the visit, ask:

- Am I to return for another visit? _____
- Am I to phone in for test results? _____
- What danger signs should I look for? _____
- When do I need to report back? _____
- What else do I need to know? _____

  _____

I

Making Wise Health Decisions

Throughout your life you will have to make health decisions for yourself and your family. The decisions you make will influence your overall well-being as well as the quality and cost of your care. In general, people who work with their doctors to make health decisions are happier with the care they receive and the results they achieve.

Why should you help make decisions with your doctor? Aren't you paying him or her to know what to do? Well, the choices aren't always black and white. There are often several approaches to diagnosing and treating a health problem, and you are more likely to feel better about the chosen approach if it is the one best suited to your needs and values. Your doctor is an expert on medicine, but you are an expert on yourself.

The best way to make health decisions is to combine the most reliable medical facts with your personal values.

Among your personal values are your beliefs, fears, lifestyle, and experiences. They all play a role in helping you make decisions about your health. Put more simply:

Medical Information + **Your Information** =

Wise Health Decisions

Skills for Making Wise Health Decisions

The following are some simple steps for you to follow when you have a health decision to make. Depending on the decision, the process may take a few minutes or hours, or as long as several weeks. Take as much time as you need to make the decision that is right for you.

1. Find out what your options are. Tell your doctor that you want to share in making a decision. Ask your doctor to clearly state the decision that needs to be made and what your choices are.

2. Get the facts. Learn all about each option by using resources like the library, the Internet, and your doctor. Make sure the information you collect is based on sound medical research, not the results of a single study or facts published by a company that will profit by your using its product.

 In this book, a special icon marks some of the health problems for which having the right information at the right time will help you make better decisions about your care. This form of information therapy is powerful medicine. Read the back cover of this book to learn more about where you can find reliable health information.

3. What do you think? Think about your own needs and values and what you hope the best possible outcome will be. Talk with family members and others who will be affected by your decision. Then sort out the information you've gathered into a list of pros and cons as you see them for each option. You may want to share your list with your doctor to make sure you have all the information you need.

4. Try on a decision. Write down what you expect will happen if you choose a particular option. Ask your doctor if what you expect is reasonable. Ask again about the side effects, pain, recovery time, or long-term outcomes of that option. Then see if you still feel it's the best choice for you.

5. Make an action plan. Once you and your doctor have made a decision, find out what you can do to make sure that you will have the best possible outcome. Write down the steps that you need to take next. Think positively about your decision, and do your part to ensure success by following your doctor's advice. Remember, when you share in making a decision, you share the responsibility for the outcome.

Work in Partnership With Your Doctor

Your relationship with your doctor greatly influences your ability to make wise health decisions and the outcome of your care. Tell your doctor that you want to be a partner in making decisions about your health. Chances are, your doctor will be happy to know that you are interested in taking an active role in your health. Common goals, shared effort, and good communication are the basis of good doctor-patient partnerships.

Skills for Becoming a Good Partner

You can hold up your end of the partnership bargain with your doctor by doing the following:

1. Take good care of yourself. Many health problems can be prevented if you protect yourself and your family by getting immunizations, being screened for health problems, and making healthy lifestyle choices. See Aging With Vitality starting on page 15 for more information about how you can have more control over your health.

2. Practice medical self-care. You can manage a lot of minor problems on your own. All it takes is for you to trust your common sense and monitor how well your efforts are working. Use this book, your own experience, and advice from others to create a self-care plan.

• Use the Healthwise Self-Care Checklist on page 1 to record your self-care plan. Note whether home treatment seems to help. If you do end up calling your doctor or advice nurse, he or she will want to know what your symptoms are; what you've tried to do for the problem; and how well what you tried to do worked.

• Plan a time to call a health professional if the problem continues. If the problem seems to be getting more severe, don't wait too long before calling for help.

3. Prepare for office visits. Most medical appointments are scheduled to last only 10 to 15 minutes. The better organized you are, the more value you can get from the visit.

• Prepare an Ask-the-Doctor Checklist like the one on page 2, and take it with you.

• Complete a self-care checklist like the one on page 1, and take it with you.

• Write down your hunches or fears about what is wrong. These are often helpful to your doctor.

• Write down the three questions that you most want to have answered. There may not be time to ask a long list of questions.

You Have the Right:

• To be spoken to in words that you understand.

• To be told what's wrong with you.

• To read your medical record.

• To know the benefits and risks of any treatment and its alternatives.

• To know what a treatment or test will cost you.

• To share in all treatment decisions.

• To refuse any medical procedure.

Adapted from the American Hospital Association's "Patient's Bill of Rights."

Calling Your Doctor

Is it okay to call your doctor? Of course it is. Often a phone call to the doctor is all you need to manage a problem at home or determine if an appointment is needed. Here's how to get the most from every call:

Prepare for your call. Write down a one-sentence description of your problem. Then list two or three questions you have about the problem.

Have your symptom list handy.

Have your calendar handy in case you need to schedule an appointment.

Leave a clear message. Tell your one-sentence description to the person who answers, and ask to talk with your doctor.

If your doctor is not available, ask the receptionist to relay your message and have someone call you back. Ask when you might expect the return call.

Follow through. When the doctor calls back, briefly describe your problem, ask your questions, and describe any major symptoms.

Some doctors are willing to answer patient questions through e-mail. If e-mail is a convenient way of communicating for you, check with your doctor to see if he or she accepts e-mail from patients.

4. Be an active participant in every medical visit.

- Be honest and straightforward. If you don't intend to take a prescribed medication, say so. If you are getting complementary treatment, such as acupuncture or chiropractic treatments, or taking herbal supplements, let your doctor know. To be a good partner, your doctor has to know what's going on.

- If your doctor recommends a drug, test, or treatment, get more information about the risks and benefits, costs, other alternatives, and the likely outcomes before agreeing to go through with it.

- Take notes. Write down the diagnosis, treatment and follow-up plan, and what you can do at home. Then read your notes back to the doctor to make sure you have it right. If you think it will help, take a friend along to write down what the doctor says while you listen.

5. Learn all you can about your health problem. Throughout this book, special icons mark topics for which more information will help you make better decisions about your care. The information at your disposal—whether you get it from your doctor, the library, or the Internet—is a powerful tool for helping you make wise health decisions.

If you have a complicated problem or want to know more about your health options:

- Start by asking your doctor if he or she has information about your problem that you could take home. Some doctors offer video- or audiotapes, brochures, or reprints from medical journals.

- If your health plan has an advice line, call and ask if they can help you get more information.

- If you use the Internet to find health information, start by searching sources such as the Agency for Healthcare Research and Quality (AHRQ), the Centers for Disease Control and Prevention (CDC), or a national organization that represents a particular disease. Your health plan may also provide health information on its Web site. See Health Information at Home starting on page 392 for tips on finding reliable information.

- The back cover of this book offers tips to help you get more information about health problems and your testing and treatment choices.

- If you have questions or concerns about the information you find, discuss them with your doctor.

A Letter to Your Doctor

If you want your doctor to hear you, write him or her a letter. Good times to write a letter include:

- Before a visit, when you will be discussing a major procedure such as surgery:

  - To ask questions you especially want answered.

  - To express concerns about a procedure or to state your preferences about treatment.

- After a visit or treatment that did not go well for you, to state your concerns and to request a different approach in the future.

- After a visit or treatment that did go well for you, to thank your doctor for what he or she did and to reinforce anything that the doctor did that made a difference to you.

Keep your letter to one page. Present your main concerns or questions clearly. Respect your doctor's expertise and appreciate what has been done well. Suggest a specific plan for dealing with any concerns.

Finding a Doctor Who Will Be a Partner

A primary care physician (family doctor or internist) who knows and understands your needs can be your most valuable health partner. A host of specialists who work on separate health problems may not see your whole health picture or get a good understanding of what's important to you. In choosing a doctor there are lots of questions to ask, but these three matter the most:

• Is the doctor well trained and experienced?

• Will the doctor be available when needed?

• Will the doctor work in partnership with me?

Training and Experience

If you are generally in good health, a good choice for a primary care physician is a board-certified family practice doctor or an internist. These doctors have broad knowledge about many common medical problems. A geriatrician is a doctor who is board-certified in the care of older adults. A doctor becomes board-certified by completing training in a particular specialty area and passing an examination to demonstrate that he or she has the skills and experience needed to practice that medical specialty.

Availability

Because health problems rarely develop when it's convenient, it helps to have a doctor who can be contacted whenever he or she is needed. Before you select a doctor, call or visit his or her office. Tell the clinic receptionist that you are looking for a new doctor. Ask these questions:

• Is the doctor accepting new patients?

• What are the office hours?

• If I called right now for a routine visit, how soon could I be seen?

• How much time is allowed for a routine visit?

• If I cancel an appointment, will I be charged for it?

• Will the doctor discuss health problems over the phone?

• Does the doctor work with nurse practitioners or physician assistants? (These health professionals have special training in managing minor and routine health problems. They can often see you sooner, take care of minor health problems, and communicate with your regular doctor about any concerns.)

• Who fills in for the doctor when he or she is not available?

• What hospitals does the doctor use?

• Is the doctor eligible for maximum payments under my health plan, and will the office complete insurance forms for me?

Partner Potential

During your first visit, tell your doctor that you would like to share in making treatment decisions.

Pay attention to how you feel during the visit.

• Does the doctor listen well?

• Does the doctor speak to you in terms you can understand?

• Does the doctor spend enough time with you?

• Do you think you could build a good working relationship with the doctor?

If the answers are no, look for another doctor. It may take more than one visit for you to decide if you will be able to work with a doctor.

Is It Time for a Change?

If you are unhappy with how your doctor treats you, it may be time for a change. Before you start looking for a new doctor, tell your current doctor how you would like to be treated. Your doctor would probably be pleased to work with you as a partner if only you would tell him or her that's what you want. Otherwise, your doctor may think that you, like many people, want him or her to do all the work.

Skills for Reducing Costs (But Not Quality)

Making wise health decisions can help you reduce your health care costs. The goal is to get just the care you need, nothing more, and certainly nothing less.

It is likely that you will be faced with one or more of the following health decisions at some time. Use the Skills for Making Wise Health Decisions described on page 3 to help you decide if the services or treatments in question are right for you.

1. Should I see a doctor about a health problem? If your symptoms and the guidelines in this book suggest that you should see a doctor, don't put it off. Ignoring problems often leads to complications that are more expensive to treat.

2. Should I have a test (X-rays, blood test, CT or MRI scan, etc.) to diagnose my health problem? Don't agree to any medical test until you understand how it will help you. See page 12 for more information. The only good reason to do a test is because the benefits to you outweigh the risks and costs. No test can be done without your consent.

3. Should I take medication to treat my health problem? Always ask your doctor about any medication he or she prescribes for you. Ask what would happen if you chose not to take a medication. Ask whether there are alternatives to taking medication. See page 13 for more information.

4. Should I have surgery to treat my health problem? Review the questions to ask about surgery on page 14. Get as much information about the surgery as you can, and consider your needs and values. If you are not convinced that the benefits to you outweigh the risks, don't have the surgery.

5. Do I need to go to the emergency room? In life-threatening situations, modern emergency services are vital. However, emergency rooms charge two to three times more for routine services than a doctor's office would. They are not set up to care for routine illnesses, and they do not work on a first-come, first-served basis. During busy times, people with minor illnesses may wait for hours. Also, your records are not available, so emergency room doctors have no information about your medical history.

Use good judgment in deciding when to use emergency medical services. Whenever you feel you can apply home treatment safely and wait to see your regular doctor, do so. However, if you believe your situation requires urgent care, by all means go to the emergency department.

6. Do I need to be hospitalized? More than half of this country's health care dollars are spent on hospitalizations. A stay in a hospital costs far more than a vacation to most luxury resorts. (And hospitals are a lot less fun.)

Skills to Use in the Hospital

When you need to be in the hospital, there are things you can do to improve the quality of the care you receive. However, if you are very sick, ask your spouse or a friend to help watch out for your best interests.

- Ask "why?" Don't agree to anything unless you have a good reason. Agree only to those procedures that make sense for you.

- Provide an extra level of quality control. Check medications, tests, injections, and other treatments to see if they are correct. Your diligence can improve the quality of the care that you receive.

- If you get an itemized bill, check it, and ask about any charges you don't understand.

Don't check in to the hospital just for tests. Ask your doctor if the tests can be done on an outpatient basis. If you agree to control your diet and activities, your doctor will usually support your request.

If you need inpatient care, get in and out of the hospital as quickly as possible. This will reduce costs and your risk of hospital-acquired infections.

Try to avoid additional days in the hospital by bringing in extra help at home. Ask about home nursing services to help while you recover.

If you have a terminal illness, know that hospitalization may not be your only choice. Many people choose to spend their remaining time at home with the people they know and love. Special arrangements can be made through hospice care programs in most communities. Look up "Hospice" in the Yellow Pages directory, or ask your doctor.

7. Should I see a specialist about my health problem? Specialists are doctors who have in-depth training and experience in a particular area of medicine. For example, a cardiologist has years of special training to deal with heart problems. A visit to a specialist often costs more than a visit to your regular doctor, and the tests and treatments that you receive may be more expensive and invasive. Of course, specialists often provide the information you need to help you decide what to do about a specific health problem and can perform certain procedures not available through your primary care doctor.

If you think you need to see a specialist and have not been referred, discuss your concerns with your primary care doctor. When you do have a referral to see a specialist, a little preparation and good communication can help you get your money's worth. Before you go see a specialist:

- Know your diagnosis or expected diagnosis.

- Learn about your basic treatment options.

- Make sure that any test results or records on your case are sent to the specialist.

- Know what your primary care doctor would like the specialist to do (take over the case, confirm the diagnosis, conduct tests, etc.).

- Ask your primary care doctor to remain involved in your care. Ask the specialist to send new test results or recommendations to both you and your regular doctor.

The Advice Nurse

Many health plans and health maintenance organizations (HMOs) offer an advice nurse telephone service. Advice nurses are registered nurses who have special training to answer your questions about health problems and help you decide how to manage minor illnesses.

A call to the advice nurse can often save you a doctor visit or help you decide if you need an urgent or routine appointment.

Advice nurses can also help when your doctor diagnoses a health problem or recommends a test or treatment that you don't fully understand. Sometimes the advice nurse can answer your questions. Other times, he or she may help you come up with questions you can ask your doctor at your next visit.

Shared Decisions About Medical Tests

Medical tests are important tools, but they have limits. Informed consumers know that medical tests have costs and risks as well as benefits.

Learn the facts:

- What is the name of the test, and why do you need it?

- If the test is positive, what will the doctor do differently?

- What could happen if you don't have the test?

Consider the risks and benefits:

- How accurate is the test? How often does it indicate a problem exists when there is none (false positive)? How often does it indicate there is no problem when there is one (false negative)?

- Is the test painful? What can go wrong?

- How will you feel afterward?

- Are there less risky alternatives?

Ask about costs:

- How much does the test cost?

- Is there a less expensive test that might give the same information? If a test seems costly, risky, or not likely to change the recommended treatment, ask your doctor if you can avoid it. Try to agree on the best approach. No test can be done without your permission, and you have the right to refuse to have a test.

Let your doctor know:

- Your concerns about the test.

- What you expect the test will do for you. Ask if that is realistic.

- Any medications (including nonprescription ones) or herbal supplements you are taking.

- Whether you have other medical conditions.

- Whether you prefer to accept or decline the test.

If you agree to a test, ask what you can do to reduce the risk of errors. Should you restrict food, alcohol, exercise, or medication before the test? After the test, ask to review the results. Take notes for your home records. If the results of the test are unexpected and the error rate of the test is high, consider redoing the test before basing further treatment on the results.

Shared Decisions About Medications

The first rule of medications is to know why you need each drug before you use it.

Learn the facts:

- What is the name of the medication, and why do you need it?

- How long does it take to work?

- How long will you need to take it?

- How and when do you take it (with food, on an empty stomach, etc.)?

- Are there nondrug alternatives?

Consider the risks and benefits:

- How much will this medication help?

- Are there side effects or other risks?

- Could this medication interact with other medications or herbal supplements that you currently take?

Ask about costs:

- How much does the medication cost?

- Is a generic form of the medication available and appropriate for you?

- Is there a similar medication that will work almost as well and be less expensive?

- Can you start with a prescription for a smaller quantity to make sure the medication agrees with you?

Let your doctor know:

- Your concerns about the medication.

- What you expect it will do. Ask if that is realistic.

- About any other medications (including nonprescription ones) or herbal supplements you are taking.

- Whether you prefer to take the medication or try other ways of treating the problem.

Shared Decisions About Surgery

Every surgery has risks. Only you can decide if the benefits are worth the risks.

Learn the facts:

- What is the name of the surgery? Get a description of the surgery.

- Why does your doctor think you need the surgery?

- Are there other options besides surgery?

- Is this surgery the most common one for this problem? Are there other types of surgery?

Consider the risks and benefits:

- How many similar surgeries has the surgeon performed? How many surgeries like this are done at this hospital?

- What is the success rate? What does success mean to your doctor? What would success mean to you?

- What can go wrong? How often does this happen?

- How will you feel afterward? How long will it be until you're fully recovered?

- How can you best prepare for the surgery and the recovery period?

Ask about costs:

- How much does the surgery cost? How can you find out?

- Can it be done on an outpatient basis, and is that less expensive?

Let your doctor know:

- How much the problem really bothers you. Are you willing to put up with symptoms to avoid surgery?

- Your concerns about the surgery.

- Whether or not you want to have the surgery at this time.

- If you want a second opinion. Second opinions are helpful if you have any doubt that the proposed surgery is the best option for your problem. If you want a second opinion, ask your primary care doctor or your surgeon to recommend another specialist. Ask that your test results be sent to the second doctor. Consider getting an opinion from a doctor who isn't a surgeon and who treats similar problems.

If I had known I was going to live this long,
I would have taken better care of myself.
Eubie Blake

2

Aging With Vitality

This chapter is all about making healthy lifestyle choices that can help you feel your best for all the years to come.

There is no doubt that your body changes as you age, but those changes don't have to lead to health problems. Even if certain health problems run in your family, you may be able to prevent them or keep them from getting worse by making healthy lifestyle choices. Research is showing that genetics play a smaller role in aging and age-related illnesses than was once thought. The lifestyle choices you make and your outlook on life often have a greater influence on your health than your genes do.

Aging with vitality means more than just staving off disease. It means having energy and enthusiasm for daily activities, maintaining relationships, contributing to your community, and nourishing your spirit. Even if you have

a chronic illness like diabetes or heart disease, you can make lifestyle choices that may help you maintain your vigor, your independence, and your zest for life.

Perhaps the most important message to keep in mind as you read this chapter is that your body will benefit from healthy lifestyle choices no matter when you make them. With the right attitude and enough support, you can develop new habits that will have a positive effect on your health and well-being. It's never too late to get started.

Keys to Healthy Aging

There is no magic to vitality and health in old age. The best approach to good health at any age is to develop good health habits and stick with them. Let these keys be your general guide.

Keep Your Body Moving

Keeping physically fit may be the single most important thing you can do to maintain your health. Find an activity that you enjoy, such as walking, swimming, or dancing, and do it regularly. If exercise is already a part of your life, keep up the good work. If you aren't physically active, there's good news: exercise doesn't have to be vigorous to improve your health. Many everyday activities, such as gardening and housework, raise your heart rate and, if done regularly, will keep your heart and lungs healthy, make your muscles stronger, and improve your flexibility. For more specific information about staying fit, see Fitness starting on page 285.

Eat Right

What you choose to eat affects many aspects of your health. Your diet plays an important role in helping you:

- Get the nutrition your body needs.
- Maintain a healthy weight.
- Prevent problems such as constipation, heart disease, diabetes, and certain cancers.
- Treat diseases such as diabetes and high blood pressure.

For more information about how you can evaluate and improve your diet, see Nutrition starting on page 301.

Maintain a Healthy Body Weight

Healthy bodies come in all shapes and sizes. People tend to focus on how much they weigh, but your weight may say very little about your overall health. Other important measurements of health include:

- Your fitness level.
- The quality of your diet and your eating habits.
- Whether you use tobacco or drink alcohol to excess.
- Whether you have a chronic condition like high blood pressure, high cholesterol, heart disease, or diabetes.
- How fat is distributed on your body (people who have more fat around their waists are at higher risk for heart disease than are people who have more fat on their hips and thighs).
- Your self-esteem and body image.

 No matter what your shape or size, you can improve your health by eating a balanced diet, getting regular exercise, and learning to feel good about your body. You can improve your health without changing your weight. The amount you weigh now could be, or could become, a <u>healthy weight</u> for you.

Body Mass Index

Your body mass index (BMI) is based on your height and weight. A healthy BMI for an adult is between 18.5 and 24.9. Disease risk increases both above and below this BMI range. A person whose BMI is 30 or higher is said to be obese.

Use the following table to look up the upper and lower weight limits for your height. The height is given in inches and the weight in pounds.

Height	Healthy weight based on BMI of 18.5 to 24.9
58	89–120
59	92–124
60	95–128
61	98–132
62	102–137
63	105–141
64	108–146
65	112–150
66	115–155
67	119–160
68	122–164
69	126–169
70	130–174
71	133–179
72	137–184
73	141–190
74	145–195
75	149–200
76	153–206

What Is a Healthy Weight?

If you think that your current weight puts you at risk for health problems, talk to your health professional about different ways you can manage your weight. Most people are concerned about being overweight, but for some people being underweight is a health concern. Being **obese** (having a body mass index of 30 or greater; see the chart on page 17) can increase your risk of developing joint problems, high blood pressure, high cholesterol, heart disease, type 2 diabetes, sleep apnea, some cancers, and other long-term illnesses. Losing as little as 5 to 10 percent of your body weight can do good things for your health, such as lowering your blood pressure, reducing other risk factors for heart disease, and lowering your blood sugar level if you have diabetes.

Set Realistic Goals

Before you start a weight management program, think about your goals and expectations and whether you are ready to make changes in your lifestyle. Diets often fail because goals are set too high and the focus is only on how much you weigh. Realistic goals for weight management should include:

- Reducing your risk for health problems.

- Increasing your fitness level by becoming more physically active.

- Making positive lifestyle changes that will become lifelong habits.

Tools for Achieving a Healthy Weight

Set your body in motion.

Regular physical activity makes you feel stronger and more energetic. It also improves your overall health. Physical activity makes your body burn more calories, not just while you're exercising, but throughout the day. So if you exercise regularly and eat a healthy diet, you will find it easier to manage your weight. In addition, regular exercise builds muscle. Increasing the amount of lean muscle in your body is healthier for you and will make your body look more toned. For tips on making regular physical activity a part of your healthy lifestyle, see Fitness starting on page 285.

Plan your meals.

People who eat regular meals find it easier to maintain a healthy weight than do people who overeat, skip meals, or snack. Skipping meals usually leads to feelings of deprivation, which can lead to overeating at the next meal or eating a less-than-nutritious snack.

Meals that are planned are usually more balanced than those that are grabbed at the last minute. Taking time to plan what you eat will improve your diet and can help you control your weight.

Focus on reducing fat.

Eat a variety of nutritious, low-fat foods. Rather than counting the exact number of calories you eat, focus on eating more fruits, vegetables, and whole grains and less fat.

A low-fat diet (less than 30 to 35 percent of total calories from fat) will help you control your weight and reduce your risk of developing heart disease, high blood pressure, cancer, and other diseases. For tips on how to cut fat from your diet, see page 307.

Enjoy your food.

You can enjoy all the foods you love and still control your weight. The key is to be sensible about how much you eat and to balance your calorie intake with calorie burn-off (daily activities and exercise). Here are some tips:

- Enjoy your steak (or cake) twice as much: eat half in the restaurant and take the rest home to enjoy the next day.

- When dining out, plan what you are going to eat before you go to the restaurant. Stick with your plan.

- Have one helping of your favorite food and enjoy every bite.

- Craving an ice cream cone? Walk to the ice cream shop, have a single dip, and walk home.

All foods can fit into a healthy diet; the proper balance of those foods is what's most important. For more guidance on how to include a variety of foods in your diet, see the Food Guide Pyramid on page 304.

Be Tobacco-Free

In addition to exercising regularly and eating a healthy diet, being tobacco-free is one of the most important things you can do to improve your own health and the health of those around you. Tobacco use increases your risk for many health problems, including cancer, heart disease, and stroke. Your tobacco use puts others at risk as well. Secondhand smoke (the smoke other people breathe from your burning cigarettes and exhaled smoke) causes lung and other cancers, heart disease, and a long list of other health problems in nonsmokers.

It's never too late to quit. No matter how much tobacco you use or how long you've been using it, once you stop, it doesn't take long for your body to start to heal and for your risk of developing other health problems to decrease.

- When you quit smoking, your risk of heart attack is cut in half within 1 year after you quit. Five years after quitting, your risk is about the same as that of a person who never smoked.

- While the lung damage that smoking causes is not reversible, quitting smoking prevents more lung damage from occurring. Coughing and shortness of breath will decrease.

- When you give up tobacco, damage to your lips, tongue, mouth, and throat is reduced. Your risk for mouth and throat cancer decreases.

- If you have asthma, you will have fewer and less severe asthma attacks after you quit smoking.

- After quitting smoking, a man may have fewer problems getting and maintaining an erection.

Quitting is not easy. If you have already tried to quit, you know how difficult it is. But don't give up—with the right attitude and enough help, you'll eventually succeed.

Cigars and Smokeless Tobacco

Many people who smoke cigars feel it is safe because they do not inhale the cigar smoke. Think again. Holding cigars and cigar smoke in your mouth increases your risk for cancers of the mouth, tongue, throat, and voice box (larynx).

Smokeless tobacco, or snuff, can be chewed, inhaled, or held in your cheek. There is a direct link between using these products and developing mouth and throat cancer.

Here are some facts you should know about cigars and smokeless tobacco:

- They contain nitrosamines, which cause cancer.

- They contain nicotine, which raises your heart rate and blood pressure.

- They may produce leukoplakias (wrinkled, thick, white patches) on the inside of your mouth. Leukoplakias can develop into mouth cancer.

Tips for Quitting

 No one can tell you when or how to quit smoking or chewing tobacco. Only you know why you use tobacco and what will be most difficult as you try to quit. The important thing is that you try. Believe that you will succeed, if not the first time, then the second time, or twenty-second time.

Prepare

- List the reasons why you want to quit using tobacco: to improve your own health and your family's health, to save money, or whatever. Read through the list every day, and keep it handy as a reminder of how important quitting is.

- Figure out why you smoke. Do you use tobacco to pep yourself up? To relax? Do you like the ritual of smoking or chewing? Do you use tobacco out of habit? If specific situations trigger your desire to use tobacco, changing your routine so that you can temporarily avoid those situations may help you stop.

- Decide how and when you will quit. About half of ex-tobacco users quit "cold turkey." The other half cut down more slowly. If you plan to go through a quit smoking program, choose a reliable one. Good programs have at least a 20 percent success rate after 1 year. Great programs have a 50 percent success rate. A higher success rate may be too good to be true.

- Plan things to do to distract yourself when you get the urge to smoke or chew. Urges don't last that long: take a walk, brush your teeth, have a mint, drink a glass of water, or chew gum.

- Find something healthy to replace what smoking or chewing does for you. For example, if you like to have something to do with your hands, pick up something else: a coin, worry beads, a pen, or a pencil. If you like to have something in your mouth, substitute sugarless gum or minted toothpicks.

- Plan a healthful reward for yourself for when you have stopped using tobacco. Take the money you save by not buying tobacco and spend it on yourself.

Act

- Set a quit date and stick to it. Choose a time that will be busy but not stressful.

- Remove ashtrays and all other reminders of using tobacco. Dry-clean your clothes to get rid of the tobacco smell. Have your teeth cleaned. Choose non-smoking sections in restaurants. Avoid alcohol. Do things that reduce the likelihood of using tobacco, like taking a walk or going to a movie.

- Ask for help and support. Choose a trusted friend, preferably another former tobacco user, to give you a helping hand over the rough spots.

- Know what to expect. The worst will be over in just a few days, but physical withdrawal symptoms may last 1 to 3 weeks. After that, it is all psychological. See Mind-Body Wellness starting on page 337 for relaxation tips.

- Keep low-calorie snacks handy for when the urge to munch hits. Your appetite may perk up, but most people gain fewer than 10 pounds when they quit using tobacco. The health benefits of quitting outweigh the risk of gaining a few extra pounds.

- Get out and exercise. It will distract you, help keep off unwanted pounds, and release tension.

Aids for Quitting Tobacco Use

Nicotine replacement products can help you break the habit of using tobacco and prevent nicotine withdrawal symptoms. The products deliver nicotine to the bloodstream without the dangerous tars, carbon monoxide, and other chemicals released by tobacco and smoke. You gradually reduce the amount of nicotine you give yourself until your body is no longer dependent on nicotine.

Nicotine replacement treatment comes in four forms: chewing gum, skin patches, nasal sprays, and inhalers.

All nicotine replacement products cause side effects. You may need to try more than one product before finding the one that works best for you.

Using a nicotine replacement product works best if you also enroll in a tobacco cessation program. Such programs help you deal with the habit of using tobacco, while the nicotine replacement product helps you manage your cravings for nicotine and overcome your addiction to it.

Medications that do not contain nicotine are available to help control irritability and cravings when you quit using tobacco. These medications are available only with a doctor's prescription. First try to stop using tobacco without medications. Many people are successful without them.

• Don't be discouraged by slipups. It often takes several tries to quit using tobacco for good. If you do slip up, forgive yourself and learn from the experience. You will not fail as long as you keep trying. Good luck!

Use Alcohol and Drugs Wisely

Alcohol and drug use can be very hard on your body. Alcohol, in particular, increases your risk for accidents and injuries by impairing your mental alertness, judgment, memory, and physical coordination. What's more, many of the prescription and nonprescription medications that older adults take increase the intoxicating effect of alcohol.

Long-term overuse of alcohol increases your risk for many illnesses, including liver disease, high blood pressure, and certain cancers. It can also put your relationships and livelihood in jeopardy.

Limit your consumption of alcoholic beverages to no more than 2 drinks per day if you are a man and no more than 1 drink per day if you are a woman. One drink equals 12 ounces of beer, 5 ounces of wine, or 1½ ounces of hard liquor.

Never use prescription or nonprescription medications along with alcohol.

Many medications, even as they are doing good, also have some risks. Go over your list of medications with your doctor regularly. Review all the prescription and nonprescription medications you take, and determine whether they are necessary. However, don't stop taking a medication unless your doctor tells you it is all right to do so. For more tips on good medication management, see page 378.

If alcohol or drug abuse is a problem for you or someone close to you, now is the time to seek help. For more information about alcohol and drug problems, see page 319.

Keep Up With Shots and Screenings

Immunizations provide protection against many serious diseases. Chances are, you have been immunized against the major childhood illnesses, or you are immune because you had the diseases when you were a child.

However, there are several immunizations that need to be updated throughout your life or given for the first time later in life. If your doctor does not suggest them to you, make a note to mention them at your next visit.

Tetanus

Tetanus (lockjaw) is a bacterial infection that can be fatal. The bacteria enter the body through a deep cut or puncture wound. The only sure protection against tetanus is immunization. Many cases of tetanus occur in adults over age 50 who have forgotten to keep their tetanus immunizations up to date.

Routine boosters are recommended every 10 years throughout your life to maintain immunity. If you are age 50 or older and have not had boosters every 10 years, now is a good time to talk to your doctor about updating your tetanus boosters. If you suffer a puncture wound or deep cut, get a booster shot if you haven't had one in the past 5 years.

Influenza

Influenza (flu) is a contagious viral illness that causes fever and chills, head and muscle aches, fatigue, weakness, sneezing, and runny nose. (See Influenza on page 147.)

Older people are more likely to develop complications of influenza, such as pneumonia and dehydration.

To protect yourself, get a flu shot each autumn if any one of the following applies to you:

• You are age 50 or older.

• You have a chronic lung disease, such as asthma or emphysema.

• You have heart disease.

• You have diabetes.

• You have sickle cell anemia or another red blood cell disorder.

• You have an illness that has weakened your immune system or are taking medication that weakens the immune system.

Health Screening Schedule

Recommended Time Intervals Between Preventive Services
(For more information about this chart, see page 25.)

Preventive Service	Age 50–64	Age 65+	Comments
Blood pressure (p. 165)	1–2 years	1–2 years	More often if your blood pressure is high.
Cholesterol (p. 312)	5 years	5 years	More often if you have risk factors for heart disease (see p. 313). Talk with your doctor about screening after age 65 even if your cholesterol levels have been normal.
Colorectal cancer screening (pp. 70 to 71) • Blood in stool test (fecal occult blood test) • Flexible sigmoidoscopy • Colonoscopy	 1 year 3–5 years 10 years (5 if high-risk)	 1 year 3–5 years 10 years (5 if high-risk)	Screening may involve one or more of these tests. Talk with your doctor about which tests and screening schedules are most appropriate for you. More frequent screening with flexible sigmoidoscopy or colonoscopy is recommended if you have risk factors for colorectal cancer (see p. 70).
Hearing test	Assess during other regular visits.		
Vision test	2–5 years	1–2 years	More often for people who have eye diseases or diabetes.
Glaucoma test	Usually done as part of regular eye exams.		
Dental exam	6 months	6 months	
Men Only			
Prostate cancer screening (p. 272)	1 year	1 year	May include digital rectal exam (DRE) or prostate-specific antigen (PSA) test. Talk with your doctor to determine whether screening is appropriate for you.

Health Screening Schedule

Recommended Time Intervals Between Preventive Services
(For more information about this chart, see page 25.)

Preventive Service	Age 50–64	Age 65+	Comments
Women Only			
Clinical breast exam (p. 256)	1–2 years	1–2 years	Discuss appropriate frequency with your doctor.
Mammogram (p. 255)	1–2 years	1–2 years	Discuss appropriate frequency and whether to discontinue the exam after age 70 with your doctor.
Pelvic exam (p. 258)	1 year	1 year	
Pap test (p. 258)	1–3 years	1–3 years	May discontinue after age 65 if prior exams were normal and you have no significant risk factors for cervical cancer. If you have had a hysterectomy, talk to your health professional about whether and how often you need a Pap test.
Immunizations			
Tetanus booster (p. 22)	10 years	10 years	
Flu shot (p. 22)	1 year	1 year	Given in fall. Recommended before age 50 if you have chronic lung disease, heart disease, diabetes, or an impaired immune system.
Pneumococcal vaccine (p. 25)		Once	Recommended before age 65 if high-risk. Booster may be needed if high-risk.

• You have frequent contact with people who could develop complications if they caught the flu from you (for example, nursing home residents, people over age 65, and people who have weakened immune systems).

• You want to reduce your risk of getting the flu.

Side effects of the flu shot, such as a low-grade fever and minor aches, are usually mild and do not last long. Don't get a flu shot if you are allergic to eggs: the virus in the vaccine is grown in eggs, and you may develop an allergic reaction.

Pneumococcal Infection

Most people think of pneumococci as the bacteria that cause pneumonia, but pneumococci can also infect the blood (bacteremia) or the covering of the brain (meningitis). Older people have a higher risk than younger people of developing pneumonia and other pneumococcal infections.

A one-time-only dose of the pneumococcal vaccine is recommended for people age 65 and older. You can get the pneumococcal vaccine at the same time as your yearly flu shot. Get a pneumococcal vaccine if:

• You are healthy, over 65, and have never received the shot.

• You have a chronic illness, such as cancer, an immune system disorder, diabetes, or heart, lung, or kidney disease.

If you received the pneumococcal vaccine before age 65 and it has been more than 5 years since you last had the shot, ask your doctor if you need a booster shot.

Side effects of the shot often include mild swelling and pain at the injection site.

Other Immunizations

Immunization against hepatitis A is recommended in some parts of the country. Ask your health professional if you should receive this vaccine.

If you are in close contact with people who have contagious diseases or you are planning travel to areas where illnesses such as hepatitis A, typhoid, cholera, and yellow fever are common, contact your local health department to find out if you need to be immunized. While there is no vaccine to prevent malaria, your doctor can prescribe medication for you to take to prevent the disease if you are traveling to an area where malaria is known to occur.

Periodic Medical Exams and Screening Tests

Another way to protect your health is to detect diseases early, when they may be easier to treat. You can do this in two ways: by getting periodic medical exams from a health professional and by becoming a good observer of changes in your own body.

The Health Screening Schedule on pages 23 and 24 will help you decide which tests are right for you and how often you should have them. Recommended immunizations are also listed. The recommendations apply to people of average risk in each age group. If you are at high risk for certain diseases, you may need more frequent exams and tests. Factors that may help your doctor determine your level of risk include your overall health, your family history (whether your close relatives have had certain diseases), and lifestyle factors, such as whether you use tobacco, how often you exercise, and your sexual history.

The most appropriate schedule of preventive exams is one you and your doctor agree upon, based on your age, your risk factors for disease, how healthy you are, and how important periodic health screening is to you.

Self-Exams

Periodic self-exams are also an important part of staying healthy. See Breast Self-Exam on page 256. Turn to page 247 to learn how to look for changes in your skin that may be early signs of skin cancer.

Tuberculin Test

A tuberculin test is done to determine if you have been infected with the bacteria that cause tuberculosis (TB). See page 144.

Whether you need to be tested depends on how common TB is in your area and your risk of coming in contact with the bacteria that cause TB. If you think you may have been exposed to TB and wish to be tested, contact your doctor or the local health department.

Manage Stress

Stress is practically unavoidable, but it doesn't have to have a negative impact on your health and well-being.

By learning how to deal with stress in ways that make you feel more in control, you may be able to improve your health, your relationships, and your outlook on life.

 It shouldn't surprise you that some of the key factors in helping you manage stress are eating a healthy diet, getting regular exercise and enough sleep, avoiding drugs and tobacco, and drinking alcohol only in moderation. All these lifestyle factors work together.

For more information about how stress can affect your health and how you can identify and deal with the sources of stress in your life, see Mind-Body Wellness starting on page 337.

Practice Safety

Accidents do happen, but they don't have to happen to you. Many older adults are injured in car accidents, fires, and falls. Follow these safety precautions to reduce the risk of fire in your home and to make the roads safer for you and your fellow drivers. For tips on preventing falls, see page 48. For information about using prescription and nonprescription medications safely, see Managing Your Medications beginning on page 378.

Fire Safety

- Post emergency telephone numbers near telephones.

- Have an emergency exit plan in case of fire. Practice the plan.

- Install smoke detectors in or near every bedroom and on every level of your home. Test the alarms once a month, and change the batteries at least once a year.

- Keep multipurpose fire extinguishers in the kitchen and near fireplaces or woodstoves. Shake the extinguisher once a month to make sure the chemicals don't settle to the bottom. Have the extinguisher inspected yearly. Practice using the fire extinguisher in a non-emergency situation, and have it recharged after you use it.

- Turn off appliances after use. Replace frayed or damaged electrical cords on appliances.

- Don't run electrical cords under rugs or furniture. Keep cords away from bathtubs, showers, and sinks.

- Install special safety outlets in your bathroom. Ask for a ground fault circuit interrupter.

- Never smoke in bed or when you are sleepy.

- Don't tuck in electric blankets, and don't cover them with other blankets. Turn the temperature down before you go to bed.

- Avoid using electric, kerosene, and propane heaters. If you must use them, keep them away from curtains, rugs, and furniture.

- Clean woodstove and fireplace chimneys at least once a year.

- Keep objects such as kitchen towels and paper wrappers away from the stove top. Roll up loose long sleeves when cooking.

- Select a stove with controls that clearly show when the burners are on.

- If your clothing catches fire:

  - Do not run, because running will fan the flames. Stop, drop, and roll on the ground to smother the flames. Or smother the flames with a blanket, rug, or coat.

  - Use water to douse the fire and cool your skin.

Automobile Safety

- Always wear a seat belt, especially if your car has air bags.

- Never drink and drive.

- Check with your doctor or pharmacist about driving while on medications, especially if you take insulin or an oral diabetes medication. Medications, including some nonprescription drugs, can cause dizziness, drowsiness, impaired judgment, and balance problems.

- Be sure that your car is properly tuned and equipped with emergency supplies.

- Consider updating your driving skills by taking a driver's safety course. (AARP offers a good one, as do many hospitals.)

- Have your vision checked regularly, and always wear prescription eyewear when driving.

- Wear high-quality sunglasses to reduce glare.

- If your night vision is limited, don't drive at night.

- If your hearing is limited, keep a window open and the radio volume low.

Stay Mentally Active

The "use it or lose it" approach definitely applies to brain power. Memory loss and decreased mental function are not inevitable aspects of aging. The brain benefits from exposure to stimulating environments and activities, and this stimulation can help you regain your memory and stay sharp.

Learn something new every day. Take classes or read books about new subjects. Read, write, talk, and think about what interests you. For more information about preventing memory loss, see page 331.

Nurture the Ties That Bind

People who have many social ties are healthier than people with few social connections. Examples of social ties are being married, having contact with friends and relatives, belonging to a church or social group, and volunteering to help others.

Create a support network of family and friends who will help see you through a crisis. Find a friend you can confide in. Be a confidant for someone else.

Combine physical and social health by joining a walking group or exercise class.

Know Where Your Help Is

The best way to stay independent is to know when to ask for help. Become familiar with your community's support services for seniors, such as transportation, financial counseling, and Meals on Wheels. See your local senior center or Area Agency on Aging for information on available services. Also see Staying Independent starting on page 357.

Accentuate the Positive

The pictures we have in our minds and the verbal messages or self-talk we give ourselves affect both our minds and bodies.

Expect good things to happen. Count your blessings and express thanks. Add humor, laughter, and fun into every day. Also see Mind-Body Wellness starting on page 337.

Celebrate Your Wisdom

Victor Hugo said, "One sees a flame in the eyes of the young, but in the eyes of the old, one sees light." More than anything else, the world needs wisdom. Recognize your purpose for living. Think about your values and beliefs. Help others to gain wisdom too. Consider becoming a mentor. You could be the one to make all the difference in the world to someone else.

Be prepared.
Boy Scout Motto

3

First Aid and Emergencies

This chapter will inform you about what you can do to avoid injuries, be prepared for emergencies, and handle minor first aid situations.

Review this chapter before you need it. Then, when you are faced with an emergency, you will know where to turn. Your confidence in dealing with both major and minor emergencies will be reassuring to an injured person.

For your own safety and to help you respond quickly in case of an emergency, do the following:

• Keep first aid supplies on hand. See the Self-Care Supplies chart on page 376.

• Know who to call in an emergency. Keep emergency contact numbers next to every phone in your home.

• Keep in touch with neighbors, relatives, or friends every day if you live alone. Ask them to check up on you if they haven't heard from you.

• Wear a medical ID bracelet or necklace that gives information about any medical conditions or drug allergies you have and any medications you are taking.

• Consider registering with a medical alarm service, which provides a necklace or other item you can wear that allows you to get immediate help, 24 hours a day, with the push of a button.

Dealing With Emergencies

If you are faced with an emergency, try to stay calm. Take a deep breath and count to 10. Tell yourself you can handle the situation.

Assess the danger. Protect yourself and the injured person from fire, explosions, or other hazards. If you suspect that the injured person has a spinal injury, do not move the person unless the danger is immediate and life-threatening.

Prepare for the Emergency Room

• If possible, call ahead to let emergency room staff know you are coming.

• Call your doctor, if possible. He or she may meet you at the emergency room or call in important information.

• If you think you may have to wait to be seen by a doctor, take this book and your home medical records with you. While you are waiting you can:

 - Use page 1, the Healthwise Self-Care Checklist, to help you think through the problem and report symptoms to the doctor.

 - Use page 2, the Ask-the-Doctor Checklist, to organize questions for the doctor.

 - Review the medical test checklist on page 12.

 - Use your home medical records (see page 380) to prepare to discuss your medications, past test results, or treatments. Information about your allergies, medications, and health conditions may be critical.

If the person is unconscious or unresponsive, check the ABCs: Airway, Breathing, Circulation. If the person is not breathing, see Rescue Breathing and CPR on page 37.

Identify and prioritize the injuries. Treat the most life-threatening problems, like bleeding and shock, first. Check for broken bones and other injuries. If you need emergency assistance, call 911 or other emergency services, such as the local fire department, sheriff, or hospital.

Legal Protection

If you are needed in an emergency, give what help you can. Most states have a Good Samaritan law to protect people who help in an emergency. You cannot be sued for giving first aid unless it can be shown that you are guilty of gross negligence.

Bites and Stings

Insect and spider bites and bee, yellow jacket, and wasp stings usually cause a localized reaction with pain, swelling, redness, and itching. In most cases, bites and stings do not cause reactions all over the body. In some parts of the world, mosquitoes may spread illnesses, including encephalitis and malaria.

Some people have severe skin reactions to insect or spider bites or stings, and a few have severe allergic reactions (called anaphylaxis) that affect the whole body. Symptoms of a severe allergic reaction may include hives all over the body, shortness of breath and tightness in the chest, dizziness, wheezing, swelling of the tongue and face, lightheadedness, confusion, and shock. Anaphylactic reactions are not common but can be life-threatening and require emergency care.

Spider bites are rarely serious, although any bite may be serious if it causes a person to have an allergic reaction.

Black widow spider bites may cause chills, fever, nausea, muscle spasms, and severe stomach pain. A bite from a brown recluse (fiddler) spider or a hobo (Northwestern brown) spider may result in intense pain and a blister that turns into a larger, open sore. Other symptoms (headache, dizziness, drowsiness, nausea) may occur after the bite.

Ticks are small, spiderlike insects that bite into the skin and feed on blood. Most ticks do not carry diseases, and most tick bites do not cause serious health problems. However, it is important to remove a tick from your body as soon as you find one.

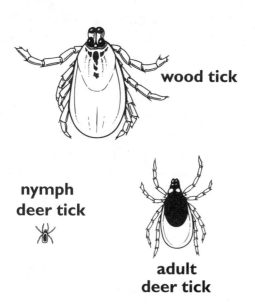

wood tick

nymph deer tick

adult deer tick

Adult deer ticks are about the size of an apple seed. All ticks grow larger as they fill up with blood.

Many of the diseases ticks may pass on to humans (including Rocky Mountain spotted fever, relapsing fever, Colorado tick fever, and Lyme disease) have the same initial flulike symptoms. Sometimes a rash or craterlike sore may accompany the flulike symptoms. An expanding red rash is an early symptom of Lyme disease. It may appear 1 day to 1 month after you have been bitten by a deer tick.

Jellyfish are common on some ocean beaches. If touched, their tentacles release a stinging venom that causes a painful reaction.

Prevention

• To avoid bee stings, wear white or light-colored, solid fabrics. Bees are attracted to dark colors and flowered prints. Also avoid wearing perfumes and colognes when you are outside.

• Before going outdoors in tick-infested areas, put on light-colored clothing and tuck your pant legs into your socks.

• Wear gloves and tuck your pants into your socks when working in woodpiles, sheds, and basements where spiders are found.

• Apply an insect repellent containing DEET to clothing and exposed areas of skin every few hours when you are in areas infested with insects, spiders, or ticks. Apply the repellent carefully around your eyes and mouth. Wash the repellent off after you go inside. Alpha Keri and Skin-So-Soft bath oils and lotions also seem to repel insects.

Animal and Human Bites

When they are bitten by an animal, most people want to know if they need a rabies shot. The main wild animal carriers of rabies are bats, raccoons, skunks, and foxes. Pet dogs, cats, and ferrets that have been vaccinated rarely have rabies. However, many stray animals have not been vaccinated. Also keep in mind that animals you encounter in other countries— even if they are people's pets—may not have been vaccinated against rabies. Rabies is rare in the U.S., but it is fatal if you are not vaccinated soon after exposure. The vaccination is no more painful than a typical injection.

Bites that break the skin can cause bacterial infections, including tetanus if you have not kept up with your tetanus booster shots. Cat and human bites are particularly prone to infection. Human bites can also spread diseases like hepatitis B and HIV infection.

Treat all bites as you would a puncture wound (see page 43). If you are bitten by someone's pet, find out whether the animal has been vaccinated for rabies. If you are bitten by a wild animal, contact your doctor and the local health department. If you are bitten by another person and the bite has broken the skin, call your doctor.

- To limit your risk of being stung by a jellyfish:

  - Watch for signs that are posted during a jellyfish invasion, and stay out of the water when jellyfish are present. If you do go in the water, wear a wet suit to reduce your risk of being stung. Don't rely on clothing or on coating the skin with petroleum jelly to prevent stings.

  - Watch out for jellyfish in the water, particularly when there are strong onshore winds.

  - Watch out for beached jellyfish. Their tentacles may still sting.

Home Treatment

For insect and spider bites and stings:

- Remove a bee stinger by scraping or flicking it out. Don't squeeze the stinger; you may release more venom into the skin. If the stinger isn't visible, assume there isn't one.

- Apply a cold pack or ice cube to the bite or sting. Some people also find that applying a paste of baking soda, meat tenderizer, or activated charcoal mixed with a little water helps relieve pain and decreases the reaction.

- If you are bitten by a black widow, brown recluse, or hobo spider, apply ice to the bite and call your doctor immediately. Do not apply a tourniquet.

- Take an oral antihistamine (such as Benadryl or Chlor-Trimeton) to relieve pain, swelling, and itching if you have many bites. Applying calamine lotion or hydrocortisone cream to the bites may also help.

- Carry an emergency kit containing a syringe and adrenaline (epinephrine) if you have had a severe allergic reaction to insect venom in the past. Ask your doctor or pharmacist how and when to use the kit.

- Trim your fingernails to prevent scratching, because scratching can lead to infection.

For tick bites:

- Check regularly for ticks when you are out in the woods, and thoroughly examine your skin and scalp when you return home. Check your pets too. The sooner ticks are removed, the less likely they are to spread infection.

- Remove a tick by gently pulling on it with tweezers, as close to the skin as possible. Fine-tipped tweezers may work best. Pull straight out and try not to crush the tick's body. Once the tick has been removed, wash the area where the tick was attached and apply an antiseptic. Save the tick in a jar for tests in case you develop flulike symptoms later.

For jellyfish stings:

- Rinse the area immediately with salt water. Do not use fresh water, and do not rub; doing so will release more venom into the wound.

- Spray or rinse the tentacles with household vinegar for at least 30 seconds to prevent further stings. You can sprinkle unseasoned meat tenderizer or baking soda on the tentacles if you don't have vinegar.

- If it is available, apply shaving cream to the tentacles. The tentacles will stick to the shaving cream and can then be easily scraped off with a safety razor, the edge of a sand shovel, or the edge of a credit card. Protect your hand with a towel or glove.

- Rinse eye stings with a saline solution, such as Artificial Tears. Do not put vinegar, alcohol, or any other "stinger solution" in the eyes. The skin around the eye can be dabbed with a cloth saturated in vinegar, but you must be extremely careful not to get any of the vinegar in the eye.

- Ice packs may help relieve the pain, and antihistamines (such as Benadryl or Chlor-Trimeton) or 1% hydrocortisone cream may help relieve itching.

- Clean any open sores 3 times per day. Apply an antiseptic ointment, and cover the sores with a light bandage.

- Carry an allergy kit if you have had any sort of allergic reaction or toxic reaction to a jellyfish sting in the past.

When to Call a Health Professional

Call 911 or other emergency services immediately if you develop signs of a severe allergic reaction after you are bitten or stung by an insect, spider, or jellyfish. Signs of a severe allergic reaction include:

- Wheezing or difficulty breathing.

• Swelling around the throat, lips, tongue, or face, or significant swelling around the site of the bite or sting (for example, your entire arm or leg is swollen).

• Signs of shock. See Shock on page 60.

Call your doctor:

• If you have been bitten by the same type of spider or insect that previously caused a serious reaction.

• If a blister appears at the site of a spider bite, or if the surrounding skin becomes discolored.

• If you develop flulike symptoms or an expanding red rash after spending time in an area that may have been infested with ticks.

• If there is some swelling around the site of a jellyfish sting, or if the surrounding skin becomes discolored.

• If you develop a spreading skin rash, hives, or itching after being bitten or stung.

• If your symptoms have not improved after 2 to 3 days, or if you develop signs of infection. See Signs of a Wound Infection on page 59.

• If you have had a serious allergic reaction and want to talk to your doctor about adrenaline kits or allergy shots (immunotherapy) for insect or jellyfish venom.

Breathing Emergencies

Who needs to be trained to help a person who is having a breathing emergency? You do. If you drive a car, shop at the mall, or go anyplace where a person may be in a life-threatening situation, you need to know how to respond. An added benefit is the confidence you will have when you know you can help a person when it matters most.

The guidelines presented in this book are not meant to replace formal training from a certified instructor. They are here for you to use to refresh your memory between trainings or to read aloud to a person who is performing a rescue procedure. (Note, however, that your first responsibility as a helper is to call 911 or other emergency services and to make the area safe for the victim and the rescuer.)

Choking Rescue Procedure (Heimlich Maneuver)

Choking is usually caused by food or an object stuck in the windpipe. A person who is choking cannot talk, cough, or breathe, and may turn blue or dusky. The Heimlich maneuver can help dislodge the food or object.

WARNING: Do not begin the choking rescue procedure unless you are certain that the person is choking.

If the person who is choking is standing or sitting:

- Stand behind the person and wrap your arms around his or her waist. If the person is standing, place one of your feet between the person's legs so you can support the person's body if he or she loses consciousness.

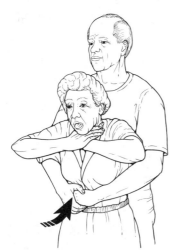

Give quick upward thrusts to dislodge the object.

- Make a fist with one hand. Place the thumb side of your fist against the person's abdomen, just above the navel but well below the breastbone (sternum).

- Grasp your fist with the other hand. Give a quick upward thrust into the person's abdomen. This may cause the object to pop out.

- Repeat thrusts until the object pops out or the person loses consciousness.

- **If you choke while you are alone**, do abdominal thrusts on yourself, or lean over the back of a chair and press forcefully to pop out the object.

If the person who is choking loses consciousness, gently lower him or her to the ground. **Call 911 or other emergency services.**

- Begin standard CPR (cardiopulmonary resuscitation), including chest compressions. See page 37.

- Each time the airway is opened during CPR, look for an object in the mouth or throat. If you see an object, remove it.

- Do not perform blind finger sweeps.

- Do not perform abdominal thrusts, such as the Heimlich maneuver.

- Continue performing CPR until the person is breathing on his or her own or until an ambulance arrives.

Rescue Breathing and CPR

Warning: CPR (cardiopulmonary resuscitation) that is done improperly or on a person whose heart is still beating can cause serious injury. Do not perform CPR unless:

1. The person has stopped breathing.

2. The person does not show signs of circulation, such as breathing, coughing, or movement, in response to rescue breathing.

3. No one with more training in CPR is present.

For basic life support, think **ABC:** **A**irway, **B**reathing, and **C**irculation, in that order. You must give rescue breaths before you can begin the chest compressions, which will help circulate blood for a person whose heart has stopped beating.

Step 1: Check for consciousness. Tap the person on the shoulder and shout, "Are you okay?"

If the person does not respond, **call 911 or other emergency services immediately**. Have someone else make the call if possible. Then proceed to Step 2.

Step 2: Check for breathing. Look, listen, and feel for breathing for 5 seconds. Kneel next to the person with your head close to his or her head.

- Look to see if the person's chest rises and falls.

- Listen for breathing sounds, wheezing, gurgling, or snoring.

- Put your cheek near the person's mouth and nose to feel whether air is moving out.

If the person is not breathing (or if you can't tell), roll the person onto his or her back. If the person may have a spinal injury, stabilize the head and neck as you gently roll the person onto his or her back.

Step 3: Begin rescue breathing.

- Place your hand on the person's forehead and pinch the person's nostrils shut using your thumb and forefinger. With your other hand, lift the person's chin to keep the airway open.

- Take a deep breath and place your mouth over the person's mouth, making a tight seal. As you slowly blow air into the person, watch to see if his or her chest rises.

- If the first breath does not go in, try tilting the person's head again and give another breath.

- Slowly blow air in until the person's chest rises. Take 1 to 2 seconds to give each breath. Between rescue breaths, remove your mouth from the person's mouth and take a deep breath. Allow the person's chest to fall as the air goes out of his or her mouth.

- Give the person 2 full breaths. Then check for circulation.

Step 4: Check for circulation. Look for signs of circulation, such as breathing, coughing, or leg or arm movement, in response to rescue breathing.

If there **are no signs of circulation**, begin chest compressions. See Step 5.

If there are signs of circulation, continue to give rescue breaths until help arrives or until the person starts to breathe on his or her own. Give 2 rescue breaths every 15 seconds.

If the person starts breathing again, he or she still needs to be seen by a health professional.

Step 5: Begin chest compressions.

- Kneel next to the person. Use your fingers to locate the end of the person's breastbone (sternum), where the ribs come together. Place 2 fingers at the tip of the person's sternum. Place the heel of the other hand directly above your fingers (on the side closest to the person's face).

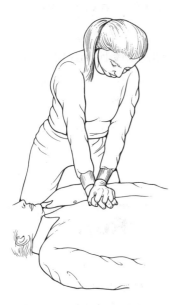

Chest compressions: Keep your shoulders directly over your hands with your elbows straight as you give chest compressions.

- Place your other hand on top of the one that you just put in position. Lock the fingers of both hands together, and raise the fingers so they don't touch the person's chest.

- Straighten your arms, lock your elbows, and center your shoulders directly over your hands.

- Press down in a steady rhythm, using your body weight and keeping your elbows locked. The force from each thrust should go straight down onto the sternum, compressing it 1½ to 2 inches. Give 1 thrust per second. It may help to count "one and two and three and

four . . . ," giving 1 downward thrust each time you say a number. Lift your weight, but not your hands, from the person's chest each time you say "and." Give 15 compressions.

- After 15 compressions, give 2 full, slow breaths.

- Repeat the 15 compressions/2 breaths cycle 4 times (1 minute); then check again for signs of circulation. If there are still no signs of circulation, continue to give chest compressions and rescue breaths until help arrives or until the person's circulation and breathing are restored.

Bruises

Bruises (contusions) occur when small blood vessels under the skin tear or rupture. Blood seeps into the surrounding tissues, causing the black-and-blue color of a bruise.

Bruises usually develop after a bump or fall. People who take aspirin or blood thinners (anticoagulants) may bruise easily. A bruise may also develop after blood is drawn. Sun damage and aging weaken the tiny veins in the skin. The weakened veins are easily broken, so you bruise more easily as you age. The bruises also take longer to heal.

A black eye is a type of bruise. If you have a black eye, apply home treatment for a bruise and inspect the eye for blood. If there is loss of vision or any change in your vision, or if you cannot move your eye in all directions, see a doctor.

Home Treatment

- Apply ice or cold packs for 10 minutes every 1 to 2 hours. Do this for the first 48 hours to help vessels constrict and to reduce swelling. The sooner you apply ice, the less bleeding there will be. See Ice and Cold Packs on page 62.

- If possible, elevate the bruised area above the level of your heart. Blood will leave the area, and there will be less swelling.

- Rest the injured body part so you don't injure it further.

- If the area is still painful after 48 hours, apply warm towels, a hot water bottle, or a heating pad.

- If you bruise easily, ask your doctor or pharmacist to review your medications to see if bruising may be a side effect.

When to Call a Health Professional

- If signs of infection develop. See Signs of a Wound Infection on page 59.

- If pain increases, or if your ability to use or move the bruised body part decreases.

- If a blow to the eye causes:

  - Blood in the colored part of the eye or blood in the white part of the eye. See Blood in the Eye on page 205.

  - Extreme sensitivity to light.

  - Loss of vision or any change in your vision.

  - Inability to move the eye normally in all directions.

  - Severe pain in the eyeball rather than in the eye socket.

- If you suspect a medication may be causing bruises.

- If you suddenly begin to bruise easily or if you have unexplained recurrent or multiple bruises.

- If unexplained bruising develops while you are ill.

Burns

Burns are classified as first-, second-, or third-degree depending on their depth, not the amount of pain or the size of the burned area. A first-degree burn involves only the outer layer of skin. The skin is dry, painful, and sensitive to touch. A mild to moderate sunburn is an example of a first-degree burn.

A second-degree burn involves several layers of skin. The skin becomes swollen, puffy, weepy, or blistered.

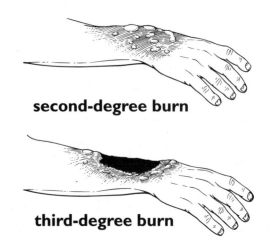

second-degree burn

third-degree burn

A third-degree burn involves all layers of skin and may include any underlying tissue or organs. The skin is dry, pale white or charred black, and swollen, and sometimes breaks open. Nerves are destroyed or damaged, so there may be little pain except on the edges of the burn, where there may be second-degree burns.

Chemical burns occur when something caustic, such as a cleaning product, gasoline, or turpentine, is splashed into an eye or onto the skin. The vapors or fumes from strong chemicals can also burn or irritate the eyes, the skin, the respiratory passages, and the lungs.

A chemically burned eye becomes red and watery and may be sensitive to light. If the damage is severe, the eye will look whitish. Chemically burned skin may become red, blistered, or blackened, depending on how strong the caustic material is.

Electrical burns are a medical emergency. An electrical burn may look minor on the outside, but electricity can cause serious internal damage, including burns and heart rhythm disturbances.

Prevention

- See the fire safety tips on page 27.
- Set your water heater to 120° or lower.
- To prevent kitchen burns:
  - Use caution when handling hot foods and beverages.
  - Turn pot handles toward the back of the stove.
  - Smother burning food or grease with a pot or pot lid.
- To prevent chemical burns to your eyes, wear goggles or safety glasses when working with substances that may burn your eyes.
- To prevent electrical burns, replace frayed power cords on electrical appliances, unplug lamps before replacing light bulbs, and turn off the power at the circuit breaker when replacing bulbs in ceiling or wall sockets. Keep appliances away from water. During a lightning storm, take cover inside a car, large building, or house, or seek low ground.

Home Treatment

Third-degree burns require immediate medical treatment. Call a health professional and apply home treatment:

- Make sure the source of the burn has been extinguished.
- Have the person lie down to prevent shock.
- Cover the burned area with a clean sheet.
- Do not apply any salve, medication, or ice to the burn.

First- and second-degree burns can be treated at home as follows:

- Run cool tap water over the burn until the pain stops (10 to 30 minutes). Cool water is the best immediate treatment for minor burns. The cold lowers skin temperature and lessens the severity of the burn. Do not use ice or ice water, because it may further damage the injured skin.

- Remove rings, bracelets, watches, or shoes from the burned limb. Swelling may make these items difficult to remove later, and if left on, they may damage nerves or blood vessels.

- Clean the burned area with mild soap and water. If the burned skin or blisters have broken open, a bandage is needed. Otherwise, don't cover the burn unless clothing rubs on it. If clothing rubs the burned area, cover the burn with a gauze pad taped well away from the burn. Do not encircle a hand, arm, or leg with tape. Keep the bandage clean and dry. Change it once a day and anytime it gets wet or dirty.

- Do not put salve, butter, grease, or oil on a burn. They increase the risk of infection and don't help the burn heal.

- After 2 to 3 days of healing, apply aloe to soothe minor burns.

- If the burn causes blisters to form:

  - Take acetaminophen or ibuprofen to help relieve pain. Aspirin is not recommended because it can affect the swelling and bleeding in the burned area.

  - Do not break blisters. If blisters break, clean the area by running tap water over it and applying a mild soap.

  - Apply an antibiotic ointment, such as Polysporin or Bacitracin, and cover the burn with a sterile dressing. Don't touch the burned area with your hands or any unsterile objects.

Remove the dressing every day, clean the burned area with water and mild soap, and cover it again.

For chemical burns:

- Call the local poison control center for specific advice. Have the chemical's container or its label available when you call.

- Immediately flush your eye or skin with a large amount of water. Use a cold shower for skin burns. For eye burns, fill a sink or dishpan with water, immerse your face in the water, and open and close your eyelids with your fingers to force the water to all parts of the eye. Or flush your eye under a running faucet or shower. A sink with a sprayer also works well. Many first aid kits include an eye wash.

- Continue flushing for 30 minutes or until the pain stops, whichever takes longer.

For electrical burns:

- Do not approach a person who has been electrocuted until you are sure the area surrounding the person is safe. Disconnect the power source if possible. If you feel tingling in your lower body, turn around and hop to a safe place.

- Do not attempt to move wires off of a person unless you are sure the power has been disconnected.

- If it is safe to approach the person, check ABCs (Airway, Breathing, Circulation). If necessary, begin rescue breathing and CPR. See page 37.

• Keep the person warm and lying down.

• Cover burns with dry, sterile dressing.

When to Call a Health Professional

Call 911 or other emergency services immediately:

• If a person who has been burned or electrocuted stops breathing or has no pulse. After calling 911, begin rescue breathing and CPR if necessary. See Breathing Emergencies on page 36.

• If a person who has been burned or electrocuted fell and may have a spinal injury or another serious injury.

• If a strong chemical such as acid or lye is splashed into your eye.

Call your doctor:

• If you have an electrical burn. Even an electrical burn that looks minor can be serious and needs to be evaluated.

• If you have a third-degree burn.

• If you are in doubt about the extent of a burn or in doubt whether it is a second- or third-degree burn.

• If a second-degree burn involves the face, ears, eyes, hands, feet, genitals, or a joint.

• If a burn encircles an arm or leg, or if it covers more than 25 percent of the body part involved.

• If a large area of skin (more than 25 percent of any part of the body) or any part of the face has been exposed to a strong acid or to a caustic substance, such as lye or Drano.

• If a chemically burned eye still hurts after 20 minutes of home treatment.

• If a chemically burned eye appears to be damaged. Symptoms include:

- Persistent redness.

- Discharge or watering.

- Any visual impairment, such as double vision, blurring, or sensitivity to light.

- A grayish or white discoloration over the colored part of the eye.

• If your skin shows signs of a chemical burn (see page 40).

• If pain lasts longer than 48 hours.

• If signs of infection develop (see Signs of a Wound Infection on page 59).

Cuts and Puncture Wounds

When you have a cut (laceration), the first steps are to stop the bleeding and determine whether medical evaluation is needed.

If the cut is bleeding heavily or spurting blood, see Stopping Severe Bleeding on page 44.

Bleeding from minor cuts will usually stop on its own or after you apply a little direct pressure.

To decide whether stitches are needed, see Are Stitches Necessary? on page 45. If stitches are needed, apply home treatment and seek medical care as soon as possible, certainly within 8 hours. If stitches are not needed, you can clean and bandage the cut at home.

Stopping Severe Bleeding

• Elevate the site that is bleeding.

• Remove any visible objects from the surface of the wound. Do not attempt to clean out the wound.

• Press firmly on the wound with a clean cloth or the cleanest material available. If there is an object deep in the wound, apply pressure around the object, not directly over it.

• Apply steady pressure for a full 15 minutes. Don't peek after a few minutes to see if bleeding has stopped. If the bleeding does not seem to be slowing down during this time, **call 911 or other emergency services** and continue to apply pressure to the wound. If blood soaks through the cloth, apply another cloth without lifting the first one.

• If bleeding decreases after you apply pressure for 15 minutes, but minimal bleeding starts again once you release the pressure, apply direct pressure to the wound for another 15 minutes. Direct pressure may be applied up to 3 times (a total of 45 minutes) for minimal bleeding. If bleeding (more than just oozing small amounts of blood) continues after 45 minutes of direct pressure, call a health professional.

• Watch for signs of shock. See page 60.

Puncture wounds are caused by sharp, pointed objects (including teeth) that penetrate the skin. They become infected easily because they are difficult to clean and provide a warm, moist place for bacteria to grow.

Home Treatment

For cuts:

• Stop any bleeding from a cut by applying direct, continuous pressure over the wound for 15 minutes.

• Wash the cut well with soap and water.

• If you think the cut may need stitches, see a health professional (see page 45). If the cut does not need stitches, proceed with home treatment.

• Consider bandaging the cut, especially if it is an area that may get dirty or irritated.

• Apply antibiotic ointment (such as Polysporin or Bacitracin) to keep the cut from sticking to the bandage. Do not use rubbing alcohol, hydrogen peroxide, iodine, or mercurochrome; these may harm tissue and slow healing.

• Use an adhesive bandage (such as a Band-Aid) to provide continuous pressure and to protect the cut from further irritation. Always put an adhesive strip across a cut rather than lengthwise. A butterfly bandage (made at home or purchased) can help hold cut skin edges together. Small cuts that are not in easily irritated locations may be bandaged or left uncovered.

For puncture wounds:

- If the object that caused the wound is small, remove it and make sure that it is intact. If the object is large or made a deep wound, leave it in place and call a health professional immediately.

- Allow the wound to bleed freely for a minute or two to clean itself out, unless the bleeding is heavy or the blood is squirting out. If bleeding is heavy, see Stopping Severe Bleeding on page 44.

- Clean the wound thoroughly with soap and water.

- Watch for signs of infection. See Signs of a Wound Infection on page 59. If the wound closes, an infection under the skin may not be detected for several days.

When to Call a Health Professional

- If the person has signs of shock, even if bleeding has stopped. See Shock on page 60.

- If a cut continues to bleed through bandages after you apply direct pressure for 15 minutes. See Stopping Severe Bleeding on page 44.

- If a puncture wound is in your head, neck, chest, or abdomen, unless you are certain it is minor.

- If the skin near the wound is blue, white, or cold; if you have numbness, tingling, or loss of feeling; or if you are unable to move a limb normally below the wound.

Are Stitches Necessary?

For best results, cuts that need stitches should be sutured within 8 hours. Wash the cut well with soap and water and stop the bleeding. Then pinch the sides of the cut together. If it looks better, you may want to consider stitches. If stitches are needed, avoid using an antibiotic ointment until after a health professional has examined the cut.

Stitches may be needed for:

- Cuts more than ¼ inch deep that have jagged edges or gape open.

- Deep cuts over a joint, such as an elbow, knuckle, or knee.

- Deep cuts on the hand or fingers.

- Cuts on the face, eyelids, or lips.

- Cuts in any area where you are worried about scarring.

- Cuts that go down to the muscle or bone.

- Cuts that continue to bleed after 15 minutes of direct pressure.

Cuts like these that are sutured usually heal with less scarring.

Stitches may not be needed for:

- Cuts with smooth edges that tend to stay together when you move the affected body part.

- Shallow cuts less than ¼ inch deep and less than 1 inch long.

- If part of a bone is poking out of or visible in the wound.

- If you are unable to remove an object from the wound, or if you think part of the object may still be in the wound.

- If bleeding that can be controlled by applying direct pressure continues longer than 45 minutes.

- If a cut needs stitches. Stitches usually need to be done within 8 hours.

- If a deep puncture wound to the foot occurred through a shoe or if the object that punctured the skin was dirty.

- If a cut has removed all layers of skin.

- If a puncture wound was caused by a cat or human bite.

- If you have a cut or puncture wound and your tetanus shots are not up to date. See page 22. If you need a tetanus booster shot, you should have it within 2 days of being injured.

- If signs of infection develop (see page 59).

Fainting and Unconsciousness

Fainting is a short-term loss of consciousness, usually lasting only a few seconds. It is most often caused by a momentary drop in blood flow to the brain. When you fall or lie down, blood flow is improved and you regain consciousness.

Fainting is a mild form of shock and is usually not serious. If it happens more than once, there may be a more serious problem, and it should be checked out by a doctor. Dizziness and fainting can also be brought on by sudden emotional stress or injury. See Dizziness and Vertigo on page 216.

An **unconscious** person is completely unaware of what is going on and is unable to make purposeful movements. Fainting is a brief episode of unconsciousness; a coma is a deep, prolonged state of unconsciousness.

Causes of unconsciousness include stroke, seizures, heat stroke, diabetic coma, insulin shock, head injury, lack of oxygen (due to suffocation, choking, drowning, etc.), alcohol or drug overdose, shock, bleeding, irregular heartbeat, and heart attack.

Home Treatment

- Make sure the unconscious person can breathe. Check for breathing, and if necessary, begin rescue breathing. See Breathing Emergencies on page 36.

- Check for signs of circulation, such as coughing, normal breathing, or movement in response to rescue breaths. If there are none, call for help and start cardiopulmonary resuscitation (CPR). See page 37.

- Keep the person lying down.

- Look for a medical alert bracelet, necklace, or card that identifies a medical problem such as epilepsy, diabetes, or drug allergy.

- Treat any injuries.

- Do not try to give the person anything to eat or drink.

When to Call a Health Professional

Call 911 or other emergency services if a person remains unconscious for longer than a few seconds.

Call your doctor:

- If a person completely loses consciousness, even if the person is now awake.

- If unconsciousness follows a head injury and the person is now awake. A person with a head injury needs to be carefully observed. See Head Injuries on page 51.

- If a person has fainted more than once.

- If a person has "blank spells," even if the person doesn't fall.

- Whenever a person with diabetes loses consciousness, even if he or she is now awake. He or she may have insulin shock (low blood sugar) or be in a diabetic coma (too much sugar in the blood).

Falls

Many older adults are concerned about falling. Falling can cause serious injuries, especially in older adults who may have weak bones. The injuries caused by falling may take longer to heal than they would in a younger person.

Taking a Pulse

The pulse is the rate at which a person's heart beats. As the heart pumps blood through the body, you can feel a throbbing in the arteries wherever they come close to the skin's surface. Most of the time, the pulse is taken at the wrist, neck, or groin.

- Count the pulse after a person has been sitting or resting quietly for 10 minutes or more.

- Place two fingers gently against the wrist as shown (don't use your thumb).

- If it is hard to feel the pulse in the wrist, locate the carotid artery in the neck, just to either side of the windpipe. Press gently.

- Count the beats for 30 seconds; then double the result to calculate beats per minute.

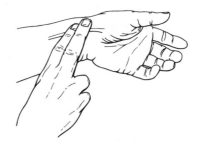

The normal resting pulse for an adult is 50 to 100 beats per minute. Certain illnesses can cause your pulse to change, so it is helpful to know what your resting pulse rate is when you are well. When you have a fever, your pulse rate rises about 10 beats per minute for every degree of fever.

Many falls are related to poor eyesight or household hazards, such as loose rugs, slippery sidewalks, poorly placed electrical cords, and dark stairways. Falls may also be caused by health problems or medications that make you dizzy, unsteady on your feet, or sleepy. Any fall that was caused by dizziness, a seizure, or loss of consciousness needs to be evaluated by a doctor.

Prevention

• Exercise regularly to keep your muscles and bones strong and flexible. This may help prevent falls and will also help you recover faster from a fall.

• Have your hearing and eyesight tested regularly. Inner ear problems can affect your balance. Vision problems make it difficult for you to see potential hazards.

• See a doctor about anything that makes it hard for you to walk, such as joint pain or foot problems.

• Talk to your doctor or pharmacist to find out whether any of the medications you take have side effects like drowsiness or dizziness. Take medications only as directed.

• Limit your alcohol intake.

• Turn on lights when you walk through the house at night. Use night-lights in the bedroom, bathroom, and hallways.

• Install light switches at both ends of stairs and halls. Install handrails on both sides of stairs.

Splinting

Splinting immobilizes a limb that may be broken or severely sprained to prevent further injury and ease pain until you can see a health professional. There are two ways to immobilize an injured body part: tie the injured limb to a stiff object, or fasten it to some other part of the body.

For the first method, tie rolled-up newspapers or magazines, a stick, a cane, or anything that is stiff to the injured limb with a rope, a belt, or anything else that will work. Do not tie too tightly.

Position the splint so the injured limb cannot bend. A general rule is to splint from a joint above the injury to a joint below it. For example, splint a broken forearm from above the elbow to below the wrist.

For the second method, tape a broken toe or finger to the one next to it, or immobilize an arm by tying it across the person's chest. Again, do not tie too tightly.

These splinting methods are temporary measures you can use until you can see a health professional. They are not substitutes for proper medical evaluation and care.

• Add grab bars in the shower, tub, and toilet areas. Use nonslip adhesive strips or a mat in the shower or tub. Consider sitting on a bench or stool in the shower.

- Consider using an elevated toilet seat.

- Wear nonslip, low-heeled shoes or slippers that fit snugly. Don't walk around in stocking feet.

- Keep telephone and electrical cords out of pathways.

- Tack down rugs and glue down vinyl flooring so they lie flat. Remove or replace rugs or runners that tend to slip, or attach a nonslip backing to them. Make certain carpet is firmly attached to the stairs.

- Purchase a step stool with high and sturdy handrails. Do not stand on a chair to reach things. Store frequently used objects where you can reach them easily.

- Use a bright color to paint the edges of outdoor steps and any steps that are especially narrow or are higher or lower than the rest.

- Paint outside stairs with a mixture of sand and paint for better traction.

- Keep entrances and sidewalks clear and well lit, and remove snow and ice promptly.

- Many hip fractures happen when older adults with bone or joint problems get up from a sofa or low chair. Avoid sitting in sofas and chairs that put your hips lower than your knees. When getting up from a sofa or chair, use the armrest or the edge of the chair for support; put your feet flat on the floor, toes facing forward; stand up slowly and hold on to the chair or sofa until you have your balance.

- Use helping devices such as canes or chairs that raise or tilt to help you get up.

- If you feel dizzy or lightheaded, sit down or stay seated until your head clears. Stand up slowly to avoid unsteadiness.

Home Treatment

If you fall and you are not seriously injured, you may be able to treat yourself at home. To get up from the floor safely, roll to your hands and knees and crawl to a piece of furniture that will support your weight, such as a sofa or an armchair. Use the furniture to pull yourself up gently. Sit for a minute before trying to stand up.

If you have any minor injuries, such as a bruise or sprain, see the appropriate home treatment section in this chapter.

When to Call a Health Professional

Call 911 or other emergency services immediately:

- If a person remains unconscious after a fall. See Fainting and Unconsciousness on page 46.

- If a fall causes a person to have a seizure.

- If you are not able to get up after a fall.

Call a health professional:

- If a person lost consciousness because of a fall but has now regained consciousness.

- If a person fell while having a seizure but the seizure has now stopped. If the seizure is related to a chronic condition and a doctor has recommended treatment, begin the treatment.

- If a fall causes severe bleeding or bruising. See Shock on page 60.

- If you think you may have a broken bone. See page 60.

- If you develop pain in your hips, lower back, or wrists after a fall. These areas are especially likely to fracture in older adults.

- If you think a fall was caused by a medical problem or the side effects of a medication.

Frostbite

Frostbite is freezing of the skin or underlying tissues that occurs as a result of prolonged exposure to cold.

Frostbitten skin is pale or blue, is stiff or rubbery to touch, and feels cold and numb. Frostbite is rated by its severity:

First degree ("frostnip"): Skin is whitish or red and tingling or burning, but there is little likelihood of blistering if the skin is rewarmed promptly.

Second degree: Outer skin feels hard and frozen, but tissue underneath is normal. Blistering is likely.

Third degree: The skin is white or blotchy and blue. Skin and tissue underneath are hard and very cold. Blistering always occurs.

Prevention

Stay dry and out of the wind in extreme cold, and cover areas of exposed skin. Keep your body's core temperature up:

- Wear layers of clothing. Wool and polypropylene are good insulators. Wear windproof, waterproof outer layers. Wear wool socks and waterproof boots that fit well.

- Wear a hat to prevent heat loss from your head. Wear mittens rather than gloves.

- Keep protective clothing and blankets in your car in case of a breakdown in an isolated area.

- Drink plenty of fluids, especially water, to prevent dehydration.

- Don't drink alcohol or caffeinated beverages and don't smoke when you are out in extreme cold.

Home Treatment

- Get inside or take shelter from the wind.

- Check for signs of hypothermia (see page 55), and treat it before treating frostbite.

- Protect the frozen body part from further exposure to the cold. Don't rewarm the area if refreezing is possible. Wait until you reach shelter.

- Warm small areas (ears, face, nose, fingers, toes) with warm breath or by tucking hands or feet inside warm clothing next to bare skin.

• Don't rub or massage the frozen area, because doing so will further damage tissues. Avoid walking on frostbitten feet if possible.

• Keep the frostbitten body part warm and elevated. Wrap it with blankets or soft material to prevent bruising. If possible, immerse it in warm water (104° to 108°) for 15 to 30 minutes.

• Blisters may appear as the skin warms. Do not break them. The skin may turn red, burn, tingle, or be very painful. Taking aspirin or acetaminophen may help relieve the pain.

When to Call a Health Professional

• If the skin is white or blue, hard, rubbery, and cold, which indicates third-degree frostbite. Careful rewarming and antibiotic treatment are needed to prevent permanent tissue damage and infection.

• If blisters develop (second- or third-degree frostbite). Do not break the blisters. The risk of infection is very high.

• If signs of infection develop. See Signs of a Wound Infection on page 59.

Head Injuries

Most bumps to the head are minor and heal as easily as bumps anywhere else. Minor cuts on the head often bleed heavily because the blood vessels of the scalp are close to the skin's surface.

Head injuries that do not cause visible external bleeding may still have caused life-threatening bleeding and swelling inside the skull. The more force involved in a head injury, the more likely a serious injury to the brain has occurred. Anyone who has experienced a head injury should be watched carefully for 24 hours for signs of a serious head injury.

Prevention

• Make your home safe from falls by removing hazards that might cause a fall. See Falls on page 47.

• Wear your seat belt when you are in a motor vehicle.

• Wear a helmet while biking, skiing, snowboarding, horseback riding, or whenever you are doing an activity in which there is a risk of falling.

• Wear a hard hat if you work in an industrial area.

• Don't dive into shallow or unfamiliar water.

• If you keep firearms in your home, store them unloaded and uncocked, and lock them up. Store and lock ammunition in a separate place.

Home Treatment

• If the person with a head injury is unconscious, check his or her ABCs (airway, breathing, and circulation; see Breathing Emergencies on page 36). Assume that the person has a spinal injury; do not move the person without first protecting his or her neck from movement. Check for other injuries as well. The alarm from seeing a head injury may cause you to miss other injuries that need attention.

- If there is bleeding, apply firm pressure directly over the wound with a clean cloth or bandage for 15 minutes. If the blood soaks through, apply additional cloths over the first one. See Stopping Severe Bleeding on page 44.

- Apply ice or cold packs to reduce the swelling. A "goose egg" may appear anyway, but ice will help ease the pain.

- For the first 24 hours after a head injury, watch the person for signs of a serious head injury. Check for the following symptoms every 2 hours:

  - Confusion or difficulty speaking. Ask the person his or her name, address, age, the date, etc.

  - Numbness or weakness on one side of the body.

  - Blurred or double vision that does not clear, or significant changes in pupil size or reaction.

  - Lethargy, abnormally deep sleep, or difficulty waking up.

  - Vomiting that continues after the first 2 hours, or violent vomiting that persists after the first 15 minutes.

  - Seizures or convulsions.

- Continue observing the person every 2 hours during the night. Wake the person up and check for any unusual symptoms. **Call 911 or go to an emergency room immediately** if you cannot wake the person or if he or she has any signs of a serious head injury.

When to Call a Health Professional

Call 911 or other emergency services immediately:

- If the injured person stops breathing. Begin rescue breathing. Start CPR if the person has no signs of circulation, such as normal breathing, coughing, or movement, in response to rescue breaths. See Breathing Emergencies on page 36.

- If the injured person has any of the symptoms of a serious head injury outlined in Home Treatment.

- If the person loses consciousness at any time after being injured.

- If the injured person shows signs of a serious spinal injury. These signs include:

  - Paralysis in any part of the body.

  - Severe neck or back pain.

  - Weakness, tingling, or numbness in the arms or legs.

  - Loss of bowel or bladder control.

Call a health professional if a person suffers a head injury and:

- Has blood (not caused by a cut or direct blow) or clear fluid draining from the ears or nose.

- Becomes confused or does not remember being injured.

- Develops a severe headache.

- Vomits.

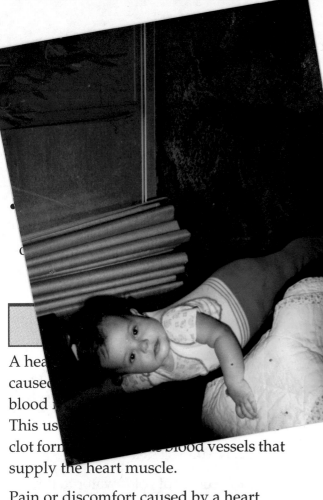

stages of a heart attack and seek emergency care. Medical treatment is needed to prevent death. Sometimes medications can be given to avoid the heart muscle damage caused by a heart attack.

When to Call a Health Professional

Call 911 or other emergency services immediately if you think you may be having a heart attack. Do not try to drive yourself to the hospital. After calling 911, chew and swallow 1 adult aspirin (unless you are allergic to or unable to take aspirin).

Symptoms of a heart attack include squeezing or crushing chest pain that feels like someone is sitting on your chest. The pain or discomfort may increase in intensity or occur with any of the following symptoms:

• Rapid or irregular heartbeat

• Sweating

• Shortness of breath

• Pain in the abdomen, upper back, neck, jaw, and one or both shoulders or arms

• Nausea or vomiting

• Lightheadedness

Call your doctor if you have chest pain or discomfort and there is no obvious cause (such as a pulled muscle or broken rib).

A heart attack is caused by a blood clot. This usually happens when a blood clot forms in the blood vessels that supply the heart muscle.

Pain or discomfort caused by a heart attack may occur in the chest, abdomen, upper back, neck, jaw, and one or both shoulders or arms.

The pain of a heart attack usually lasts longer than 10 minutes and often occurs with other symptoms, such as sweating, shortness of breath, or nausea. The pain of a heart attack will not usually go away with rest.

Many people mistake heart attack symptoms for other problems, such as indigestion, heartburn, or a pulled muscle. It is important to recognize the signals your body sends during the early

Heat Exhaustion and Heat Stroke

Heat exhaustion usually occurs when you are sweating a lot and do not drink enough to replace the lost fluids. Symptoms include:

- Fatigue, weakness, headache, dizziness, or nausea.
- Cool, moist, pale, or flushed skin.

Heat exhaustion can sometimes lead to **heat stroke**, which requires emergency treatment. Heat stroke occurs when your body fails to regulate its own temperature and the temperature continues to rise, often to 105° or higher. You may stop sweating entirely if you have heat stroke. Symptoms include:

- Confusion, delirium, or unconsciousness.
- Skin that is red, hot, and dry, even in the armpits.

Prevention

- Avoid strenuous physical activity outdoors during the hottest part of the day.
- Wear light-colored, loose-fitting clothing and a hat with a brim to reflect the sun.
- Avoid sudden changes of temperature. Air out a hot car before getting into it.
- If you take diuretics, ask your doctor if you can take a lower dose during hot weather.

- Drink 8 to 10 glasses of water per day. If you exercise or work strenuously in hot weather, drink more liquid than your thirst seems to require. Make sure you drink before you become thirsty.

Home Treatment

- Stop your activity. Get out of the sun to a cool spot, and drink lots of cool water, a little at a time. If you are nauseated or dizzy, lie down.

- Heat exhaustion can sometimes lead to heat stroke, particularly in older adults. If a person's temperature exceeds 102.3°, call for immediate help and try to lower the temperature as quickly as possible:

  - Remove unnecessary clothing.

  - Apply cool (not cold) water to the person's whole body; then fan the person. Apply ice packs to the person's groin, neck, and armpits. Do not put the person in ice water.

  - If you can get the person's temperature down to 102°, take care to avoid overcooling. Stop cooling the person once his or her temperature is lowered to 98.6°.

  - Do not give aspirin or acetaminophen to reduce the temperature.

  - Watch for signs of heat stroke (confusion or unconsciousness; red, hot, dry skin).

  - If the person stops breathing, start rescue breathing (see page 37).

When to Call a Health Professional

Call 911 or other emergency services if the person's body temperature reaches 102.3° and keeps rising, or if signs of heat stroke develop. Signs of heat stroke include:

- Confusion, delirium, or unconsciousness.
- Skin that is red, hot, and dry, even in the armpits.

Hypothermia

Hypothermia occurs when body temperature drops below normal and the body loses heat faster than heat can be produced by metabolism, muscle contractions, and shivering.

Early symptoms indicating mild to moderate hypothermia include:

- Shivering.
- Cold, pale skin.
- Apathy or listlessness.
- Impaired judgment.
- Clumsy movement and speech.

Later symptoms of severe hypothermia include:

- Cold abdomen.
- Slow pulse and breathing.
- Weakness or drowsiness.
- Confusion.
- Unconsciousness.

Shivering may stop if the body temperature drops below 90°.

People who have heart disease or diabetes, or who are inactive as a result of arthritis, stroke, or other conditions, are at increased risk for hypothermia. Certain medications, including those used to treat high blood pressure, antidepressants, narcotics, barbiturates, sleeping pills, and antianxiety drugs, increase a person's risk for hypothermia.

Some older adults, especially those who have chronic health problems, may be less likely to notice cool temperatures, and their bodies may not maintain a normal body temperature as well as a younger person's body would. Frail and inactive people can develop hypothermia indoors if they are not dressed warmly or cannot warm the area adequately.

Hypothermia is an emergency. It can quickly lead to unconsciousness and death if the heat loss continues. Early recognition of hypothermia is important. If a person starts to shiver violently, stumble, or respond incoherently to questions, suspect hypothermia and warm the person quickly.

Prevention

Whenever you plan to be outdoors for several hours in cold weather, take the following precautions:

- Dress warmly, and wear windproof, waterproof clothing. Wear fabrics that remain warm even when they get wet, such as wool or polypropylene.

- Wear a warm hat. An unprotected head loses a great deal of the body's total heat.

- Keep protective clothing and blankets in your car in cold weather in case of a breakdown in an isolated area.

- Head for shelter if you get wet or cold.

- Eat well before going out, and carry extra food. Drink plenty of fluids, especially water, to prevent dehydration.

- Don't drink alcohol while in the cold. It makes your body lose heat faster. It may also make you less likely to notice that you are becoming chilled.

To prevent hypothermia indoors:

- Keep your thermostat set at 65° or higher. If keeping the whole house heated is a problem, arrange to keep just a few rooms heated and close off the others.

- If you must keep your home below 65°, wear several layers of warm clothing and a hat.

- Eat regularly. Your body needs food to produce heat.

- Get up and move around regularly if you are indoors during cold weather. If moving around is a problem, do chair exercises or other activities that will get your blood moving.

- Wear warm clothes to bed, and use warm bedding.

Home Treatment

The goal of home or "in-the-field" treatment is to stop additional heat loss and slowly rewarm the person.

- For a mild case of hypothermia, get the person out of the cold and wind. Give the person dry or wool clothing to wear. If the person is indoors, increase the temperature in the room.

- For a moderate case of hypothermia, remove cold, wet clothes first. Then warm the person with your own body heat by wrapping a blanket or sleeping bag around both of you.

- Give warm liquids to drink and high-energy foods, such as candy, to eat. Do not give food or drink if the person is disoriented or unconscious. Do not give alcoholic or caffeinated beverages.

- Rewarming the person in warm water can cause shock or a heart attack. However, in emergency situations when help is not available and other home treatments are not working, you can use a warm bath (100° to 105°) as a last resort.

When to Call a Health Professional

Call 911 or other emergency services if the person seems confused or loses consciousness and remains unconscious.

Call your doctor:

- If the person's body temperature remains below 96° after 2 hours of warming.

- If the victim is a frail or weak older person. It's a good idea to call regardless of the severity of the symptoms.

Nosebleeds

Most nosebleeds are not serious and can usually be stopped with home treatment. Some common causes of nosebleeds are low humidity, colds and allergies, injuries to the nose, medications (especially aspirin), and high altitude. Blowing or picking your nose can also cause a nosebleed.

Prevention

• Low humidity is a common cause of nosebleeds. Humidify your home, especially the bedrooms. Keep bedrooms cool (60° to 65°) when you are sleeping.

• If your nose becomes very dry, breathe moist air for a while (such as in the shower), and then put a little petroleum jelly on the inside of your nose to help prevent bleeding. Using a saline nasal spray may also help. See page 384.

• Limit your use of aspirin and other nonsteroidal anti-inflammatory drugs (NSAIDs), which can contribute to nosebleeds.

Home Treatment

• Sit up straight and tip your head slightly forward. Tilting your head back may cause blood to run down your throat.

• Gently blow all the clots out of your nose. Pinch your nostrils shut between your thumb and forefinger or apply

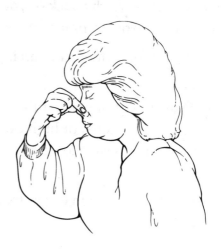

To stop a nosebleed, tilt your head forward and pinch your nostrils together below the bridge of your nose. Hold for at least 10 minutes, using a clock to time yourself.

firm pressure against the bleeding nostril for 10 full minutes. Resist the urge to peek after a few minutes to see if your nose has stopped bleeding.

• After 10 minutes, check to see if your nose is still bleeding. If it is, hold it for 10 more minutes. Most nosebleeds will stop after you apply direct pressure for 10 to 30 minutes.

• Stay quiet for a few hours, and do not blow your nose for at least 12 hours after the bleeding has stopped.

When to Call a Health Professional

• If the bleeding hasn't stopped after you have applied direct pressure for 30 minutes. Watch for signs of shock. See Shock on page 60.

- If blood runs down the back of your throat even when you pinch your nose.

- If your nose is deformed after an injury and may be broken.

- If you take blood thinners (anti-coagulant medications) or high doses of aspirin and you start to have nosebleeds.

- If nosebleeds recur often (more than four in a week).

Objects in the Eye

A speck of dirt or small object in the eye will often wash out with your tears. If the object is not removed, it may scratch the eye (corneal abrasion). Most corneal scratches are minor and heal on their own in 1 to 2 days.

When an object is thrown forcefully into the eye (from a machine, for example), it is possible that the eyeball will be punctured and emergency care will be needed.

Chemicals can get splashed into the eye and burn the eye. See Burns on page 40 for more information.

Prevention

Wear safety glasses or goggles when you mow the lawn, work with power tools, play racket sports, or do anything that might cause an object to strike your eye forcefully.

Home Treatment

- Wash your hands before touching your eye.

- Don't rub your eye; you could scratch your cornea.

- Do not try to remove an object that is over the colored part of your eye or stuck in the white of the eye. Try flushing it out with water or saline solution. If that doesn't work, call a health professional.

- If the object is at the side of the eye or on the lower lid, moisten a cotton swab or the tip of a twisted piece of tissue and touch the end to the object. The object should cling to the swab or tissue. Some minor irritation may occur after you have removed the object.

- Gently wash the eye with cool water. It may help to use an eyedropper.

- Never use tweezers, toothpicks, or other hard items to remove an object from your eye.

When to Call a Health Professional

Call 911 or other emergency services if your eyeball seems to be punctured.

Call your doctor:

- If the object is over the colored part of your eye or is embedded in the eye. Do not pull out an object that is stuck in your eye.

- If there is blood over or in the colored part of your eye.

• If you cannot remove the object.

• If pain is severe or persists; if it feels like there is still something in your eye; if your eye is extremely sensitive to light; or if your vision is blurred after the object has been removed. Your cornea may be scratched. Keep your eye closed.

Scrapes

Scrapes or abrasions happen when the skin is rubbed against a hard or rough surface. Most scrapes are shallow and don't extend far into the skin. However, because the skin gets thinner as a person ages, a scrape can cause an older person's skin to tear or peel in a thin layer. Open or peeling skin is prone to infection.

Home Treatment

• Scrapes are usually very dirty. Remove large pieces of debris with tweezers. Then scrub vigorously with soap and water and a washcloth. Thorough cleaning is necessary to prevent infection and scarring. Using a water sprayer from the kitchen sink is a good way to wash a scrape.

• Apply steady pressure with a clean bandage or cloth to stop bleeding.

• Apply ice to reduce swelling and bruising.

• If the skin on the injured area has peeled, try to gently replace the skin and then bandage it in place.

• If the scrape is large or in an area that may be rubbed by clothing, apply an antibiotic ointment to the scrape and cover it with a nonstick bandage (such as Telfa).

When to Call a Health Professional

• If your tetanus shots are not up to date. See page 22.

• If bleeding continues after 30 minutes of direct pressure.

• If you cannot clean the scrape well because it is too large, deep, or painful or has dirt and debris embedded under the skin.

• If signs of infection develop. See Signs of a Wound Infection on page 59.

Signs of a Wound Infection

The following are signs that a cut or wound has become infected:

• Increased pain, swelling, redness, warmth, or tenderness

• Red streaks extending from the area

• Discharge of pus

• Fever of 100° or higher with no other cause

• Swollen lymph nodes in the neck, armpits, or groin

Shock

Shock may develop as a result of sudden illness or injury. When the circulatory system is unable to get enough blood to the vital organs, the body goes into shock. Sometimes even a mild injury will lead to shock.

The signs of shock include:

• Cool, pale, clammy skin.

• Weak, rapid pulse.

• Shallow, rapid breathing.

• Low blood pressure.

• Thirst, nausea, or vomiting.

• Confusion or anxiety.

• Faintness, weakness, dizziness, or loss of consciousness.

Shock is a life-threatening condition. Prompt home treatment can save the person's life.

Home Treatment

• After calling for emergency care, have the person lie down and elevate his or her legs 12 inches or more. If the injury is to the head, neck, or chest, keep the person's legs flat. If the person vomits, roll him or her to one side to let fluids drain from the mouth. Use care if there could be a spinal injury.

• Control any bleeding (see Cuts and Puncture Wounds on page 43) and splint any fractures (see page 48).

• Keep the person warm but not hot. Place a blanket underneath the person, and cover the person with a sheet or blanket, depending on the weather. If the person is in a hot place, try to keep him or her cool.

• Take and record the person's pulse every 5 minutes. See Taking a Pulse on page 47.

• Comfort and reassure the person to relieve anxiety.

When to Call a Health Professional

Call 911 or other emergency services if a person develops signs of shock.

Strains, Sprains, Fractures, and Dislocations

A **strain** is an injury caused by over-stretching or tearing a muscle or tendon. A **sprain** is an injury to the ligaments or soft tissues around a joint. A **fracture** is a broken bone. A **dislocation** occurs when one end of a bone is pulled or pushed out of its normal position.

All four injuries cause pain and swelling. Unless a broken bone is obvious, it may be difficult to tell if an injury is a strain, sprain, fracture, or dislocation. Injuries may involve all four. Rapid swelling often indicates a more serious injury. Immediate care is needed if part of a bone is poking out of or visible in the wound, or if a limb turns white, cold, or clammy below the injured area.

Most minor strains and sprains can be treated at home, but severe sprains, fractures, and dislocations need professional care. Apply home treatment while you wait to see your doctor.

A **stress fracture** is a weak spot or small crack in a bone caused by repeated overuse. Stress fractures in the small bones of the foot are common in people who train intensely for running and other events. The most common symptom of a stress fracture is persistent pain at the site of the fracture. The pain may improve during exercise but will be worse before and after the activity. There may not be any visible swelling.

Prevention

It may not always be possible to prevent accidents that cause sprains, strains, fractures, or dislocations. However, you will improve your chances of avoiding serious injury if you keep your muscles strong and flexible with regular, moderate exercise; wear protective gear; and use equipment that is in good repair.

Other tips for preventing accidents include the following:

• Make sure you can always see where you are going.

• Don't carry objects that are too heavy.

• Use a step stool to reach objects that are above your head. Don't stand on chairs, countertops, or unstable objects.

Also read about preventing falls on page 47.

Home Treatment

Generally speaking, whether the injury affects soft tissue or bone, the basic treatment is the same: **RICE**, which stands for rest, ice, compression, and elevation, to treat the acute pain or injury. Begin the RICE process immediately for most injuries.

R. Rest. Do not put weight on the injured joint for at least 24 to 48 hours.

• Use crutches to support a badly sprained knee or ankle.

• Support a sprained wrist, elbow, or shoulder with a sling, which will help the injury heal faster.

• Rest a sprained finger by taping it to the healthy finger next to it. This works for toes too. Always put padding between the two fingers or toes you are taping together.

Injured muscles, ligaments, or tendons need time and rest to heal. Stress fractures need rest for 2 to 4 months.

I. Ice. Cold reduces pain and swelling and promotes healing. Heat feels nice, but it does more harm than good if it is applied less than 48 hours after an injury.

Apply ice or cold packs immediately to prevent or minimize swelling. For difficult-to-reach injuries, a cold pack works best. See Ice and Cold Packs on page 62.

C. Compression. Wrap the injured area with an elastic (Ace) bandage or compression sleeve to immobilize and compress the area. Don't wrap it too tightly, because doing so can cause more swelling. Loosen the bandage if the area

Ice and Cold Packs

Ice can relieve pain, swelling, and inflammation from injuries and other conditions such as arthritis. Apply ice as long as you have symptoms. Use one of the following:

- Ice towel: Wet a towel with cold water and squeeze it until it is just damp. Put the towel in a plastic bag and freeze it for 15 minutes. Remove the towel from the bag and place it on the affected area.

- Ice pack: Put about a pound of ice in a plastic bag. Add water to barely cover the ice. Squeeze the air out of the bag and seal the bag. Wrap the bag in a wet towel and apply it to the affected area.

- Cold pack: see Self-Care Supplies on page 376.

Ice the area at least 3 times a day. For the first 48 hours, ice for up to 10 minutes once an hour. After that, a good pattern is to ice for up to 10 minutes in the morning, in the late afternoon, and about half an hour before bedtime. Also ice after any prolonged activity or vigorous exercise.

To protect the skin, always keep a damp cloth between your skin and the cold pack. Do not apply ice for longer than 10 minutes at a time. Do not fall asleep with the ice on your skin.

below the wrap feels numb, cool, or tingly, or starts to swell. A tightly wrapped sprain may fool you into thinking you can keep using the joint. With or without a wrap, the joint needs total rest for 1 to 2 days.

E. Elevation. Elevate the injured area on pillows while you apply ice and anytime you are sitting or lying down. Try to keep the injury at or above the level of your heart to help minimize swelling.

You may apply a hot water bottle, warm towel, or heating pad to the injury after the first 48 to 72 hours as long as all the swelling is gone. Some experts recommend applying warmth and ice alternately.

You may be able to prevent further damage with some of the following:

- Splint an arm, leg, finger, or toe that you suspect is broken. Use a splint or a sling for a short period of time (a few hours) while waiting to see your doctor. See Splinting on page 48.

- Remove all rings, watches, and bracelets immediately if the sprain is to a finger, hand, or wrist. Swelling is likely to occur, making removal of the item more difficult later. See Removing a Ring on page 63.

- Take aspirin, ibuprofen, naproxen sodium, or ketoprofen to help ease inflammation and pain.

- Start gentle exercise as soon as the initial pain and swelling have gone away. If you have a broken bone or a severe sprain, your doctor may put the limb in a cast.

When to Call a Health Professional

- If an injured limb is deformed, if part of a bone is poking out of or visible in the wound, or if the skin over the site of a suspected fracture is broken.

- If there are signs of nerve or blood vessel damage. These signs include:

  - Numbness, tingling, or a pins-and-needles sensation.

  - Skin that is pale, white, or blue, or feels colder than the skin on the limb that is not hurt.

  - Inability to move the limb normally because of weakness, not just pain.

- If you cannot bear weight on or straighten the injured limb, or if an injured joint wobbles or feels unstable.

- If pain is severe or lasts longer than 24 hours.

- If swelling develops within 30 minutes of the injury or does not improve after 48 hours of home treatment.

- If signs of infection develop following an injury. See Signs of a Wound Infection on page 59.

Stroke

A stroke occurs when a blood vessel (artery) that supplies blood to the brain bursts or becomes blocked by a blood clot. Within minutes, the nerve cells in that area of the brain are damaged and die. As a result, the part of the body controlled by those cells cannot function properly.

Removing a Ring

To remove a ring from a sprained or swollen finger:

- First, try soapy water. Using ice water will decrease the swelling.

- Stick one end of a slick piece of string, such as dental floss, under the ring toward the hand.

- Starting at the side of the ring closest to the knuckle, wrap the string snugly around the finger toward the nail, wrapping past the knuckle. Each wrap should be right next to the one before.

- Grasp the end of the string that is under the ring and pull the string toward the ring to start unwrapping. Push the ring along ahead of the string as you go, until the ring passes the knuckle.

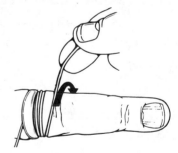

Wrap toward the end of the finger.

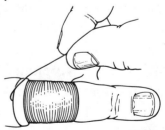

Pull the ring over the wrapped joint.

Call 911 or other emergency services immediately if you think you may be having a stroke. Do not try to drive yourself to the hospital. If medical treatment is sought as soon as stroke symptoms are noticed, fewer brain cells may be permanently damaged by the stroke.

The effects of a stroke may range from mild to severe and may be temporary or permanent. A stroke can affect vision, speech, behavior, thought processes, and the ability to move parts of the body.

Sometimes it can cause a coma or death. The effects of a stroke depend on:

• Which brain cells are damaged.

• How much of the brain is affected.

• How quickly blood supply is restored to the affected area.

People who have had a stroke often need to go through rehabilitation to regain their strength and mobility. They may also need to relearn how to do some everyday tasks.

A person may have one or more **transient ischemic attacks (TIAs)** before having a stroke. TIAs are often called mini-strokes because their symptoms are similar to those of a stroke. The difference between a TIA and a stroke is that TIA symptoms usually end after 10 to 20 minutes (although symptoms can sometimes last up to 24 hours). A TIA can occur months before a stroke occurs. It is a warning signal that a stroke may soon follow. The first TIA should always be treated as an emergency, even if the symptoms go away quickly.

 Strokes and TIAs may be the result of reduced blood flow to the brain due to a blockage in an artery in the neck. Your doctor may recommend a surgical procedure called <u>carotid endarterectomy</u> to remove the blockage. Getting all the facts and thinking about your own needs and values will help you make the best decision about carotid endarterectomy.

Prevention

You can prevent a stroke by controlling your risk factors. Some ways you can control your risk factors include the following:

• Have regular medical checkups. Work with your doctor to control high blood pressure, high cholesterol, heart disease, diabetes, or other disorders that affect your blood vessels.

• Don't smoke. Smoking is a leading cause of stroke. If you do smoke, quit. Stopping smoking can reduce your risk of stroke to the same level as that of nonsmokers within 5 years.

• Maintain a healthy weight.

• Exercise regularly and take steps to reduce stress.

• Eat a nutritious, well-balanced diet that is low in cholesterol, saturated fats, and salt. Make sure you include fruits and vegetables in your diet to provide your body with enough potassium and vitamins B, C, E, and riboflavin. Include whole grains in your diet.

MORE INFO **For more information, see the back cover.**

• Limit your alcohol intake. Heavy drinking may raise your blood pressure, making you more prone to having a stroke.

• Avoid taking birth control pills if you have other risk factors for stroke. If you smoke or have high cholesterol, migraine headaches, or a history of blood clots, taking birth control pills increases your risk of having a stroke.

Home Treatment

• Know the warning signs of a stroke (see When to Call a Health Professional). Seek emergency care if they occur.

• Involve family members and friends in your recovery process. Also see Caregiver Secrets starting on page 367.

• Learn to recognize signs of depression. Depression is common in people who have had strokes. It can be treated. See Depression on page 325.

When to Call a Health Professional

Call 911 or other emergency services immediately if you have any of the following warning signs of stroke:

• Any new weakness, numbness, or paralysis in your face, arm, or leg, especially on only one side of your body

• Blurred or decreased vision in one or both eyes that does not clear with blinking

• New difficulty speaking or understanding simple statements

• Sudden, unexplainable, and intense headache that is different from any headache you have had before

• Severe dizziness, loss of balance, or loss of coordination, especially if another warning sign is present at the same time

If a symptom was definitely there and then went away after a few minutes, call your doctor immediately. Symptoms that go away in a few minutes may be caused by a TIA. A TIA is a strong sign that a major stroke may soon occur and should be treated as an emergency.

4

Digestive and Urinary Problems

The cause of digestive and urinary problems can be hard to pinpoint. Sometimes serious problems and minor ones start with the same symptoms. Fortunately, most digestive and urinary problems are minor, and home treatment is all that is needed.

Use the chart on page 68 to find the symptoms that most closely match the ones you are having. Some illnesses that can cause digestive and urinary problems are covered more thoroughly in other chapters. Use the chart or the index to find those topics.

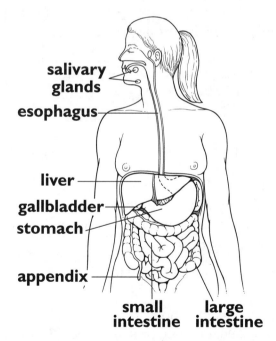

Organs of the digestive tract

Abdominal Pain

You can get clues about the cause of abdominal pain and how serious the problem may be by noting the following:

- The severity of the pain. A visit to a health professional is usually needed when severe abdominal pain comes on suddenly and continues, or when new or different pain becomes more severe over several hours or days.

- The location of the pain. See the illustration on page 69.

Digestive and Urinary Problems

Symptoms	Possible Causes
Nausea or vomiting	See Nausea and Vomiting, p. 84; Hepatitis, p. 85; medication reaction—call your doctor or pharmacist; Adverse Drug Reactions, p. 390.
Bowel Movements	
Frequent, watery stools	Diarrhea, p. 75; Stomach Flu and Food Poisoning, p. 88; Antibiotics, p. 388.
Stools are dry and difficult to pass	Constipation, p. 72.
Bloody or black, tarry stools	Ulcers, p. 89; Diarrhea, p. 75.
Pain during bowel movements; bright red blood on surface of stools or on toilet paper	Rectal problems, p. 86; Constipation, p. 72.
Blood in stool; bleeding from rectum; persistent change in bowel movements; thin, pencil-like stools	Colorectal Cancer, p. 70.
Abdominal Pain	
Pain and tenderness localized to one place with possible nausea, vomiting, and fever	Urinary Tract Infections, p. 94; Gallbladder Disease, p. 77; Kidney Stones, p. 96; also see p. 67.
Bloating and gas with diarrhea, constipation, or both	Irritable Bowel Syndrome, p. 81.
Pain in abdomen, possibly with vomiting or fever	Diverticular Disease, p. 76; Gallbladder Disease, p. 77.
Burning or discomfort behind or below breastbone	Heartburn, p. 78; Ulcers, p. 89; Chest Pain, p. 140.
Urination	
Pain or burning while urinating	Urinary Tract Infections, p. 94; Kidney Stones, p. 96; Prostate problems, pp. 269 to 273; Sexually Transmitted Diseases, p. 279.
Loss of bladder control	Urinary Incontinence, p. 92.
Difficulty urinating or weak urine stream (men)	Prostate problems, pp. 269 to 273.
Blood in urine	Urinary Tract Infections, p. 94; Kidney Stones, p. 96; Prostate problems, pp. 269 to 273.
Abdominal Lump or Swelling	
Painless lump or swelling in groin that comes and goes	Hernia, p. 80.

Generalized pain is pain that occurs in more than half of the abdomen. Generalized pain can occur with many different illnesses, most of which will go away without medical treatment. Stomach flu is a common problem that can cause generalized abdominal pain. **Cramping,** which can be very painful, is rarely serious if passing gas or a stool relieves it. Unless it is significantly different than usual, or it localizes to one area of the abdomen, generalized pain is usually not a cause for concern.

Localized pain is pain that is most intense in one part of the abdomen. Localized pain that comes on suddenly and persists, that gradually becomes more severe, or that gets worse when you move or cough may indicate a problem in an abdominal organ, such as appendicitis, pancreatitis, diverticulitis, an ovarian cyst, or gallbladder disease.

Any new abdominal pain that lasts more than a few days needs to be evaluated by a health professional.

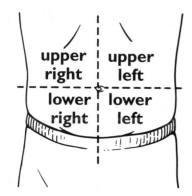

If you have abdominal pain, it helps to tell your doctor exactly where the pain is.

Home Treatment

Most abdominal pain improves with home treatment and does not require a visit to a health professional.

Specific home treatment for abdominal pain often depends on the symptoms that accompany the pain, such as diarrhea or nausea and vomiting. Be sure to review the home treatment guidelines for any other symptoms you have that are covered in this book.

If you have mild abdominal pain without other symptoms, try the following:

• Rest until you are feeling better.

• Drink plenty of fluids to avoid dehydration. You may find that taking small, frequent sips of a beverage is easier on your stomach than trying to drink a whole glass at once.

• Try eating several small meals instead of two or three large ones. Eat mild foods, such as rice, dry toast or crackers, bananas, and applesauce. Avoid other fruits, spicy foods, alcohol, and drinks that contain caffeine until 48 hours after all symptoms have gone away.

When to Call a Health Professional

Call 911 or other emergency services if you have any of the following:

• Signs of shock (see page 60)

• Pain or discomfort in the upper abdomen that occurs with squeezing or crushing chest pain or any other symptoms of a heart attack (see page 53)

- Signs of severe dehydration (see page 73)
- Severe abdominal pain following an injury to the abdomen

Call your doctor if you have:

- Ongoing severe abdominal pain.
- Localized pain that lasts longer than 4 hours.
- Generalized abdominal pain or cramping pain that has lasted longer than 24 hours and is not improving.
- Inability to keep down fluids.
- Pain that gets worse when you move or cough and does not feel like a pulled muscle.
- Any abdominal pain that has lasted longer than 3 days.

Colorectal Cancer

Cancer of the colon and rectum is the second leading cause of cancer deaths in the United States. Early in the course of the disease, when treatment is most likely to be successful, colorectal cancer has no symptoms. Later, symptoms of colorectal cancer include blood in the stool; bleeding from the rectum; a persistent change in bowel movements; thin, pencil-like stools; and lower abdominal pain.

You are at increased risk for colorectal cancer if you have a family history of the disease, if you have growths (polyps) in your colon, or if you have ulcerative colitis. High-fat and low-fiber diets have also been linked to colorectal cancer.

If you have colorectal cancer, learn as much as you can about the different treatment options. Work with your doctor to develop a treatment plan that will best meet your needs and desires. If you are not comfortable with the treatment options offered, ask your doctor about other options or consider a second opinion. Also see Winning Over Serious Illness on page 341.

Prevention

Eating a low-fat, high-fiber diet, limiting alcohol and red meat in your diet, not smoking, and getting regular physical activity may help prevent colorectal cancer. Taking calcium and folic acid supplements may also reduce your risk, but talk to your health professional before taking any supplements.

 Although screening tests don't prevent cancer, they can detect changes that may lead to cancer or detect the cancer early enough that it can be successfully treated. Screening for colorectal cancer may include tests for blood in the stool (fecal occult blood test), flexible sigmoidoscopy, and colonoscopy.

MORE INFO™ For more information, see the back cover.

The **fecal occult blood test** (FOBT) can detect hidden blood in your stool, which may indicate colon cancer or other problems. This test is inexpensive and easy to do at home, but it does not detect colon cancer as well as other screening tests do. The test for blood in the stool is very sensitive to blood from other sources, such as bleeding gums, ulcers, or red meat in your diet. Follow the package instructions exactly, and report any positive results to your doctor, even if other tests are negative.

Flexible sigmoidoscopy is a screening test for precancerous growths and cancers of the colon and rectum. The test may also be done if your doctor wants to determine the cause of rectal bleeding or persistent diarrhea or constipation. The sigmoidoscope is a flexible viewing instrument that is inserted into the rectum to examine the lower bowel. The exam takes about 10 to 15 minutes, is only mildly uncomfortable, and is very safe.

Colonoscopy is a test that allows the doctor to view the entire length of the colon and detect polyps, tumors, and areas of inflammation. Polyps found during the colonoscopy or in a previous test can be removed during the procedure. Colonoscopy is the most thorough screening method for colorectal cancer, but it is also the most invasive and most expensive. You have to take a laxative solution the day before the test to clean out your bowels, and you will be given pain medication and at least a mild sedative for the test itself. Many people worry that the procedure will be uncomfortable or embarrassing, but in reality, most don't remember the procedure well because of the sedative they are given. A colonoscopy usually takes 30 to 60 minutes.

See page 23 for the recommended schedule for colorectal cancer screening tests. You may need to have screening tests more often if you have a family history of colorectal cancer or if you have a history of colon polyps or ulcerative colitis.

When to Call a Health Professional

- Call immediately if your stools are dark red, black, or tarry. This usually means there is blood in your stool, which needs to be evaluated. Bright red blood in the stools is sometimes a sign of hemorrhoids. See Rectal Problems on page 86.

- If you have unexplained changes in bowel habits that last longer than 2 weeks, such as:

  - Constipation or diarrhea that doesn't clear up with home treatment.

  - Persistently thin, pencil-like stools.

- If you have unexplained pain in your lower abdomen.

Constipation

Constipation occurs when stools are difficult to pass. Some people are overly concerned with frequency because they have been taught that a healthy person has a bowel movement every day. This is not true. Most people pass stools anywhere from 3 times a day to 3 times a week. If your stools are soft and pass easily, you are not constipated.

Constipation may occur with cramping and pain in the rectum caused by straining to pass hard, dry stools. There may be some bloating and nausea. There may also be small amounts of bright red blood on the stools caused by slight tearing as the stools are pushed through the anus. The bleeding should stop when the constipation is relieved.

If a stool becomes lodged in the rectum, mucus and fluid may leak out around the stool, which sometimes leads to leakage of fecal material. This is called fecal incontinence. You may experience this as constipation alternating with diarrhea.

Older adults are slightly more prone to constipation than younger people are. Lack of fiber and too little water in the diet are common causes of constipation. Other causes include lack of exercise, delaying bowel movements, pain caused by a tear in the lining of the rectum, laxative overuse, and travel (if it disrupts your usual bowel movement schedule). Certain medications, such as antacids, antidepressants, antihistamines, diuretics, and narcotics, can also cause constipation. Constipation may also be a symptom of irritable bowel syndrome (see page 81).

Prevention

- Eat plenty of high-fiber foods such as fruits, vegetables, and whole grains. You can also add fiber to your diet in the following ways (also see Fiber on page 306):

  - Eat a bowl of bran cereal with 10 grams of bran per serving.

  - Add 2 tablespoons of wheat bran to cereal or soup.

  - Try a product that contains a bulk-forming agent, such as Citrucel, FiberCon, or Metamucil. If you are using a powder, start with 1 tablespoon or less. Drink extra water to avoid bloating.

- Avoid foods that are high in fat and sugar.

- Drink 1 to 2 quarts of water and other fluids every day. Drink extra fluids in the morning.

- Exercise more. A walking program is a good start. See Fitness starting on page 285.

- Set aside relaxed times for having bowel movements. Urges usually occur sometime after meals. Establishing a daily routine may help.

- Go when you feel the urge. Your bowels send signals when a stool needs to pass. If you ignore the signal, the urge will go away and the stool will eventually become dry and difficult to pass.

Home Treatment

Follow the diet outlined in Prevention to help relieve and prevent constipation. If necessary, use a stool softener or a very mild laxative such as milk of magnesia. Do not use mineral oil or any other laxative for more than 2 weeks without consulting your doctor.

When to Call a Health Professional

- If constipation and major changes in bowel movements continue after 1 week of home treatment, and there is no clear reason for such changes.

- If rectal bleeding is heavy (more than a few bright red streaks) or if the blood is reddish brown or black.

- If rectal bleeding lasts longer than 2 to 3 days after constipation has improved, or if bleeding occurs more than once.

- If you have sharp or severe abdominal pain.

- If you have rectal pain that either continues after you pass a stool or keeps you from passing stools at all.

- If you experience stool leakage.

- If your stools have become consistently more narrow.

- If you are unable to have bowel movements without using laxatives.

Dehydration

Dehydration occurs when the body loses too much water. When you stop drinking water or lose large amounts of fluids because of diarrhea, vomiting, or sweating, your body's cells reabsorb fluid from the blood and other tissues. Severe dehydration can lead to shock, which can be life-threatening.

Dehydration is dangerous for everyone, but especially for people who are weak or in frail health. Watch closely for early signs of dehydration whenever an illness causes vomiting, diarrhea, or high fever. The early symptoms of dehydration include dry mouth and sticky saliva, urinating smaller amounts than usual, and dark yellow urine.

Prevention

- Prompt home treatment for illnesses that cause diarrhea, vomiting, or fever will help prevent dehydration. See the chart on page 68.

- To prevent dehydration during hot weather or when exercising, drink 8 to 10 glasses of fluid (water and sports drinks) each day. Drink extra water before, during, and after exercise.

Rehydration Drinks

Diarrhea and vomiting can cause your body to lose large amounts of water and essential minerals called electrolytes. If you are unable to eat for a few days, you are also losing nutrients. This happens faster and is more serious in older adults who are weak or frail.

A rehydration drink (Rehydralyte, Lytren) will replace fluids and electrolytes in amounts that are best used by your body. Sports drinks and other sugared drinks will replace fluid, but most contain too much sugar (which can make the diarrhea worse) and not enough of the other essential ingredients. Plain water won't provide any necessary nutrients or electrolytes.

Rehydration drinks won't make diarrhea or vomiting go away faster, but they will prevent serious dehydration from developing.

You can make an inexpensive rehydration drink. Measure all the ingredients precisely. Small variations can make the drink less effective or even harmful. Mix:

- 1 quart water
- ½ teaspoon baking soda
- ½ teaspoon table salt
- 3 to 4 tablespoons sugar
- ¼ teaspoon salt substitute ("lite" salt), if available

Home Treatment

Treatment of mild dehydration is simple: stop the fluid loss and restore lost fluids as soon as possible.

- To stop vomiting or diarrhea, do not eat any solid foods for several hours or until you are feeling better. During the first 24 hours, take frequent, small sips of water or a rehydration drink.

- Once the vomiting or diarrhea is controlled, drink water, diluted broth, or sports drinks a sip at a time until your stomach can handle larger amounts. Drinking too much fluid too soon can cause vomiting to recur.

- If vomiting or diarrhea lasts longer than 24 hours, sip a rehydration drink to restore lost electrolytes. See Rehydration Drinks on page 74.

- Watch for signs of more severe dehydration (see When to Call a Health Professional).

When to Call a Health Professional

Call 911 or other emergency services if you develop signs of severe dehydration:

- Sunken eyes, no tears, dry mouth and tongue
- Little or no urine for 8 hours
- Skin that is doughy or doesn't bounce back when pinched
- Extreme dizziness or lightheadedness when moving from lying down to sitting upright

• Rapid breathing and heartbeat

• Sleepiness, difficulty awakening, list-lessness, and extreme irritability

Call a health professional:

• If vomiting lasts longer than 24 hours.

• If you are unable to hold down even small sips of fluid and therefore cannot drink enough to replace lost fluids.

• If severe diarrhea (large, loose stools every 1 to 2 hours) lasts longer than 2 days.

Diarrhea

Diarrhea occurs when the intestines push stools through before the water in the stools can be reabsorbed by the body or when the intestines produce extra water. This causes bowel movements to occur more frequently and stools to become watery and loose. A person who has diarrhea may also have abdominal cramps and nausea.

Viral stomach flu (gastroenteritis) or food poisoning often causes diarrhea. Many medications, especially antibiotics, can cause diarrhea; so can laxatives, if they are overused. Sorbitol (a sugar substitute) and olestra (a fat substitute used in some processed foods) may cause diarrhea. For some people, emotional stress, anxiety, or food intolerance may bring on this problem. Irritable bowel syndrome (see page 81) may also cause diarrhea.

Drinking untreated water that contains parasites, viruses, or bacteria is another cause of diarrhea. Symptoms usually develop a few days to a few weeks after you drink the contaminated water.

Prolonged diarrhea may lead to serious fluid loss and malnutrition, since nutrients are passed before the body can absorb them. See Dehydration on page 73.

Home Treatment

• Don't eat any food for several hours or until you are feeling better. Take frequent, small sips of water or a rehydration drink.

• Avoid antidiarrheal drugs for the first 6 hours. After that, use them only if there are no other signs of illness, such as fever, cramping or discomfort, or bloody stools. See Antidiarrheals on page 383.

• After the first 24 hours (or sooner, depending on how you feel), begin eating mild foods, such as rice, dry toast or crackers, bananas, and applesauce. Avoid other fruits, spicy foods, alcohol, and drinks that contain caffeine until 48 hours after all symptoms have disappeared. Avoid dairy products for 3 days after symptoms disappear.

• Take care to avoid dehydration. See page 73.

When to Call a Health Professional

- If you develop signs of dehydration (see page 73).

- If you have severe diarrhea (large, loose bowel movements every 1 to 2 hours).

- If diarrhea is accompanied by a fever of 101° or higher, chills, vomiting, or fainting.

- If diarrhea lasts longer than 2 weeks.

- If your stools are bloody or black.

- If abdominal pain increases or localizes, especially to the lower right or lower left part of your abdomen.

- If your symptoms become more severe or frequent.

- If diarrhea occurs after you drink untreated water.

Diverticular Disease

Many older adults have diverticular disease, a condition in which small sacs, called diverticula, form on the wall of the large intestine (colon). Diverticular disease can occur as diverticulosis or diverticulitis.

Most people who have **diverticulosis** have no symptoms and may never even know they have the condition. However, some people experience abdominal pain and cramping, especially on the left side. Treatment for painful diverticular disease is the same as for irritable bowel syndrome. See Home Treatment on page 82.

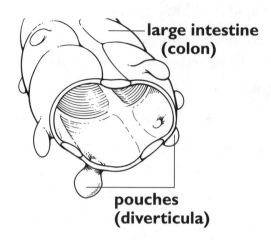

Diverticular disease occurs when pouches form in the lining of the colon.

In **diverticulitis**, the pouches in the wall of the large intestine become inflamed or infected. Fewer than 20 percent of people who have diverticulosis develop diverticulitis. Diverticulitis causes abdominal pain, often with fever and other signs of infection; a bloated sensation; diarrhea or constipation; nausea; and sometimes vomiting.

Blood vessels inside the diverticula can sometimes break and bleed. This will cause a large amount of bright red blood in the stool. Bleeding starts suddenly and usually stops on its own. Blood in the stool should always be evaluated by a health professional.

Prevention

Eating a high-fiber diet and drinking plenty of water may help prevent diverticulosis or prevent additional attacks of diverticulitis. Exercise may help prevent painful symptoms. Also see the tips for preventing constipation on page 72.

When to Call a Health Professional

• If you have been bleeding from the anus and you have signs of shock. See Shock on page 60.

• If abdominal pain that is localized to one spot lasts longer than 4 hours.

• If you have generalized, severe abdominal pain that is getting worse.

• If you have abdominal pain that gets worse when you move or cough.

• If you have cramping abdominal pain that does not get better when you have a bowel movement or pass gas.

• If you have noticed any unusual changes in your bowel movements or you have abdominal swelling.

• If you have blood in your stool.

Gallbladder Disease

The gallbladder is a small sac located under the liver. The gallbladder stores bile, a substance produced by the liver that helps the body digest fats. If there are problems with the gallbladder or if chemicals in the bile become too concentrated, stones may form in the gallbladder or the gallbladder may become inflamed. Gallstones are usually made of hardened cholesterol, but they can also be made of bilirubin, another chemical found in bile. In most cases, gallstones cause no problems, so people often don't even know that they have them.

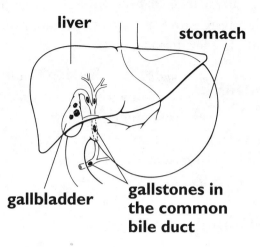

liver

stomach

gallbladder

gallstones in the common bile duct

Gallstones usually do not cause problems unless they move out of the gallbladder into the common bile duct.

In some cases, however, a stone may cause the gallbladder to become inflamed. The inflammation causes pain—usually in the upper right abdomen—that can be severe. Gallstone attacks often happen at night. They may awaken you from sleep and can last several hours. Fever and vomiting may also be present.

Gallstones can also cause problems if they start moving out of the gallbladder and become stuck in the common bile duct. If the common bile duct is blocked, inflammation of the pancreas (pancreatitis), jaundice, or infection may result.

People are more likely to develop gallbladder disease as they grow older. Gallbladder disease affects twice as many women as it does men. Other risk factors include a high-fat, high-sugar diet; obesity; lack of exercise; rapid weight loss; estrogen replacement therapy; diabetes; high cholesterol; high blood pressure; and a family history of gallbladder disease.

 Gallstones that don't cause symptoms don't require treatment. If gallstones cause pain, you may want to consider having surgery to remove your gallbladder.

Prevention

Maintain a healthy weight based on your height and age. If you need to lose weight, do so slowly and sensibly, losing no more than 1 to 1½ pounds per week.

Home Treatment

There is no home treatment for gallstones. If you think you have symptoms of gallstones, call your doctor to confirm the diagnosis. If the symptoms are mild, in most cases it is safe to wait until symptoms recur a few times before seeking treatment.

When to Call a Health Professional

- If you have continuous moderate to severe pain in the upper right part of your abdomen that occurs with a fever of 100.4° or higher and chills.

- If you have pain in the upper right part of your abdomen along with signs of jaundice, such as a yellow tint to your skin and the whites of your eyes, dark yellow or brown urine, or light-colored stools.

- If you have diabetes or a weakened immune system and you develop symptoms of gallstones.

- If you have symptoms that you think may be caused by gallstones, but there is no severe pain, fever, chills, or jaundice. If your symptoms are mild, it is probably safe to wait until your symptoms recur several times before seeking treatment.

Heartburn

Heartburn occurs when there is an abnormal backflow of stomach juices into the esophagus, the tube that leads from the mouth to the stomach. This backflow, called reflux, causes a feeling of burning, warmth, or heat beneath the breastbone. The discomfort may spread in waves upward into your neck, and you may get a sour taste in your mouth. Heartburn can last up to 2 hours or longer. Symptoms often start after you eat. They grow worse when you lie down or bend over and improve when you sit or stand up.

 Don't be concerned if you have heartburn now and then; nearly everyone does. Following the home treatment tips can prevent most cases of heartburn. However, if reflux of stomach acid into your esophagus happens regularly, you may have **gastroesophageal reflux disease (GERD)**. GERD can cause continuous irritation of the lining of the esophagus, which can lead to other health problems.

For more information, see the back cover.

It is important to visit a health professional if you have frequent heartburn and home treatment does not relieve the discomfort.

Home Treatment

Try other home treatment measures before taking antacids or stomach acid reducers to relieve heartburn. If you take medications to relieve your heartburn without doing other home treatment, your heartburn is likely to keep coming back. If symptoms are not relieved by home treatment, or if symptoms last longer than 2 weeks, call your doctor.

• Eat smaller meals, and avoid late-night snacks. Don't lie down for 2 to 3 hours after eating.

• Avoid foods that bring on heartburn. These may include chocolate, fatty or fried foods, peppermint- or spearmint-flavored foods, coffee, alcohol, and carbonated drinks.

• Limit acidic foods that can irritate your esophagus. These include citrus fruits and juices such as orange juice and tomato juice. Limit spicy foods.

• Avoid clothes with tight belts or waistbands.

• Stop smoking. Smoking promotes heartburn.

• Lose weight if you are overweight. Being overweight can worsen heartburn, and the loss of even a few pounds can help prevent heartburn.

• Raise the head of your bed 6 to 8 inches by putting blocks underneath your bed frame or placing a foam wedge under the head of your mattress. (Adding extra pillows does not work well.)

• Avoid aspirin, ibuprofen, naproxen sodium, and other anti-inflammatory drugs, which can aggravate heartburn. Try acetaminophen instead.

• Take a nonprescription product for heartburn. Antacids, such as Maalox, Mylanta, Tums, and Gelusil, neutralize stomach acid. Stomach acid reducers, such as Pepcid AC, Tagamet HB, and Zantac, reduce the amount of acid the stomach produces. Ask your pharmacist to help you choose one of these medications, and follow the package instructions and your doctor's advice for its use.

When to Call a Health Professional

Call 911 or other emergency services:

• If you have pain in the upper abdomen with chest pain that is crushing or squeezing, feels like a heavy weight on your chest, or occurs with any other symptoms of a heart attack (see page 53).

• If you have signs of shock (see Shock on page 60).

Call your doctor:

• If there is blood in your vomit or stools.

• If you suspect that a medication is causing heartburn. Antihistamines, central nervous system depressants, and anti-inflammatory drugs, including aspirin, ibuprofen, and naproxen sodium, can sometimes aggravate heartburn.

• If you are routinely having pain or difficulty when swallowing solid foods.

• If you are losing weight and you don't know why.

• If heartburn persists for more than 2 weeks despite home treatment. Call sooner if your symptoms are severe or are not relieved at all by antacids or acid reducers. Also see Ulcers on page 89.

Hernia

A hiatal hernia is a common problem that occurs when a portion of the stomach bulges into the chest cavity. Hiatal hernias often do not cause symptoms. However, sometimes a hiatal hernia will cause a backflow of stomach acid into the esophagus (the tube leading from the mouth to the stomach), which can cause heartburn and a sour taste in the mouth.

An inguinal hernia occurs when abdominal tissue bulges into the groin area through a weak spot in the abdominal wall. Inguinal hernias are more common in men than in women. In a man, an inguinal hernia may bulge into the scrotum.

A person with an inguinal hernia may sense that something has "given way." Other symptoms may include:

• A tender bulge in the groin or scrotum. The bulge may appear gradually, or it may form suddenly after heavy lifting, coughing, or straining. The bulge may disappear when the person lies down.

• Groin discomfort or pain that may extend into the scrotum. In a woman, the pain may occur in the groin or lower abdomen, just above the crease in the thigh. Discomfort may increase with bending or lifting.

• Nausea and abdominal swelling.

Inguinal hernias can be caused by increased abdominal pressure resulting from lifting heavy weights, coughing, or straining to pass stools. Sometimes a weak spot in the abdominal wall is present at birth. An inguinal hernia is called reducible if the protruding tissue can be pushed back into place in the abdomen. If the tissue cannot be pushed back into place, the hernia is called irreducible.

If an inguinal hernia is irreducible, the tissue may become trapped outside the abdominal wall. If the blood supply to the tissue is cut off (strangulated hernia), the tissue will swell and die. The dead tissue will quickly become infected, requiring immediate medical attention. Rapidly increasing pain in the groin or scrotum is a sign that a hernia has become strangulated.

A hernia can develop anywhere there is a weakness in the abdominal wall. Common places for hernias to develop are the belly button (umbilical hernia) and the site of an incision from abdominal surgery (incisional hernia).

Prevention

• Use proper lifting techniques (see page 100), and avoid lifting weights that are too heavy for you.

• Lose weight if you are overweight.

• Avoid constipation and do not strain when passing stools or urinating.

• Stop smoking, especially if you have a chronic cough.

When to Call a Health Professional

• If mild groin pain or an unexplained bump or swelling in the groin continues for more than 1 week.

• If the skin over a hernia or bulge in the groin or abdomen becomes red.

• If heartburn persists for more than 2 weeks despite home treatment. Call sooner if symptoms are severe or are not relieved at all by antacids or acid reducers. See Heartburn on page 78.

If you have been diagnosed with a hernia, call a health professional:

• If you have sudden, severe pain in the groin area, along with nausea, vomiting, and fever.

• If the hernia cannot be pushed back into place with gentle pressure when you are lying down.

 If you suspect that you have a hernia, see your doctor to confirm the diagnosis and discuss your treatment options.

Irritable Bowel Syndrome

Irritable bowel syndrome (IBS) is a common digestive disorder. Symptoms of IBS often increase with stress or after eating and include:

• Abdominal bloating, pain, and gas.

• Mucus in the stool.

• Feeling as if a bowel movement hasn't been completed.

• Irregular bowel habits, with constipation, diarrhea, or both.

The cause of IBS is unknown. Symptoms are thought to be related to abnormal muscle contractions in the intestines. However, when tests are done, they indicate no changes (no inflammation or tumors) in the physical structure of the intestines.

IBS can persist for many years. An episode may be more severe than the one before it, but the disorder itself does not worsen over time or lead to more serious diseases such as cancer. Symptoms tend to get better over time.

If you have not yet been diagnosed with IBS, try to rule out other causes of stomach problems, such as eating a new food, nervousness, or stomach flu. Try home treatment for 1 to 2 weeks. If there is no improvement, or if your symptoms worsen, call your doctor for an appointment.

 Your doctor may prescribe medication for you to take and ask you to continue home treatment. There are no tests that can diagnose <u>IBS</u>, but your doctor may recommend testing to rule out other possible causes of your symptoms. The amount of testing needed depends on your age, the pattern and severity of your symptoms, and your response to initial treatment.

Prevention

There is no way to prevent IBS. However, symptoms often worsen or improve because of changes in your diet, your stress level, medications, the amount of exercise you are getting, and other reasons that may or may not be known. Identifying the things that trigger your symptoms may help you avoid or minimize attacks.

Home Treatment

If constipation is your main symptom:

• Eat more fruits, vegetables, legumes, and whole grains. Add these fiber-rich foods to your diet slowly so that they do not worsen gas or cramps. See Fiber on page 306.

• Add unprocessed wheat bran to your diet. Start by using 1 tablespoon per day, and gradually increase to 4 tablespoons per day. Sprinkle bran on cereal, soup, and casseroles. Drink extra water to avoid becoming bloated.

• Try a bulk-forming product such as Citrucel, FiberCon, or Metamucil. If you are using a powder, start with 1 tablespoon or less per day, and drink extra water to prevent bloating.

• Use laxatives only if your doctor recommends them.

• Be more physically active. Exercise helps your digestive system work better.

If diarrhea is your main symptom:

• Using the fiber-rich food and wheat bran suggestions for relieving constipation can sometimes help relieve diarrhea by absorbing liquid in the large intestine.

• Avoid foods that make diarrhea worse. Try eliminating one food at a time; then add it back gradually. If a food doesn't seem to be related to symptoms, there is no need to avoid it. Many people find that the following foods or drinks make their symptoms worse:

   - Alcohol, caffeine, and nicotine

   - Beans, broccoli, cabbage, and apples

   - Spicy foods

   - Foods high in acid, such as citrus fruit

   - Fatty foods, including bacon, sausage, butter, oils, and anything deep-fried

Controlling Intestinal Gas

Passing intestinal gas, even as often as 20 times per day, is perfectly normal. However, if you want to reduce flatulence, there are some things you can do.

- Don't give up on beans; they are too good for you. Soak dry beans overnight, and then use fresh water for cooking them. Cook beans thoroughly. Beano, a product you can take as a tablet or put on food, may help reduce gas.

- If dairy products give you gas, switch to cultured milk products, such as yogurt or buttermilk, or add a lactase supplement, such as Lactaid, to your milk to help your digestion. See Lactose Intolerance on page 307.

- Avoid foods that contain the sweeteners fructose and sorbitol. They may increase flatulence.

- Take time to chew your food. Large lumps of food are harder to digest.

- Avoid constipation by eating a high-fiber diet and drinking plenty of water.

- Avoid dairy products that contain lactose (milk sugar) if they seem to worsen symptoms. But be sure to get enough calcium in your diet from other sources. See Lactose Intolerance on page 307.

- Avoid sorbitol (an artificial sweetener found in some sugarless candies and gum) and olestra (a fat substitute used in some processed foods, such as potato chips).

- Add more starchy foods, such as bread, rice, potatoes, and pasta, to your diet.

- If diarrhea persists, a nonprescription medication such as loperamide (the active ingredient in products such as Imodium) may help. Check with your doctor if you are using loperamide more than once a month.

To reduce stress:

- Keep a record of the life events that occur with your symptoms. This may help you see any connection between your symptoms and stressful occasions.

- Get regular, vigorous exercise such as swimming, jogging, or brisk walking to help reduce tension.

- See page 343 for more tips on managing stress.

When to Call a Health Professional

- If you have been diagnosed with irritable bowel syndrome and your symptoms get worse, begin to disrupt your usual activities, or do not respond as usual to home treatment.

- If you are becoming increasingly fatigued.

- If your symptoms frequently wake you.

- If your pain gets worse with movement.

- If you have abdominal pain and a fever of 100.4° or higher.

- If you are losing weight and you don't know why.

- If your appetite has decreased.

- If you have abdominal pain that does not get better when you pass gas or stools.

- If there is blood in your stools that is not obviously related to previously diagnosed hemorrhoids.

Nausea and Vomiting

Nausea is a very unpleasant feeling in the pit of the stomach. A person who is nauseated may feel weak and sweaty and produce lots of saliva. Intense nausea often leads to vomiting, which forces stomach contents up the esophagus and out of the mouth. Home treatment will help ease the discomfort.

Nausea and vomiting may be caused by:

- Viral stomach flu or food poisoning (see page 88).

- Stress or nervousness.

- Diabetes.

- Migraine headache (see page 185).

- Head injury (see page 51).

Nausea and vomiting can also be signs of other serious illnesses involving abdominal organs such as the liver (hepatitis; see page 85), pancreas, gallbladder (see page 77), or stomach (ulcers; see page 89).

In older adults, vomiting is often a sign of a medication reaction, especially if the person has just started taking a new medication or the dose has been changed. Antibiotics and anti-inflammatory drugs such as aspirin, ibuprofen, and naproxen sodium can cause nausea and vomiting.

Weak or frail older adults can become dehydrated quickly from fluid loss caused by vomiting. See Dehydration on page 73.

Home Treatment

- Watch for and treat early signs of dehydration. See page 73. Older adults can quickly become dehydrated from vomiting.

- After vomiting has stopped for 1 hour, drink 1 ounce of a clear liquid every 20 minutes for 1 hour. Clear liquids include apple or grape juice mixed to half strength with water; rehydration drinks; weak tea with sugar; clear broth; and gelatin dessert. Avoid citrus juices.

- If vomiting lasts longer than 24 hours, sip a rehydration drink to restore lost fluids and nutrients. See page 74.

- Rest in bed until you are feeling better.

- When you are feeling better, begin eating clear soups, mild foods, and liquids. Gelatin dessert, dry toast, crackers, and cooked cereal are good choices. Continue this diet until all symptoms have been gone for 12 to 48 hours.

Hepatitis

Hepatitis means "liver inflammation." Viruses cause hepatitis A, B, and C, the most common types of hepatitis.

Most people in the United States get hepatitis A after having personal contact with someone who is infected with the hepatitis A virus (HAV). Large groups of people can become infected with HAV if someone who has hepatitis A prepares food for them. HAV infection usually goes away without medical treatment, rarely causing long-term problems.

The hepatitis B virus (HBV) lives in blood and other body fluids. It is commonly spread during sexual contact and when people share needles to inject drugs, but it can also be spread when a person who is infected shares items like razors or tooth-brushes with others. Most adults with hepatitis B recover completely after 4 to 8 weeks. A few remain infected for months or years. Chronic infection can lead to life-threatening liver disease.

The hepatitis C virus (HCV) is spread when HCV-infected blood enters a person's body. Blood transfusions were once a common means of spreading HCV. The virus is also spread among people who share needles to inject drugs.

Many people with hepatitis C develop chronic HCV infection, which can lead to severe liver damage after many years.

Hepatitis symptoms are similar to flu symptoms. They include nausea, head-ache, sore muscles, and fatigue. Some people have pain in the upper right side of the abdomen. Jaundice may develop, causing the skin and whites of the eyes to turn yellow and making the urine dark. Call a health professional if you develop hepatitis symptoms or if you may have been exposed to hepatitis. Because all three types of viral hepatitis have similar symptoms, blood tests are needed to determine which hepatitis virus is caus-ing the infection.

Vaccines can prevent hepatitis A and B, but there is no vaccine for hepatitis C. If you are exposed to HAV or HBV before you have been vaccinated, getting a shot of immune globulin is likely to keep you from becoming infected.

 Drug treatment is available for people with chronic hepatitis (HBV or HCV) infection who are likely to develop liver problems.

When to Call a Health Professional

- If you develop signs of severe dehydration. See Dehydration on page 73.

- If vomiting occurs with:

  - A headache and severe stiff neck, drowsiness, confusion, or memory problems. See Encephalitis and Meningitis on page 189.

  - Chest pain and fever.

  - Fever and increasing pain in the lower right abdomen.

  - Fever and shaking chills.

  - Abdominal swelling.

  - Pain in the upper right or upper left abdomen.

- If vomit contains blood or material that looks like coffee grounds. You may be at risk for shock. See Shock on page 60.

- If vomiting and fever last longer than 48 hours.

- If you suspect that a medication is causing the problem. Learn which of your medications can cause these symptoms.

- If vomiting occurs after a head injury (see page 51).

- If vomiting lasts longer than 1 week.

- If nausea or vomiting is keeping you from taking medications you need to treat chronic conditions such as high blood pressure.

Rectal Problems

The rectum is the lower part of the large intestine. At the end of the rectum is the anus, where stools pass out of the body.

Rectal problems are common. Most everyone experiences itching, pain, or bleeding in the rectal or anal area at some time. These problems are often minor and will go away on their own or with home treatment.

Anal itching can have many causes. The skin around the anus may become irritated because of stool leakage. Caffeine and spicy foods can irritate the lining of the rectum, causing anal itching and discomfort. If the anus is not kept clean, itching may result. However, trying to keep the area too clean by rubbing it with dry toilet paper or using harsh soap may injure the skin.

Hemorrhoids are enlarged and inflamed veins that may develop inside or outside of the anus. Straining to pass hard stools, being overweight or pregnant, and prolonged sitting or standing can all cause hemorrhoids.

Hemorrhoids generally last several days and often come back (recur). The symptoms of hemorrhoids include bright red streaks of blood on stools or blood dripping from the anus; leakage of mucus from the anus; and irritation or itching around the anus. Sometimes an internal hemorrhoid will actually stick out of the anus, and it may have to be pushed back into place with a finger. Pain is not usually a symptom, unless a blood clot forms in a hemorrhoid or the blood supply to a hemorrhoid is cut off (strangulated or thrombosed). A clotted hemorrhoid may be extremely painful but is not dangerous. However, a strangulated hemorrhoid may need emergency treatment.

 You may want to consider surgery if you have hemorrhoids that bleed persistently, are very uncomfortable, or make it difficult to keep your anal area clean. Talk to your doctor about your options for surgery.

An **anal fissure** may cause pain during bowel movements and streaks of blood on stools. Anal fissures are long, narrow sores that usually develop when the tissue in the anal area is torn during a bowel movement.

Prevention

- Keep your stools soft. Include plenty of water, fresh fruits and vegetables, and whole grains in your diet. Include up to 2 tablespoons of bran or a commercial stool softener, such as Citrucel, in your diet each day. Regular exercise promotes smooth bowel movements. Also see Constipation on page 72.

- Try not to strain during bowel movements, and never hold your breath. Take your time, but don't sit on the toilet too long.

- Avoid sitting or standing too much. Take short walks to increase blood flow in your pelvic region.

- Keep your anal area clean, but be gentle when cleansing it. Use water and a fragrance-free soap, such as Ivory, or use baby wipes or Tucks pads.

Home Treatment

- Take warm baths. They are soothing and cleansing, especially after you have a bowel movement. Sitz baths (warm baths with just enough water to cover the anal area) are also helpful for hemorrhoids but may worsen anal itching.

- Wear cotton underwear and loose clothing to decrease moisture in the anal area.

- Apply a cold compress to your anus for 10 minutes, 4 times a day.

- Ease itching and irritation with zinc oxide, petroleum jelly, or 1% hydrocortisone cream. Use medicated suppositories such as Preparation H to relieve pain and lubricate your anal canal during bowel movements. Ask your doctor before using any product that contains a local anesthetic (these products have the suffix "-caine" in the name or ingredients). Such products cause allergic reactions in some people.

When to Call a Health Professional

- If rectal bleeding occurs for no apparent reason and is not associated with trying to pass stools.

- If rectal bleeding continues for more than 1 week or occurs more than a few times.

- If your stools become more narrow than usual (they may be no wider than a pencil).

- If pain caused by hemorrhoids is severe, or if moderate anal pain lasts longer than 1 week after home treatment.

- If any unusual material or tissue seeps or sticks out of your anus.

- If a lump near your anus gets bigger or becomes more painful and you develop a fever.

- If bloody stools are accompanied by a fever.

Stomach Flu and Food Poisoning

Stomach flu and food poisoning are different ailments with different causes. However, many people confuse the two because the symptoms are so similar.

Stomach flu is usually caused by a viral infection in the digestive system. To prevent stomach flu, you must avoid contact with the virus, which is not always easy to do. Always wash your hands after using the bathroom, changing diapers, blowing your nose, or playing with pets.

Food poisoning is usually caused by a toxin made by bacteria in food that is not handled or stored properly.

Bacteria can grow rapidly when certain foods, especially meats, dairy products, and sauces, are not handled properly during preparation or are kept at temperatures between 40° and 140°.

Suspect food poisoning when symptoms are shared by others who ate the same food or when symptoms develop after eating unrefrigerated foods. Symptoms of food poisoning may begin as soon as 1 or 2 hours or as long as 48 hours after eating. Nausea, vomiting, and diarrhea may last from 12 to 48 hours for common food poisoning.

Botulism is a rare but often fatal type of food poisoning. It is generally caused by improper home canning methods for low-acid foods like beans and corn. Bacteria that survive the canning process may grow and produce toxins in the jar. Symptoms include blurred or double vision and difficulty swallowing or breathing.

Prevention

To prevent food poisoning:

- Keep hot foods hot and cold foods cold.

- Follow the 2-40-140 rule. Don't eat meats, dressings, salads, or other foods that have been kept for more than 2 hours between 40° and 140°.

- Use a thermometer to check your refrigerator. It should be between 34° and 40°.

- Defrost meats in the refrigerator or microwave, not on the kitchen counter.

- Keep your hands and your kitchen clean. Wash your hands with hot soapy water before you handle food or utensils. After preparing raw meats, fish, poultry, shellfish, or eggs, wash your hands, cutting board, utensils, and countertop with hot soapy water.

- Cook meat until it is well done, poultry until the juices run clear, fish until it flakes with a fork, and shellfish until it is opaque.

- Do not eat raw or partially cooked eggs or uncooked foods that contain raw eggs.

- Discard any cans or jars that have bulging lids or leaks or that don't seem to be sealed well when you first open them.

- Follow home canning and freezing instructions carefully. Contact your county agricultural extension office for advice.

Home Treatment

- Viral stomach flu and food poisoning will usually go away within 24 to 48 hours. Good home care can speed recovery. See Nausea and Vomiting on page 84 and Diarrhea on page 75.

- Watch for and treat early signs of dehydration (see page 73). Weak or frail older adults can quickly become dehydrated from diarrhea and vomiting.

When to Call a Health Professional

Call 911 or other emergency services:

- If you develop signs of severe dehydration. See Dehydration on page 73.

- If you have symptoms of botulism, such as blurred or double vision or difficulty swallowing or breathing. If you still have a sample of the food that you suspect caused your symptoms, take it to the doctor for testing.

Call a health professional:

- If vomiting lasts longer than 1 day.

- If severe diarrhea (large, loose stools every 1 to 2 hours) lasts longer than 2 days.

Ulcers

A peptic ulcer is a sore or crater in the lining of the digestive tract. Most ulcers develop in the stomach, where they are called gastric ulcers, or in the upper part of the small intestine, where they are called duodenal ulcers.

Until recently, the cause of ulcers was not well understood. It is now believed that most people who develop ulcers are infected with *Helicobacter pylori (H. pylori)* bacteria. Many people who are infected with *H. pylori* do not develop ulcers unless other factors are also present. Such factors may include:

- Use of certain medications.

- Excessive alcohol use.

- Smoking.

- Physical stress, such as surgery or trauma.

- Other illnesses.

Most ulcers that are not caused by *H. pylori* infection are caused by frequent use of aspirin or other nonsteroidal anti-inflammatory drugs (such as ibuprofen, indomethacin, naproxen sodium, and Clinoril), which can damage the digestive tract's lining.

The symptoms of an ulcer are often similar to symptoms of other stomach problems like heartburn or inflammation of the stomach lining (gastritis). Symptoms may include a burning or gnawing pain between the navel and the breastbone. The pain often occurs between meals and may wake you during the night. Eating something or taking an antacid usually relieves the pain. Ulcers may also cause bloating, nausea, or vomiting after meals.

Ulcers can cause bleeding in the stomach and small intestine, which may cause stools to look dark red, black, or tarry. Without treatment, ulcers may occasionally cause a blockage between the stomach and the small intestine. An ulcer may break through (perforate) the stomach wall, causing severe abdominal pain and a rigid abdomen. Ulcers that bleed or perforate the stomach wall require immediate medical treatment.

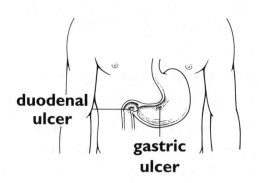

Gastric ulcers form in the stomach. Duodenal ulcers form in the upper part of the small intestine (duodenum).

 If you think you have an ulcer and your symptoms do not improve after 10 to 14 days of home treatment, make an appointment with your doctor. He or she can evaluate your symptoms and prescribe a treatment plan that may include antacids or other medications.

Prevention

You can greatly reduce the chance that you will get an ulcer if you:

- Quit smoking. People who smoke are twice as likely as nonsmokers to develop ulcers.

- Avoid aspirin, ibuprofen, and other nonsteroidal anti-inflammatory drugs (NSAIDs). If you must take these drugs regularly, take the smallest effective dose, and always take them with food. Some NSAIDs are made with a special coating that reduces the amount of stomach irritation they cause. However, this coating does not eliminate the risk of getting an ulcer if the medications are used frequently. Check with your doctor before changing your medications.

• Drink alcoholic beverages only in moderation. Never drink alcohol on an empty stomach.

• Manage stress. Although psychological stress alone does not cause ulcers to form, stressful situations may lead you to do things that increase your risk for developing ulcers, such as smoking or drinking too much alcohol. Stress may also make you more likely to develop an ulcer if you have a *H. pylori* infection in your stomach. Develop ways to help relieve stress, such as exercising, meditating, listening to music, reading, or talking to a friend or a counselor. See Mind-Body Wellness beginning on page 337.

Home Treatment

• Avoid foods that seem to bring on symptoms. Spicy or greasy foods cause problems for some people. Caffeine and alcohol may also trigger symptoms. However, it isn't necessary to eliminate any particular food from your diet if it doesn't cause problems.

• Try eating smaller, more frequent meals. If it doesn't help, return to a regular diet.

• Stop smoking. Smoking slows healing of ulcers and increases the likelihood that they will come back.

• Limit your alcohol intake. Excessive amounts of alcohol may make an ulcer heal more slowly and may make symptoms worse.

• Do not take aspirin, ibuprofen, or naproxen sodium. Try acetaminophen instead.

• Antacids, such as Tums, Maalox, and Mylanta, neutralize the acid in your stomach. Acid reducers, such as Pepcid AC, Tagamet HB, Zantac 75, and Axid AR, reduce the amount of acid your stomach produces. Proton pump inhibitors, including Prevacid, Prilosec, and Nexium, reduce the amount of stomach acid produced even more than acid reducers. Reducing the amount of acid in your stomach helps your ulcer heal. If you are taking antacids, you may need frequent, large doses to do the job. Talk with your doctor about the best dose. Also see page 382.

• Too much stress may slow ulcer healing. Practice the relaxation techniques beginning on page 344.

When to Call a Health Professional

• If you have pain in the upper abdomen with chest pain that is crushing or squeezing, feels like a heavy weight on your chest, or occurs with any other symptoms of a heart attack (see page 53).

• If you have been diagnosed with an ulcer and you have severe, continuous abdominal pain, severe vomiting, blood in vomit or stools, dizziness or lightheadedness, or signs of shock (see page 60).

- If your symptoms continue or get worse after 10 to 14 days of treatment with antacids or acid reducers.

- If you are losing weight and you don't know why.

- If you vomit often.

- If abdominal pain awakens you from sleep.

- If you have pain or difficulty when swallowing.

Urinary Incontinence

If you suffer from loss of bladder control, called urinary incontinence, you are not alone. Many older adults are coping with this problem.

Many cases of incontinence can be controlled or cured if the underlying problem is corrected. Water pills (diuretics) and many other common medications can cause temporary incontinence. Constipation, urinary tract infections, stones in the urinary tract, multiple pregnancies, and being overweight are other causes of incontinence.

The two most common types of persistent or chronic loss of bladder control are stress incontinence and urge incontinence.

Stress incontinence occurs when small amounts of urine leak out during exercise or when you cough, laugh, or sneeze. It is more common in women than in men, but it may affect some men after prostate surgery. Kegel exercises often help relieve stress incontinence. See page 93. Ask your doctor about devices that can be used to prevent urine from leaking.

Urge incontinence happens when the need to urinate comes on so quickly that you don't have enough time to get to the toilet. Causes include bladder infection, prostate enlargement, tumors that press on the bladder, Parkinson's disease, and nerve-related disorders such as multiple sclerosis or stroke.

Other types of incontinence may be caused by a blockage in the urinary tract, injury or damage to the nerves that control bladder function, or physical or mental problems that make it hard for a person to get to the bathroom or recognize the need to urinate.

Home Treatment

- Ask your doctor or pharmacist whether any of the medications you are taking can cause urinary incontinence. Your doctor may be able to prescribe a different drug that does not have this side effect. Do not stop taking any medication without first discussing it with your doctor.

- Don't let incontinence keep you from doing the things you like to do. Absorbent pads or briefs, such as Attends and

Depend, are available in pharmacies and supermarkets. No one will know you are wearing an absorbent pad.

- Avoid beverages that contain caffeine, which overstimulates the bladder. Do not cut down on fluids overall; you need fluids to keep the rest of your body healthy.

- Stop smoking. This may reduce your coughing, which may in turn reduce your problem with incontinence.

- Lose weight if you are overweight.

- Practice "double-voiding." Empty your bladder as much as possible, relax for a minute, and then try to empty it again.

- If you have stress incontinence, practice Kegel exercises daily. See Kegel Exercises on page 93.

- Urinate on a schedule, perhaps every 3 to 4 hours during the day, whether the urge is there or not. This may help you restore control.

- Wear clothing that can be removed quickly, such as pants with elastic waistbands.

- Clear a path from your bed to the bathroom, or consider placing a portable commode by your bed.

- Keep skin in the genital area dry to prevent rashes. Vaseline or Desitin ointment will help protect the skin from irritation caused by urine.

Kegel Exercises

Kegel exercises can help cure or improve stress incontinence by strengthening the muscles that control the flow of urine. No one will know you are doing them except you.

- Locate the muscles by repeatedly stopping your urine in midstream and starting again.

- Practice squeezing these muscles while you are not urinating. If your stomach or buttocks move, you are not using the right muscles.

- Hold the squeeze for 3 seconds; then relax for 3 seconds.

- Repeat the exercise 10 to 15 times per session. Do at least 3 Kegel exercise sessions per day.

 Try not to let <u>incontinence</u> embarrass you. It is not a sign of approaching senility. Take charge and work with your doctor to treat any underlying condition that may be causing the problem.

For more information about urinary incontinence, contact the National Association for Incontinence, P.O. Box 8310, Spartanburg, SC 29305, 1–800–252–3337.

When to Call a Health Professional

- If you suddenly become incontinent.

- If you are urinating frequently, but only passing small amounts of urine.

- If your bladder feels full even after you urinate.

- If you have difficulty urinating when your bladder feels full.

- If you feel burning or pain while urinating. See Urinary Tract Infections on page 94.

- If your urine looks bloody and there is no dietary reason why your urine might look this way (for example, if you had eaten beets).

- If your urine has an unusual odor.

- If urinary incontinence is disrupting your life.

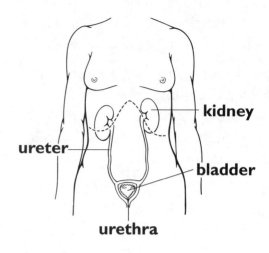

Infections can occur in any of the structures of the urinary tract.

Urinary Tract Infections

The urinary tract includes the kidneys, ureters, bladder, and urethra. The kidneys filter the blood, and the waste products from the blood become urine. The ureters carry urine from the kidneys to the bladder. The bladder holds the urine until the urine is expelled from the body through the urethra.

Urinary tract infections (UTIs), including bladder infections (cystitis) and kidney infections (pyelonephritis), are usually caused by bacteria that are normally present in the digestive system. Women get UTIs more often than men do.

Early symptoms of a UTI may include burning or pain during urination and itching or pain in the urethra. You may also have discomfort in your lower abdomen or back and a frequent urge to urinate without being able to pass much urine. Your urine may be cloudy or reddish in color and may have an unusual odor. Chills and fever may be present if the infection is severe, especially if it has spread to the kidneys.

Men with symptoms similar to those caused by a UTI may have an infection of the prostate gland or the epididymis (the tube that transports sperm from the testicle). See Prostate Infection on page 269.

Men who have enlarged prostates, women who have had multiple pregnancies, people with kidney stones or diabetes, and those who are paralyzed from the waist down may be at higher risk for chronic urinary tract infections.

Other causes of irritation to the genital area that may be associated with UTIs include having sexual intercourse, wearing tight pants, riding a bike, using perfumed soaps and powders, or even eating spicy foods.

Prevention

• Drink plenty of fluids; water is best. Aim for at least 2 quarts per day.

• Urinate frequently.

• Women should wipe from front to back after going to the toilet. This will reduce the spread of bacteria from the anus to the urethra.

• Avoid douching and bubble baths, and don't use vaginal deodorants or perfumed feminine hygiene products.

• Wash the genital area once a day with plain water or mild soap and water. Rinse well and dry the area thoroughly.

• Drink extra water before sexual intercourse and urinate promptly afterwards. This is especially important if you tend to get UTIs.

• Wear cotton underwear, cotton-lined panty hose, and loose clothing.

• Avoid alcohol, caffeine, and carbonated beverages, which can irritate the bladder.

• Include cranberry and blueberry juice in your diet. These may protect against UTIs, especially in women.

Home Treatment

Start home treatment at the first sign of genital irritation or painful urination. A day or so of self-care may clear up a minor infection. However, if your symptoms last longer than 1 or 2 days or worsen despite home treatment, call your doctor. Because the organs of the urinary tract are connected, untreated UTIs can spread, which may lead to kidney infections and other serious problems.

• Drink extra fluids (think in terms of gallons) as soon as you notice symptoms and for the next 24 hours. This will help dilute the urine, flush bacteria out of the bladder, and decrease irritation. Cranberry and blueberry juice are good choices in addition to water.

• Urinate frequently and follow the other tips outlined in Prevention.

• Check your temperature twice daily. Fever may indicate a more serious infection.

• Taking a hot bath may help relieve pain. Avoid using bubble bath and harsh soaps. Apply a heating pad over your genital area to help relieve the pain. Never go to sleep with a heating pad in place.

• Avoid sexual intercourse until your symptoms improve.

When to Call a Health Professional

- If painful urination occurs with any of the following symptoms:

  - Fever of 100.4° or higher and chills.

  - Inability to urinate when you feel the urge.

  - Pain in the back, side, groin, or genital area.

  - Blood or pus in the urine.

  - Unusual vaginal discharge.

  - Nausea and vomiting.

- If symptoms get worse despite home treatment.

- If symptoms do not improve after 24 hours of home treatment.

- If you have diabetes and you have symptoms of a urinary tract infection.

Kidney Stones

 Kidney stones can form from the minerals in urine. The most common cause of kidney stones is not drinking enough water.

As long as they stay in the kidneys, kidney stones usually cause no problems. A stone may move out of the kidney into the tube that leads to the bladder (ureter) and may block the flow of urine. This can cause severe pain.

Symptoms that may develop when a kidney stone moves through a ureter include:

- Pain in the side, groin, or genital area that begins suddenly and gets worse over 15 to 60 minutes until it is steady and nearly unbearable. The pain may stop for a while when the stone is not moving, and pain often vanishes suddenly when the stone moves into the bladder.

- Nausea and vomiting.

- Blood in the urine.

- Feeling like you need to urinate often or pain when urinating.

- Loss of appetite, diarrhea, or constipation.

Call your doctor immediately if you suspect that you are passing a kidney stone. Most small kidney stones pass without the need for any medical treatment other than pain medication. In rare cases, surgery may be needed.

5

Back and Neck Pain

Few of us are lucky enough to make it through life without having back or neck pain at some time. Because it supports the weight of your body throughout your entire life, your lower back is especially prone to injury and the effects of aging. As you grow older, it is common for back or neck pain to be caused by health problems that affect your spine or its supporting structures. These conditions can cause chronic pain. However, most back and neck problems are the result of strain or overuse. By following the home treatment guidelines in this chapter, you can recover from most back and neck pain and prevent it from recurring.

Most back pain is the result of overuse injuries caused by repeated movements or prolonged postures that strain the back. Poor body mechanics while lifting, standing, walking, sitting, or even sleeping cause many episodes of back pain.

Strains or sprains can occur if a sudden or awkward movement twists your spine beyond its usual limits. These injuries may affect the ligaments and muscles that support your spine or the sacroiliac joints (the joints between the spine and either side of the pelvis).

Back Pain

Your back is composed of the bones of the spine (vertebrae), the joints that guide the direction of movement of the spine, the discs that separate the bones of the spine and absorb shock as you move, and the muscles and ligaments that hold them all together.

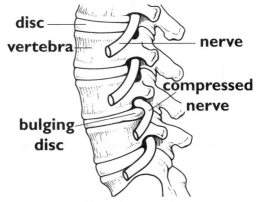

A bulging or ruptured (herniated) disc can cause pressure on a nerve.

First Aid for Back Pain

When you first feel a catch or strain in your back, try these steps to avoid or reduce pain. These are the most important home treatments for the first few days of back pain. Also see Home Treatment on page 104.

First Aid No. 1: Relax

Lie down in a comfortable position. Relax for 1 to 2 minutes.

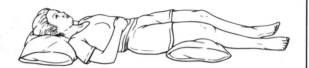

First Aid No. 2: Ice

Apply ice or a cold pack to your sore back. Do this for 10- to 15-minute periods throughout the day. Cold applied for the first 3 days limits swelling, reduces pain, and speeds healing. After 3 days, you may use heat if it helps you feel better.

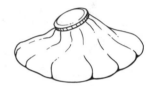

First Aid No. 3: Pelvic tilts

This exercise gently moves the spine and stretches the lower back.

Lie on your back with knees bent and feet flat on the floor.

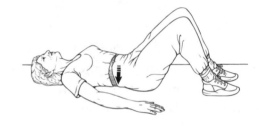

Slowly tighten your stomach muscles and press your lower back against the floor. Hold for 10 seconds (do not hold your breath). Slowly relax.

First Aid No. 4: Walk

Take a short walk (3 to 5 minutes) on a level surface every 3 hours. Walk only distances you can manage without pain, especially leg pain.

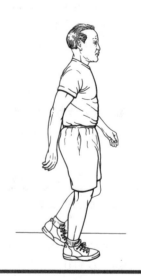

Injuries can damage the discs in the spine so that they tear, stretch, or rupture. If a tear in a disc is large enough, the jellylike material inside the disc may leak out and press against a spinal nerve. You may feel shooting pain, tingling, or numbness in the lower back, in the buttock, or down the leg (this type of pain is called sciatica). The muscles controlled by the compressed nerve may become weak.

Sciatica

Sciatica is an irritation of the sciatic nerve, which is formed by the nerve roots coming out of the spinal cord into the lower back. The sciatic nerve extends down through the buttocks and to the feet. Sciatica can occur when an injured disc presses against a spinal nerve root. Its main symptom is radiating pain, numbness, or weakness that is usually worse in the leg than in the back. In addition to the home treatment for back pain on page 104, the following may help:

- Avoid sitting if possible, unless it is more comfortable than standing.

- Alternate lying down with short walks. Increase your walking distance when you are able to do so without pain.

- Apply ice or a cold pack to the middle of your lower back.

Any of these injuries can result in several days of pain produced by swelling and inflammation in the injured tissue, followed by slow healing and a gradual reduction in pain. The goals of self-care for back pain are to relieve pain, promote healing, and avoid reinjury. Fortunately, most acute back injuries heal on their own in 6 to 12 weeks.

Back pain can also be caused by conditions that affect the bones and joints of your spine. Arthritis pain may be a steady ache, unlike the sharp, acute pain of strains, sprains, and disc injuries. If you think arthritis may be causing your back pain, combine the self-care guidelines for back pain with those for arthritis on page 111.

Osteoporosis and Paget's disease weaken the bones, including those of the spine, which can lead to broken bones and compression fractures. Compression fractures cause vertebrae to collapse. This can cause misalignment of the spine, which may lead to varying degrees of pain. **Spinal stenosis** is the narrowing of the spinal canal, which can squeeze and irritate spinal nerves or the spinal cord itself. This can cause pain, numbness, or weakness in the legs and feet.

Prevention

The keys to preventing back pain are to use good body mechanics and to practice good health habits, such as getting regular exercise, maintaining a healthy weight, and avoiding tobacco products (nicotine weakens the discs in your back). Some of the tips presented here are things you will want to do every day, not only because they are good for your back but because they are good for your overall health. The rest will come in handy if you are ever suffering from acute back pain.

Body Mechanics

Good body mechanics will reduce the stress on your back. Use good body mechanics all the time, not just when you have back pain.

Sitting

• Avoid sitting in one position for more than an hour at a time. Get up or change positions often.

• If you must sit a lot, the exercises starting on page 101 are particularly important.

• If your chair doesn't provide enough support, use a small pillow or rolled towel to support your lower back.

• When driving, pull your seat forward so the pedals and steering wheel are within comfortable reach. Stop often to stretch and walk around. If you have pain while driving, try placing a small pillow or a rolled towel behind your lower back.

Lifting

• Keep your upper back straight. Do not bend forward from the waist to lift.

• Bend your knees and let your arms and legs do the work. Tighten your buttocks and abdomen to further support your back.

• Keep the load as close to your body as possible, even if the load is light.

Leg Weakness

Many people who have low back pain say their legs feel weak. If leg weakness is related to back pain, you will be able to make your leg muscles work, but it will probably hurt.

True leg weakness means you have decreased strength in your legs, no matter how much you try to push through the pain. This may be due to a problem in the spine, such as a herniated disc.

Leg weakness should be evaluated by a doctor, especially if you are unable to bend your foot upward, get up out of a chair, or climb stairs.

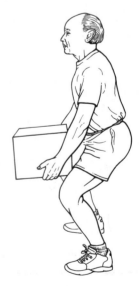

Proper lifting posture

- While holding a heavy object, turn your feet, not your back. Try not to turn or twist your body.

- If possible, don't lift heavy objects above shoulder level.

- Use a hand truck or ask someone to help you carry heavy or awkward objects.

Lying Down

If you have back pain at night, your mattress may be the problem. Try sleeping on a firmer mattress. Or, if you think your mattress is too firm, try one that's a little softer. Try these additional tips for more comfortable sleep:

- If you sleep on your back, you may want to use a rolled towel to support your lower back or put a pillow under your knees.

- If you sleep on your side, try placing a pillow between your knees.

- Sleeping on your stomach is fine if it doesn't increase your back or neck pain.

Exercise

Regular exercise that includes stretching, strengthening, and aerobic exercise helps you maintain your overall fitness and flexibility and strengthens the muscles that support your spine. Exercising also helps you maintain a healthy body weight, which reduces the load on your lower back. If you are interested in creating a personalized fitness plan, see Fitness starting on page 285.

Although there is no clear evidence that specific exercises can help prevent back pain, the exercises that follow represent a common, practical approach to helping you maintain strength and flexibility. You may choose to make the exercises a part of your regular fitness routine.

Do not do these exercises if you have just injured your back. Instead, follow the recommendations in First Aid for Back Pain on page 98.

Extension exercises strengthen the lower back muscles and stretch the stomach muscles and ligaments. Flexion exercises stretch the lower back muscles and strengthen the stomach muscles.

- You do not need to do every exercise. Do the ones that help you the most.

- If any exercise makes your back pain worse, stop the exercise and try something else. Stop any exercise that causes the pain to radiate into your buttocks or legs, either during or after the exercise.

- Start with 5 repetitions, 3 to 4 times a day, and gradually increase to 10 repetitions. Do the exercises slowly.

Extension Exercises

Press-Ups

Begin and end every set of exercises with a few press-ups.

- Lie facedown with your arms bent, palms flat on the floor.

- Lift yourself up on your elbows, keeping the lower half of your body relaxed. If it's comfortable to do so, press your chest forward.

- Keep your hips pressed to the floor. Feel the stretch in your lower back.

- Lower your upper body to the floor. Repeat this exercise slowly.

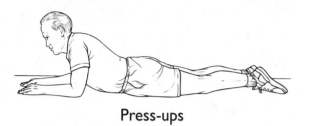

Press-ups

Shoulder Lifts

Shoulder lifts will strengthen the muscles that support the spine.

- Lie facedown with your arms beside your body.

- Lift your shoulders straight up from the floor as high as you can without pain. Keep your chin down and your eyes facing the floor. Keep your torso and hips pressed to the floor.

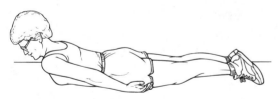

Shoulder lifts
(keep neck straight and chin down)

Backward Bend

Practice the backward bend at least once a day and whenever you work in a bent-forward position.

- Stand upright with your feet slightly apart. Back up to a countertop for greater support and stability.

- Place your hands in the small of your back and gently bend backward. Keep your legs straight and bend only at the waist. Hold the backward stretch for 1 to 2 seconds.

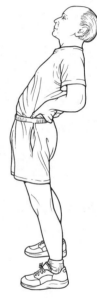

Backward bend
(keep neck straight and chin down)

Flexion Exercises

Curl-Ups

Curl-ups strengthen your abdominal muscles, which work with your back muscles to support your spine.

- Lie on your back with knees bent (60° angle), feet flat on the floor, and arms crossed on your chest. Do not hook your feet under anything.

- Slowly curl your head and shoulders up until your shoulder blades barely rise from the floor. Keep your lower back pressed to the floor. To avoid neck problems, remember to lift your shoulders, and do not force your head up or forward. Hold for 5 to 10 seconds (do not hold your breath), and then curl down very slowly.

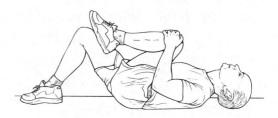

Knee-to-chest stretch

Additional Strengthening and Stretching Exercises

Prone Buttocks Squeeze

This exercise strengthens the buttocks muscles, which support the back and help you lift with your legs. You may need to place a small pillow under your stomach for comfort.

- Lie flat on your stomach with your arms at your sides.

- Slowly tighten your buttocks muscles and hold for 5 to 10 seconds (don't hold your breath). Relax slowly.

Pelvic Tilts

See instructions on page 98.

Hamstring Stretch

This exercise stretches the muscles in the back of your thigh, which will allow you to bend your legs without putting stress on your back.

- Lie on your back in a doorway with one leg through the doorway on the floor. Put the leg you want to stretch straight up, with the heel resting on the wall next to the doorway.

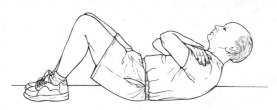

Curl-ups
(keep chin tucked in)

Knee-to-Chest Stretch

The knee-to-chest exercise stretches the lower back muscles and relieves pressure on the joints where the vertebrae come together.

- Lie on your back with knees bent and feet close to your buttocks.

- Bring one knee to your chest, keeping the other foot flat on the floor (or keep the other leg straight, if that feels better on your lower back). Keep your lower back pressed to the floor. Hold for 5 to 10 seconds.

- Relax and lower your knee to the starting position. Repeat with the other leg.

- Keep the leg straight and slowly move your heel up the wall until you feel a gentle pull in the back of your thigh. Do not overstretch.

- Relax in this position for 30 seconds; then bend the knee to relieve the stretch. Repeat with the other leg.

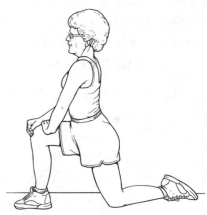

Hip flexor stretch

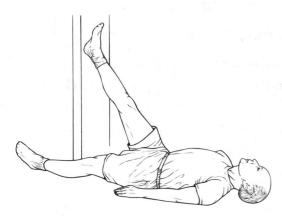

Hamstring stretch

Hip Flexor Stretch

This exercise stretches the muscles in the front of your hip.

- Kneel on one knee with your other leg bent in front of you.

- Slowly sink your hips so your weight shifts onto your front foot. The knee of your forward leg should be aligned over the ankle. Hold for 10 seconds. You should feel a stretch in the groin of the leg you are kneeling on. Repeat with the other leg.

Exercises to Avoid

Many common exercises actually increase the risk of low back pain. Avoid the following:

- Straight-leg sit-ups

- Bent-leg sit-ups when you have acute back pain

- Leg lifts (lifting both legs while lying on your back)

- Lifting heavy weights above the waist (military press, biceps curls while standing)

- Any stretching done while sitting with the legs in a V

- Toe touches while standing

Home Treatment

Immediately after an injury and for the next few days, the most important home treatment includes the following:

- Follow the First Aid for Back Pain guidelines on page 98.

- Sit or lie in positions that are most comfortable and reduce your pain, especially any leg pain. Do not sit up in bed, and avoid soft couches and twisted positions. Avoid sitting for long periods of time. Follow the body mechanics guidelines discussed earlier.

- Bed rest can help relieve back pain but may not speed healing. Unless you have severe leg pain, 1 to 3 days of bed rest should relieve the most severe pain. More than 3 days of bed rest is not recommended and could actually delay healing. For bed rest, try one of the following positions:

  - Lie on your back with your knees bent and supported by large pillows, or lie on the floor with your legs on the seat of a sofa or chair.

  - Lie on your side with your knees and hips bent and a pillow between your legs.

  - If it doesn't increase your pain, lie on your stomach.

- Take aspirin or ibuprofen regularly as directed. Call your doctor if you've been told to avoid anti-inflammatory medications. Acetaminophen may also be used. Take these medications sensibly; the maximum recommended dose will reduce the pain. Masking the pain completely might allow movement that could lead to reinjury.

- Relax your muscles. See page 345 for progressive muscle relaxation.

Back Surgery

Rest, pain relievers, and exercise can bring relief for most back problems, even disc problems.

 Most surgeries are done to treat <u>disc</u> problems that have not improved with time and exercise. Surgery may also be appropriate for spinal fracture, spinal infection, and other conditions.

Getting all the facts and thinking about your own needs and values will help you make a wise decision about back surgery.

If you do plan to have surgery, the guidelines on body mechanics and exercise in this chapter are still important. A strong, flexible back will help you recover more quickly after surgery.

- Continue daily walks (gradually increase to 5 to 10 minutes, 3 to 4 times a day).

- Try swimming, which is good for your back. It may be painful immediately after a back injury, but lap swimming or kicking with swim fins often helps prevent back pain from recurring.

- When your pain has improved, begin easy exercises that do not increase your pain. One or two of the exercises described on pages 101 to 104 may be helpful. Start with 5 repetitions 3 to 4 times a day, and increase to 10 repetitions as you are able.

When to Call a Health Professional

Call 911 or other emergency services immediately:

- If pain in the upper back occurs with chest pain or any other symptoms of a heart attack (see page 53).

- If back pain is the result of a severe injury, such as a car accident, fall, major sports injury, direct blow to the spine, forceful strike on top of the head, or a knife or gunshot wound.

- If an injured person shows signs of a spinal injury, such as:

  - Paralysis in any part of the body.

  - Severe neck or back pain.

  - Weakness, tingling, or numbness in the arms or legs.

  - Loss of bladder or bowel control.

Call a health professional:

- If you have injured your back and:

  - You cannot walk or stand.

  - You have new numbness in the buttocks, genital or rectal area, or legs.

  - You have leg weakness that is not solely due to pain. Many people with low back pain say their legs feel weak. You should see a doctor if leg weakness is so severe that you are unable to bend your foot upward, get up out of a chair, or climb stairs.

- If you have new or increased back pain with unexplained fever, painful urination, or other signs of a urinary tract infection. See page 94.

- If you have a dramatic increase in your chronic back pain, especially if it is unrelated to a new or changed physical activity.

- If you have a history of cancer or HIV infection and you develop new or increased back pain.

- If you have severe back pain that does not improve after a few days of home treatment.

- If you develop a new, severe pain in your lower back that does not change with movement and is not related to stress, muscle tension, or a known injury.

- If back pain does not improve after 2 weeks of home treatment.

Neck Pain

Most people occasionally feel pain, stiffness, or a "kink" in the neck. Pain may spread to your shoulders, upper back, or upper arms, and it may also cause headaches. Pain may limit neck movement. This usually affects one side of your neck more than the other.

Neck pain is most often caused by tension, strain, or spasm in the neck muscles or inflammation of the neck ligaments, tendons, or joints. These problems typically result from prolonged or repeated activities or movements that stress the neck. Postures that put your neck in awkward positions (such as cradling the phone between your ear and shoulder or sleeping with your neck twisted) are also common causes.

Neck Exercises

You do not need to do every exercise. Stick with the ones that help you the most. Do each exercise slowly. Stop any exercise that increases pain. Start by doing the exercises twice a day.

Dorsal glide: Sit or stand tall, looking straight ahead (a "palace guard" posture). Slowly tuck your chin as you glide your head backward over your body. Hold for a count of 5; then relax. Repeat 6 to 10 times. This stretches the back of the neck. If you feel pain, do not glide so far back. You may find this exercise easier to do while lying on your back with ice on your neck.

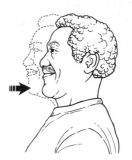

Dorsal glide

Chest and shoulder stretch: Sit or stand tall and glide your head backward as in the dorsal glide exercise. Raise both arms so that your hands are next to your ears. As you exhale, lower your elbows down and back. Feel your shoulder blades slide down and together. Hold for a few seconds. Relax and repeat 6 to 10 times.

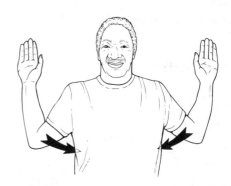

Chest and shoulder stretch

Shoulder lifts: Lie facedown with your arms beside your body. Lift your shoulders straight up from the floor as high as you can without pain. Keep your chin down and your eyes facing the floor. Keep your torso and hips pressed to the floor. Repeat 6 to 10 times.

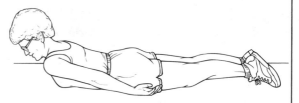

Shoulder lifts

Hands on head: Move your head backward, forward, and side to side against gentle pressure from your hands, holding each position for several seconds. Repeat 6 to 10 times.

Other causes of neck pain include:

- Injury resulting from a sudden movement of the head and neck (whiplash), a direct blow to the neck, or a fall.

- Arthritis or damage to the discs in the neck that results in a "pinched nerve." When this is the cause of neck pain, the pain usually spreads down the arm. Numbness, tingling, or weakness in the arm or hand may occur. When you have symptoms of a "pinched nerve," you need to see your doctor.

- Meningitis, a serious illness that requires emergency care. Meningitis causes a severe stiff neck with headache and fever (see page 189).

Prevention

Most neck pain can be prevented by using good posture, getting regular exercise, and avoiding prolonged periods in positions that stress the neck. You can also strengthen and protect your neck by doing neck exercises once a day. See page 107. If stress may be the cause of your neck pain, practice the progressive muscle relaxation exercises on page 345.

If your pain is **worse at the end of the day**, evaluate your posture and body mechanics during the day.

- Sit straight in your chair with your lower back supported. Avoid sitting for long periods without getting up or changing positions. Take mini-breaks several times each hour to stretch your neck muscles.

- If you work at a computer, adjust the monitor so that the top of the screen is at eye level. Use a document holder that puts the copy at the same level as the screen.

- If you use the telephone a lot, consider using a headset or speakerphone.

If your neck stiffness is **worse in the morning**, you may need better neck support when you sleep.

- Try folding a towel lengthwise into a 4-inch-wide pad and wrapping it around your neck. Pin it for good support.

- You may want to use a special neck support pillow. Look for a pillow that supports your neck comfortably when you lie on your back and on your side (try before buying). Avoid pillows that force your head forward when you are on your back.

- Avoid sleeping on your stomach with your neck twisted or bent.

- Morning neck pain also may be the result of activities done the day before or may be caused by arthritis.

Home Treatment

Much of the home treatment for back pain is also helpful for neck pain. See page 104.

- Apply ice or a cold pack to the sore area. If the pain is near your shoulder or upper back, it will usually help more to ice the back of your neck.

- Use aspirin, ibuprofen, or aceta-minophen to help relieve pain.

- Walking helps relieve and prevent neck pain. The gentle swinging motion of your arms often relieves pain. Start with short walks of 5 to 10 minutes, 3 to 4 times a day.

- If neck pain occurs with headache, see Tension Headaches on page 189.

- Once the pain starts to get better, do the exercises on page 107.

When to Call a Health Professional

Call 911 or other emergency services immediately:

- If neck pain occurs with chest pain or other symptoms of a heart attack (see page 53).

- If you have neck pain after a severe injury, such as a car accident, fall, major sports injury, direct blow to the spine, forceful strike on top of the head, or a knife or gunshot wound.

- If an injured person shows signs of a spinal injury, such as:

  - Paralysis in any part of the body.

  - Severe neck or back pain.

  - Weakness, tingling, or numbness in the arms or legs.

  - Loss of bladder or bowel control.

Call a health professional:

- If a stiff neck occurs with headache and fever (see Encephalitis and Meningitis on page 189).

- If neck pain extends or shoots down one arm, or you have numbness or tingling in your hands.

- If neck pain starts within 2 weeks of an injury.

- If you develop new weakness or continuous numbness in your arms or legs.

- If you are unable to manage your pain with home treatment.

- If neck pain has lasted 2 weeks or longer without improvement despite home treatment.

I don't deserve this award, but then I have
arthritis and I don't deserve that either.
Jack Benny

6

Bone, Muscle, and Joint Problems

Problems with bones, muscles, and joints are the main reasons why older people become less active. However, you don't have to take these problems sitting down!

As your bones, muscles, and joints age, the following changes happen:

• Your muscle strength declines.

• Your bone mass decreases.

• Your joints become less flexible, and your range of motion decreases.

You may be able to prevent these changes, or at least lessen their effects on your life, by making wise lifestyle choices. Exercising regularly—even walking or doing chair exercises—will help keep you strong and flexible. Eating a healthy diet, taking medications as prescribed to maintain the health of your bones, and treating injuries and minor

inflammation before chronic pain becomes a problem are the best ways to ensure that your bones, muscles, and joints will support you in your favorite activities.

Arthritis

Arthritis refers to a variety of joint problems that cause pain, swelling, and stiffness. Simply put, arthritis means inflammation of a joint. Arthritis can occur at any age, but it affects older people the most.

 There are more than 100 different types of arthritis. The chart on page 112 describes three common kinds of arthritis. Osteoarthritis is the most common type and can usually be successfully managed at home. Rheumatoid arthritis and gout can improve with a combination of self-care and professional care.

Common Types of Arthritis			
Type	**Cause**	**Symptoms**	**Comments**
Osteoarthritis	Breakdown of joint cartilage	Pain and stiffness; common in knees, fingers, hips, feet, and back	Most common after age 50
Rheumatoid arthritis	Inflammation of the membrane (synovium) lining the joint	Pain, stiffness, warmth, and swelling in multiple joints on both sides of body; common in hands, wrists, feet, elbows, knees, and neck	Onset most often around age 40; more common in women
Gout (p. 120)	Buildup of uric acid crystals in the joint fluid	Sudden onset of burning pain, stiffness, and swelling; common in big toe, ankle, knee, wrist, and elbow	Most common in men ages 30 to 50; rare in women before menopause; may be aggravated by alcohol, exposure to cold, and minor injury

Joint infections, sometimes called septic arthritis, can cause joints to become swollen, red, hot, and painful. Joint infections require immediate treatment.

Little is known about what causes most types of arthritis. Some seem to run in families; others seem to be related to imbalances in body chemistry or immune system problems. Many arthritis problems are the result of injury or long-term "wear and tear" on the joints.

Prevention

It may not be possible to prevent arthritis, but you can prevent a lot of pain by being kind to your joints. This is especially important if you already have arthritis.

- If activities that jar your body (such as running) cause pain, try activities that involve less impact (such as swimming).
- Control your weight.

Joint Replacement Surgery

When severe arthritis pain and loss of function interfere with your quality of life and do not respond to home treatment and medications, joint replacement surgery may be appropriate. Hip and knee joints are the most commonly replaced joints. Joint replacement surgery relieves pain and may improve your ability to use the joint, but it will not restore the joint to how it was before arthritis developed.

 Getting all the facts and thinking about your own needs and values will help you make the best decision about joint replacement surgery

- Joint replacement surgery is seldom urgent. Get a second opinion; delaying surgery for a few weeks or months will make little difference.

- Surgery is most helpful if a single joint is causing most of your problems.

- Replacement joints do not last forever. A second replacement joint may be needed in 15 to 20 years.

- The chance of success is better if you are in good shape. A regular exercise program and weight control are important both before and after the surgery.

- Exercise and stretch regularly. Exercise nourishes joint cartilage and removes waste products from your joints. It also strengthens the muscles around your joints, providing support for the joints and reducing injuries caused by fatigue. Stretching maintains your range of pain-free motion.

- Stop or modify any activity that causes pain. Don't use pain relievers to mask pain while you continue to overuse a joint.

Home Treatment

- Take a warm shower or bath to help relieve morning stiffness. Keep moving afterwards to keep stiffness from coming back.

- Apply moist heat to a sore joint for 20 to 30 minutes, 2 to 3 times a day. Or, if cold works better for you, use ice or a cold pack on the joint for 10 minutes several times a day. Some people find that alternating hot and cold helps relieve pain.

- Rest sore joints. Avoid activities that put weight or strain on your joints for a few days. Take short rest breaks from your regular activities throughout the day.

- Put each of your joints gently through its full range of motion once or twice each day.

- Exercise regularly to help maintain strength and flexibility in your muscles and joints. Strengthening exercises prevent the muscle loss that leads to weakness. Try low-impact activities, such as swimming, water aerobics, biking, or walking.

- Take acetaminophen to relieve pain caused by osteoarthritis. Anti-inflammatory medications, such as aspirin, ibuprofen, or naproxen sodium, may help ease pain but can cause stomach upset. Do not take more than one kind of anti-inflammatory medication at the same time.

- Enroll in an arthritis self-management program. Participants in these programs usually have less pain and fewer limitations on their activities.

- See Dealing With Chronic Pain on page 119.

- Avoid fraud. There is no "miracle cure" for arthritis. Avoid products and services that promise one.

When to Call a Health Professional

- If you have fever or a skin rash along with severe joint pain.

- If a joint is so painful that you cannot use it.

- If there is sudden, unexplained swelling, redness, warmth, or pain in one or more joints.

- If sudden back pain occurs with weakness in the legs or loss of bowel or bladder control.

- If joint pain continues for more than 6 weeks and home treatment is not helping.

- If you experience side effects (such as stomach pain, nausea, persistent heartburn, or dark, tarry stools) from aspirin or other arthritis medications. Do not exceed recommended doses of non-prescription medications without your doctor's advice.

- If you have been diagnosed with arthritis but the pain or impaired movement is not responding to the treatment your doctor recommended or is not following the expected course.

Bunions and Hammer Toes

A **bunion** is an enlargement of the joint at the base of the big toe. A bunion develops when the big toe bends toward and sometimes overlaps the second toe. A **hammer toe** is a toe that bends up permanently at the middle joint. These foot problems sometimes run in families. Both conditions are usually irritated by wearing high-heeled shoes or shoes that are too short or narrow.

Morton's neuroma is a foot problem that results from prolonged pressure on the nerves in the foot. It causes pain or numbness and tingling in the ball of the foot and the toes.

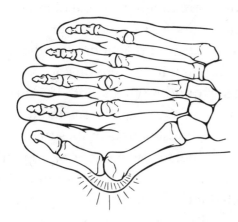

A bunion is an enlargement of the joint at the base of the big toe.

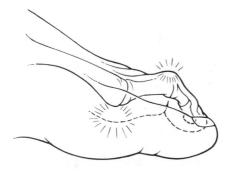

A hammer toe is a toe that bends up permanently at the middle joint.

Prevention

- Make sure your shoes fit properly. As you age, your feet may get a little bigger. Have your feet measured to make sure you are buying the right size. Shop for shoes at the end of the day, because the feet tend to swell during the day.

- Wear shoes with low or flat heels and roomy toe areas. Tennis or basketball court shoes are often best. Tight or high-heeled shoes increase the risk of bunions, hammer toes, and Morton's neuroma and irritate the affected joint once a problem has already developed.

Home Treatment

Once you have a bunion or hammer toe, there is usually no way to completely get rid of it, short of surgery. Home treatment will help relieve discomfort and keep the problem from getting worse.

- Wear low-heeled shoes that have roomy toe areas.

- Cushion the protruding joint with moleskin or doughnut-shaped pads to prevent rubbing and irritation.

- Cut out the area over the bunion or hammer toe from an old pair of shoes, and wear them around the house. Or wear comfortable sandals that don't press on the area.

- Try taking aspirin, ibuprofen, or acetaminophen to relieve pain. Ice or cold packs may also help.

When to Call a Health Professional

- If severe pain in your big toe comes on suddenly. See Gout on page 120.

- If your big toe starts to overlap your second toe.

- If you have diabetes, poor circulation, or peripheral vascular disease. In people with these conditions, irritated skin over a bunion or hammer toe can easily become infected.

- If you develop a sore over the bunion or hammer toe.

- If pain does not respond to home treatment in 2 to 3 weeks.

If severe pain interferes with walking or daily activities, you may want to consider surgical treatment. Surgery may not cure the problem completely. The more information you gather about the risks and benefits of surgery for bunions and hammer toes, the easier it will be for you to make a wise health decision.

Bursitis and Tendon Injury

A bursa is a small sac of fluid that helps the tissues surrounding a joint slide over one another easily. Injury or overuse of a joint or tendon can result in pain, redness, heat, and inflammation of the bursa, a condition known as bursitis. Bursitis often develops quickly, over just a few days, often after an injury, overuse, or prolonged direct pressure on a joint.

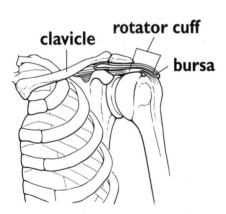

Common causes of shoulder pain are bursitis, tendon injury, and muscle tension.

Tendons are tough, ropelike fibers that connect muscles to bones. Injury or overuse can cause pain, tenderness, and inflammation in the tendons or the tissues surrounding them. Both bursitis and tendon injury can be related to job, sports, or household activities that require repeated twisting or rapid joint movements. Areas that are commonly affected include the shoulders, elbows, wrists, hips, knees, and feet. The same prevention and home treatment work for both bursitis and tendon problems.

Prevention

- Stretch and warm up well before exercising, and increase the intensity of the activity gradually. Cool down afterward by doing gentle stretches.

- Avoid repetitive twisting movements and activities that put strain on a single joint, such as a one-handed backhand stroke in tennis.

- Prevent additional flare-ups by avoiding or modifying the activities that cause the problem.

Home Treatment

Bursitis or mild tendon injury will usually improve in a few days or weeks if you avoid the activity that caused it.

The most common mistake in recovery is thinking the problem is gone when the pain is gone. Chances are, the problem will recur if you do not take steps to strengthen and stretch the muscles around the joint and change the way you do some activities.

- As soon as you notice pain, apply ice or cold packs for 10-minute periods, once an hour or as often as you can for 48 hours. Continue applying ice (10 minutes, 3 times a day) as long as it relieves pain. See Ice and Cold Packs on page 62. Although heat may feel good, ice will reduce inflammation and promote healing.

- Rest the affected area. Change the way you do the activity that causes pain so that you can do it without pain. To maintain fitness, substitute activities that don't stress the area.

- Aspirin, ibuprofen, or naproxen sodium may help ease pain and inflammation, but don't use medication to mask pain while you continue to overuse a joint.

- To prevent stiffness, gently move the joint through as full a range of motion as you can without pain. As the pain subsides, continue range-of-motion exercises, and add exercises that strengthen the affected muscles.

- Gradually resume the activity that caused the pain at a lower intensity. Increase the intensity slowly and only if pain does not recur. Warm up before and stretch after doing the activity. Apply ice to the injured area after exercise to prevent pain and swelling.

When to Call a Health Professional

- If there is fever, rapid swelling, or redness, or if you are unable to use a joint.

- If severe pain continues when the joint is at rest and you have applied ice.

- If the pain persists for 2 weeks or longer despite home treatment.

- If you experience side effects (such as stomach pain, nausea, persistent heartburn, or dark, tarry stools) from aspirin or other arthritis medications. Do not exceed recommended doses of nonprescription medications without your doctor's advice.

Carpal Tunnel Syndrome

The carpal tunnel is a narrow passageway between the bones and ligaments in the wrist. The median nerve, which controls sensation in the fingers and some muscles in the hand, passes through this tunnel along with some of the finger tendons. Carpal tunnel syndrome (CTS) develops when there is pressure on the median nerve where it goes through the carpal tunnel.

Doing activities that use the same finger or hand movements over and over can cause CTS. Other causes include being overweight, having a ganglion cyst on the tendon sheath in the wrist, or having rheumatoid arthritis. Previous wrist injuries, diabetes, thyroid disease, and pregnancy also may increase your risk for CTS.

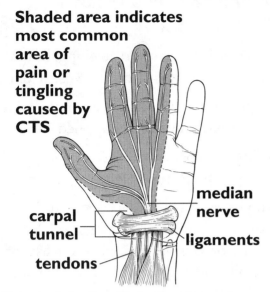

Shaded area indicates most common area of pain or tingling caused by CTS

carpal tunnel

tendons

median nerve

ligaments

Pain and tingling in the hand may be caused by pressure on a nerve in the wrist.

Pressure on the median nerve causes the following symptoms of CTS:

- Numbness or tingling in the fingers of one or both hands, except for the little finger

- Numbness or pain in your hand or wrist that wakes you up at night

- Numbness or pain that gets worse when you use your hand or wrist, especially when you grip an object or flex your wrist

- Occasional aching pain in your forearm from your hand to your elbow

- A weak grip

Prevention

- Stop any activity that you think may be causing finger, hand, or wrist numbness or pain. If symptoms improve when you stop an activity, resume that activity gradually and with greater efforts to keep your wrist straight or only slightly bent.

- Switch hands and change positions often when you are doing repeated motions. Take frequent breaks.

- Keep your arm, hand, and finger muscles strong and flexible and maintain your overall fitness.

- Avoid using too much salt if you tend to retain fluid.

Home Treatment

- Follow the prevention tips listed earlier.

- Follow the home treatment tips for bursitis and tendon injury starting on page 116.

- Avoid sleeping on your hands.

- Ask your health professional about using a wrist splint to relieve pressure on your wrist.

- Other lifestyle changes, such as losing weight, quitting smoking, reducing your alcohol intake, and controlling diabetes or thyroid problems, may help relieve symptoms of CTS that are related to swelling.

- Vitamin B_6 has not been shown to be an effective treatment for CTS.

Dealing With Chronic Pain

There is no magic solution to chronic pain, whether the pain is caused by arthritis, osteoporosis, back problems, cancer, or any other condition. Nothing offers complete and total relief. However, the following tips may help. Also see page 344.

1. Experiment with heat, cold, and massage. Find out what works best for you. Touch is important too. Ask for and give lots of hugs.

2. Continue to exercise. Find gentle, enjoyable exercises that don't aggravate your pain. Do the stretching exercises beginning on page 292 every day.

3. Try to relax. Severe pain makes your body tense, and the tension may make the pain worse. See the relaxation techniques on page 344. It takes practice to learn any relaxation skill. Give each method a 2-week trial. If one doesn't work for you, try another.

4. Do something to distract yourself. Focusing all your attention on your pain makes it seem all-consuming. Refocus your attention away from the pain and onto something else. Sing a song, recite a poem, or concentrate on a vision. See Visualization on page 338.

5. Expose yourself to humor. A good, hearty belly laugh can provide your body with natural pain relief. Laughter is the best medicine.

6. Practice positive self-talk. Refuse to entertain negative, self-defeating thoughts or feelings of hopelessness. See pages 338 and 341.

7. Consider alternative therapies such as biofeedback or acupuncture in addition to your regular medical care. See Complementary Medicine beginning on page 347.

8. Join a support group. By being around others who share your problem, you and your family can learn skills for coping with pain. To find a group near you, contact the American Chronic Pain Association, P.O. Box 850, Rocklin, CA 95677, 1-916-632-0922.

9. Consider going to a pain clinic. Be wary of clinics that promise complete relief from pain or that use only one method of treatment. Approved programs are registered with The Rehabilitation Accreditation Commission (CARF), 4891 East Grant Road, Tucson, AZ 85712, 1-520-325-1044.

10. Appeal to a higher power. If you believe in a higher power, ask for support and relief from the pain.

When to Call a Health Professional

- If tingling, numbness, weakness, or pain in your fingers and hand has not gone away after 2 weeks of home treatment.

- If you have little or no feeling in your fingers or hand.

- If you cannot do simple hand movements, or you accidentally drop things.

- If you cannot pinch your thumb and first finger together or you cannot use your thumb.

- If you have problems at work because of hand or wrist pain.

 Most cases of <u>carpal tunnel syndrome</u> are treated without surgery. If you are considering surgery, gather as much information as possible about its risks and benefits. Getting all the facts and thinking about your own needs and values will help you work with your doctor to make a wise health decision.

Gout

Gout is a form of arthritis that develops when excess uric acid in the blood builds up and forms crystals in one or more joints. Gout attacks can come on suddenly. Sometimes a minor injury can trigger an attack. The affected joint becomes tender, hot, swollen, red, and very painful. The pain often reaches its peak in a matter of hours. A low fever of 99° to 101° is common.

Gout attacks most often affect the big toe joint. Attacks may also involve the ankles, knees, elbows, fingers, and other joints. Gout attacks can last from several days to weeks. Between attacks, months or years can go by with no symptoms. If gout is not treated, attacks may gradually occur more often, last longer, and become more severe. Medication may be prescribed to prevent gout attacks.

Gout is far more common in men than in women. Other risk factors for gout include having a family history of gout, being obese, drinking excessive amounts of alcohol (particularly beer), taking aspirin regularly, and going on very low-calorie diets.

Prevention

Although you may not be able to prevent gout from developing, you can help reduce the frequency and severity of future attacks.

- Maintain a healthy body weight by eating a well-balanced, low-fat diet. If you are trying to lose weight, avoid fasting and very low-calorie diets.

- Avoid or cut back on alcoholic beverages, especially beer. Alcohol increases uric acid production.

- Drink at least 8 to 10 glasses of water each day. This will help your kidneys flush uric acid through your system.

- Do not take aspirin or water pills (diuretics).

- If your doctor has prescribed medication to prevent gout attacks, take it regularly and exactly as directed.

Home Treatment

- As soon as you know you are having a gout attack, go to bed, elevate the affected joint, and apply a warm compress to the joint. Stay in bed until the most severe symptoms have subsided. This may help prevent a second attack. Create a tent over the affected joint to reduce pressure from bedsheets.

- Take ibuprofen, ketoprofen, or naproxen sodium to relieve pain. Do not take aspirin, because it can make a gout attack worse.

- If your doctor has prescribed medication for use during a gout attack, take it as prescribed. Avoid using more than the prescribed dose. Stop taking the drug and call your doctor if reactions such as nausea, vomiting, diarrhea, or abdominal cramping occur.

When to Call a Health Professional

Call your doctor if you have a sudden onset of severe joint pain, especially with swelling, tenderness, and warmth over a joint.

Heel Pain and Plantar Fasciitis

Plantar fasciitis is a condition that occurs when the thick, fibrous tissue (plantar fascia) that covers the bottom of the foot becomes inflamed and painful. Athletes, middle-aged people, and those who are

overweight tend to develop plantar fasciitis. Prolonged standing and repetitive movements such as running and jumping can lead to heel pain and plantar fasciitis.

An excessive inward rolling of the foot (called pronation) during walking or running can also cause heel pain and plantar fasciitis. Pronation can be caused by wearing shoes that are worn out or have poor arch support, having tight calf muscles, or running downhill or on uneven surfaces.

Achilles tendon injury can cause pain in the back of the heel.

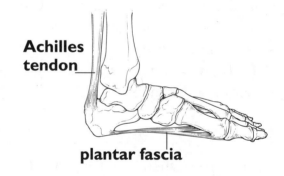

Foot or heel pain is often caused by inflammation of the Achilles tendon or the plantar fascia.

A **heel spur** is a calcium buildup that most often develops where the plantar fascia attaches to the heel bone. Heel spurs usually do not cause pain and do not need to be treated. The pain many people attribute to heel spurs is in most cases caused by plantar fasciitis, rather than by the heel spur itself. Heel spurs may also be a natural result of aging. As a person ages, the fatty pads that cushion the heels get thinner, which makes heel pain more likely.

Prevention

- Stretch your Achilles tendon and calf muscles several times a day (see Calf Stretch on page 297). Stretching is important for both athletes and nonathletes.

- Maintain a reasonable weight for your height.

- Always wear shoes with well-cushioned soles and good arch supports.

- Establish good exercise habits. If you walk or jog, increase your distance slowly, limit your training on hilly terrain, and walk or run on grass or dirt rather than on concrete.

Home Treatment

Treat heel pain when it first appears to keep plantar fasciitis or other problems from becoming chronic.

- Reduce weight-bearing activity to a level that does not cause pain. Try low-impact activities such as cycling or swimming to speed healing. You may need to check with your doctor about when you can gradually resume high-impact activities.

- Apply ice to your heel. See Ice and Cold Packs on page 62.

- You may wish to put nonprescription arch supports in your shoes.

- Do not go barefoot until the pain is completely gone. Wear shoes or arch-supporting sandals during all weight-bearing activities, even going to the bathroom during the night.

- Take aspirin, ibuprofen, or naproxen sodium to relieve pain.

- Stretch your calf muscles. See page 297.

- For Achilles tendon problems or plantar fasciitis, try putting heel lifts or heel cups in both shoes. Use them only until the pain is gone.

When to Call a Health Professional

- If heel pain occurs with fever, redness, or heat in your heel, or if there is numbness or tingling in your heel or foot.

- If a heel injury results in pain when you put weight on your heel.

- If pain continues when you are not standing or bearing any weight on your heel.

- If heel pain persists for 1 to 2 weeks despite home treatment.

 Your doctor may recommend other treatments for plantar fasciitis, such as taping, exercises, shoe inserts, or steroid injections. Surgery is usually done only as a last resort when other treatments fail to relieve pain.

MORE INFO **For more information, see the back cover.**

Caregiver's Tips for Bone, Muscle, and Joint Problems

- Encourage the person to exercise regularly. Walking, lifting light weights (or cans of soup), or even simple range-of-motion or chair exercises are good choices. People who are bedridden because of illness lose muscle strength very quickly. As soon as the person is feeling better, encourage the person to start rebuilding strength. Be patient. It can take several weeks for a person to get strong again.

- Encourage the person to do as much as possible for him- or herself. Look for devices that make daily activities, such as dressing, bathing, cooking, eating, or doing household chores, easier on sore joints.

- Look for ways to distract the person from the pain. Engage the person in conversation, games, puzzles, or hobbies. Also see Dealing With Chronic Pain on page 119.

- Be alert for signs of depression. Pain can cause depression, and depression can worsen pain, creating a vicious cycle. See page 325.

Knee Problems

The knee is a vulnerable joint. It is basically just two long leg bones held together with ligaments and muscles. Injuries are the most common cause of knee problems.

Overuse injuries, such as bursitis, tendon injury, or wearing of the cartilage behind the kneecap (patellofemoral pain syndrome), happen when you repeat the same activity again and again. The repeated activity—stair climbing, bicycle riding, jogging, or jumping—stresses the knee joint and surrounding tissues, which then become irritated and inflamed.

Receiving a direct blow to the knee or twisting or bending your knee abnormally can cause strained, sprained, or torn ligaments; damaged knee cartilage (such as a torn meniscus); a fracture; or a dislocated knee or kneecap. These injuries can cause sudden and severe pain. Bruising and swelling can be severe and may develop within a few minutes of the injury. If nerves or blood vessels are injured or pinched during the injury, your knee or lower leg may feel numb, tingly, weak, or cold; or it may look pale or blue.

A previous injury may have something to do with a new knee problem. For example, if your knee pain is worse in the morning and improves during the day, it may be caused by osteoarthritis, which often develops at the site of a previous injury.

Other possible causes of knee pain include rheumatoid arthritis, gout, and lupus. Pain that occurs in one knee with redness, swelling, warmth, fever, chills, or pus may be caused by an infection in the joint or in one of the bursae that cushion the knee joint. Occasionally knee pain is related to a problem elsewhere in the body, such as a "pinched nerve" or a problem in the hip.

Prevention

• The best way to prevent knee problems is to strengthen and stretch your leg muscles, especially those in the front and back of the thigh (quadriceps and hamstrings). See page 298.

• Avoid activities that stress your knees, such as deep knee bends and running downhill.

• Wear shoes with good arch supports. Replace running or walking shoes as soon as they start to wear out.

• Avoid wearing high-heeled shoes.

• Also see Bursitis and Tendon Injury on page 116.

Home Treatment

• Apply ice to your knee. See Ice and Cold Packs on page 62.

• Rest your knee, and reduce by at least 50 percent the activities that cause knee pain.

• Ask your health professional about wearing a brace, an elastic or neoprene sleeve, or a band with a hole for the kneecap that holds the kneecap in place

to ease pain during activity. You can buy one at a pharmacy, sporting goods store, or medical supply store.

• Stretch the front and back of your thigh muscles (quadriceps and hamstrings) after exercise, when they are warm.

• Also read about home treatment for Strains, Sprains, Fractures, and Dislocations (page 61) and Bursitis and Tendon Injury (page 116).

• If knee pain is not related to exercise or a recent or past injury, see Arthritis on page 111.

When to Call a Health Professional

• If your knee feels unstable, gives out, or cannot bear weight.

• If you felt or heard a "pop" in your knee at the time of an injury.

• If your knee begins to swell within 30 minutes of an injury.

• If you have signs of damage to the nerves or blood vessels, such as numbness, tingling, a pins-and-needles sensation below the injury, or pale or bluish skin.

• If your knee looks deformed.

• If you are unable to straighten or bend your knee, or if the joint locks.

• If your knee is red, hot, swollen, or painful to touch.

• If pain is severe enough that you are limping, or if pain does not improve within 2 days.

Muscle Cramps and Leg Pain

Leg and muscle cramps are common in older adults. Nighttime leg cramps are especially common. Cramps have no clear cause, although they may occasionally be related to low levels of calcium or potassium in the blood. If you take water pills (diuretics) for high blood pressure or heart failure, you may have lower levels of potassium in your bloodstream, or you may be slightly dehydrated. Either circumstance may contribute to muscle cramps.

Arthritis can also cause leg pain (see page 111). Leg pain that runs from the buttocks down the back of the leg and into the foot may be caused by sciatica (see page 99).

Leg pain can be caused by an inflammation of a vein in the leg. See Thrombophlebitis on page 170.

Decreased blood flow to the leg muscles (called **intermittent claudication**) caused by hardening of the arteries is another possible cause of leg cramps. Symptoms may include cramping pain in the calf that comes on with activity or exertion and is relieved by rest. Symptoms often occur after you walk a certain distance.

Shinsplints cause pain in the front of the lower leg. Their cause is unclear, but they tend to develop after activities in which the legs are overused.

Prevention

- Warm up well and stretch before any activity. Also stretch after exercise to keep hot muscles from shortening and cramping.

- Drink extra fluids before and during exercise, especially during hot or humid weather.

- Include plenty of calcium and potassium in your diet. Bananas, orange juice, and potatoes are good sources.

- If leg cramps wake you at night, take a warm bath before bedtime, and keep your legs warm while sleeping.

- Try wearing elastic stockings during the day.

Home Treatment

- If there is pain, swelling, or heaviness in the calf of only one of your legs, or if you have other symptoms that cause you to suspect thrombophlebitis (blood clot and inflammation in a vein), call your doctor before you try home treatment. See page 170.

- Gently stretch and massage the cramping muscle. Don't massage if you suspect thrombophlebitis.

- Drink more fluids. Cramps are often related to dehydration.

- The best treatment for shinsplints is ice, pain relievers (aspirin, ibuprofen, or acetaminophen), and 1 to 2 weeks of rest, followed by a gradual return to exercise.

When to Call a Health Professional

• If you have symptoms of thrombo-phlebitis, such as:

- Continuous leg or calf pain.

- Swelling of one leg.

- Any redness that is tender to the touch.

- Fever.

• If you have signs of impaired blood flow, such as:

- Pain that comes on after you walk a certain distance and that goes away with rest.

- Sudden onset of moderate to severe pain with coldness or pale skin in the lower part of the leg.

- Pale or blue-black skin on one or both legs or feet or the toes.

• If muscle cramps are not relieved by home treatment.

Osteoporosis

Osteoporosis is a disease that causes a person's bones to become so weak that they can break during normal daily activities. Osteoporosis affects 20 million older Americans. Women are four times more likely to develop osteoporosis than men are.

Osteoporosis is more common after menopause, when a woman's estrogen levels decline. Other factors that increase the risk of osteoporosis in both men and women include slender body frame, Asian or European heritage, family history of osteoporosis, and lack of weight-bearing exercise. Women who smoke or drink excessive amounts of alcohol are at greater risk, as are those who have difficulty digesting dairy products. Men who have low testosterone levels are at increased risk. Elevated thyroid hormone levels (hyperthyroidism) may also contribute to osteoporosis.

Osteoporosis usually develops over many years without symptoms. By the time a person notices symptoms of osteoporosis—such as loss of height, a curved upper back (dowager's hump), back pain, or broken bones—the disease has done a lot of damage and is likely to impact the person's everyday life. However, early diagnosis and treatment of osteoporosis can limit the effect the disease has on a person's life.

Prevention

Weakening bones are a natural part of growing older. But if you start healthy habits early in life, you may be able to delay the development of osteoporosis.

• Get regular weight-bearing exercise, such as walking, jogging, climbing stairs, dancing, or weight lifting. Weight-bearing exercise helps keep bones strong. See Fitness starting on page 285.

What Are Your Risks for Osteoporosis?

Risk Factors: Circle points that apply to you.   **Points**

Age 35 to 64 2

Age 65 to 79 5

Age 80 or older 8

White or Asian 1

Small-boned 2

Slender 2

Mother, grandmother, or sister with osteoporosis 2

After menopause 1

Have had ovaries removed 1

Never been pregnant 1

Have breast-fed 1

Allergic to milk 1

Smoke cigarettes 1

Drink 4 or more caffeinated drinks per day 1

Drink more than 1 ounce of alcohol per day 1

Risk Factor Score (Add risk factor points.)   _____

Prevention Factors: Circle points that apply to you.

Exercise (walking or equivalent)

Walk $\frac{1}{2}$ to 1 mile a day 1

Walk 1 to 2 miles a day 2

Walk 3 or more miles a day 3

Diet

Eat or drink at least 3 dairy products per day 1

Get 1,000 to 1,500 mg of calcium per day 1

Take estrogen replacement therapy 2

Get 30 minutes of sunshine or take 400 International Units of
   vitamin D per day 1

Prevention Factor Score (Add prevention factor points.)   _____

Subtract your **Prevention Factor Score** from your **Risk Factor Score**
to get your overall **Osteoporosis Risk Score**.   _____

     Low Risk: Less than 9 points   **High Risk:** 16–20 points

     Medium Risk: 9–15 points   **Very High Risk:** 21 or more points

- Eat a healthy diet that includes plenty of calcium and vitamin D. Both are needed for building healthy, strong bones. See page 310 for tips on getting more calcium in your diet. You can get a boost of vitamin D by drinking fortified milk or by spending 10 to 15 minutes in the sun each day. (If you have dark skin, you will need more time in the sun.) Take supplements of calcium and vitamin D if you think you are not getting enough in your diet.

- Don't smoke.

- Limit your alcohol intake to 1 drink per day or less.

- Cut down on caffeine. Caffeine in coffee and soft drinks increases calcium loss from your body and puts you at risk for osteoporosis.

- There are medications, including estrogen, that can help prevent osteoporosis. Talk with your doctor about whether these are appropriate for you.

 Special X-rays that measure bone density can tell you how much bone loss has occurred as a result of osteoporosis. If you are at high risk for osteoporosis, or if you are a woman over 65, a bone density measurement may provide you with important information to help you and your doctor decide whether you need treatment for osteoporosis.

When to Call a Health Professional

- If you think you have a broken bone, if you notice swelling, or if you cannot move a part of your body normally.

- If you have sudden, severe pain or problems bearing weight on the injured part of your body.

- If you notice that one of your arms or legs looks deformed or misshapen. This may mean you have a broken bone.

- If you want to discuss your risk for developing osteoporosis.

Weakness and Fatigue

Weakness is a lack of physical strength and a feeling that extra effort is required to move your arms, legs, or other muscles.

Fatigue is a feeling of tiredness, exhaustion, or lack of energy.

Unexplained muscle weakness is usually more serious than fatigue. It may be caused by diabetes (see page 176), thyroid problems (see page 181), stroke (see page 63), or other problems related to the brain and spinal cord. Call your doctor immediately if you have unexplained muscle weakness.

Fatigue, on the other hand, can usually be treated with self-care. Most fatigue is caused by lack of exercise, stress or overwork, lack of sleep, depression, worry, or boredom. Colds and flu may sometimes cause fatigue and weakness, but the symptoms disappear as the illness runs its course.

Prevention

- Regular exercise is your best defense against fatigue. If you feel too tired to exercise vigorously, try taking a short walk.

- Eat a well-balanced diet. Also consider taking a basic vitamin supplement. See page 310.

- Make sure you are getting enough sleep. See Sleep Problems on page 333.

- Deal with emotional problems instead of ignoring or denying them. See Mental Health beginning on page 317 and Mind-Body Wellness starting on page 337.

- Take steps to control stress. See page 343.

Home Treatment

- Follow the prevention guidelines and be patient. It may take a while before you feel energetic again.

- Listen to your body. Alternate rest with exercise.

- Limit medications that might contribute to fatigue, especially tranquilizers and cold and allergy medications.

- Reduce your use of caffeine, nicotine, and alcohol.

- Cut back on watching television. Take up new activities, spend time with friends, or travel to break the fatigue cycle.

When to Call a Health Professional

- If you have unexplained muscle weakness in one area of your body. See Stroke on page 63.

- If severe or persistent fatigue causes you to limit your usual activities for longer than 2 weeks despite home treatment.

- If you experience sudden, unexplained weight loss or gain.

- If you do not feel more energetic after 4 weeks of home treatment.

- If fatigue gets worse despite home treatment.

Fibromyalgia and Polymyalgia Rheumatica

MORE INFO

Fibromyalgia is a condition that causes chronic muscle and soft tissue pain and tenderness on both sides of the body, above and below the waist. Fibromyalgia does not damage the body, destroy the joints, or cause internal organ problems, but the pain may be severe enough to interfere with work and other activities.

The cause of fibromyalgia is not known. People who have fibromyalgia have multiple tender points in specific areas of their bodies. They often have trouble sleeping because of the pain. There may also be stiffness, weakness, and fatigue. Fibromyalgia is more common in women than in men. Regular exercise, such as walking, biking, or swimming, is the cornerstone of treatment. Medications are sometimes prescribed to help treat the symptoms. If stress makes your symptoms worse, see page 343.

Polymyalgia rheumatica means "many aching muscles." It is a condition that causes pain and stiffness in muscles and other soft tissues, especially in the neck, shoulders, and hips. There may be inflammation and swelling in the joints, fatigue, and sometimes fever.

The main treatment for polymyalgia rheumatica is medication. The condition is believed to be related to inflammation in small blood vessels and is related to temporal arteritis (see page 191).

Keep breathing.
Sophie Tucker

7

Chest, Lung, and Respiratory Problems

Chest, lung, and respiratory problems can be as simple as a minor cold or as life-threatening as a heart attack. For most respiratory problems, including allergies, colds, sore throats, sinusitis, and tonsillitis, this chapter will help you decide what to do at home and when to call your doctor.

Start this chapter with a look at the chart on the next page. If you don't find what you're looking for, please check the index.

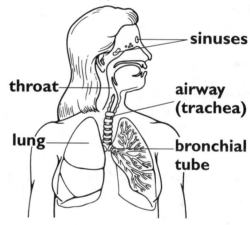

Respiratory problems can occur in the upper respiratory tract (nose, sinuses, throat, or trachea) or in the lower respiratory tract (bronchial tubes or lungs).

Allergies

Allergies come in many forms. The most common allergies are respiratory allergies, such as hay fever, which are caused by particles in the air you breathe. Symptoms of a respiratory allergy include itchy, watery eyes; sneezing; runny, stuffy, or itchy nose; and fatigue. The symptoms are a lot like cold symptoms, but they usually last longer. Dark circles under the eyes (allergic shiners) or postnasal drip may also accompany hay fever.

Chest, Respiratory, Nose, and Throat Problems

Symptoms	Possible Causes
Chest and Respiratory	
Wheezing or difficult (rapid, shallow, labored) breathing	Allergies, p. 131; Asthma, p. 135; Bronchitis, p. 138; Pneumonia, p. 151.
Cough, fever, yellow, green or rust-colored sputum, and difficulty breathing	Bronchitis, p. 138; Pneumonia, p. 151.
Chronic shortness of breath	Emphysema, p. 145.
Chest pain or discomfort with sweating or rapid pulse	Possible heart attack. Call for help. See p. 53. See Chest Pain, p. 140.
Burning, pain, or discomfort behind or below the breastbone	Heartburn, p. 78; Chest Pain, p. 140.
Coughing	Coughs, p. 143.
Pounding or racing heartbeat; heart skipping or missing a beat	Irregular Heartbeat, p. 167.
Nose and Throat	
Stuffy or runny nose with watery eyes, sneezing	Allergies, p. 131; Colds, p. 141.
Cold symptoms with fever, headache, severe body aches, fatigue	Influenza, p. 147.
Thick green, yellow, or gray nasal discharge with fever and facial pain	Sinusitis, p. 152.
Sore throat	Sore Throat, p. 153.
Sore throat with white spots on tonsils, swollen lymph nodes, and fever	Strep Throat, p. 153.
Hoarseness, loss of voice	Laryngitis, p. 149.

You can often discover the cause of an allergy by noting when symptoms occur. Symptoms that occur at the same time each year, especially during spring, early summer, or early fall, are often caused by tree, grass, or weed pollen. Allergies that persist all year long may be caused by dust, mites in household dust, cockroaches, mold spores, or animal dander. An animal allergy is often easy to detect: symptoms clear up when you stay away from the animal or its bedding.

Life-Threatening Allergic Reactions

A few people have severe allergies to insect stings or to certain foods or drugs, especially antibiotics such as penicillin. For these people, the allergic reaction is sudden and severe and may cause difficulty breathing and a drop in blood pressure. This type of reaction is called anaphylactic shock, or anaphylaxis.

An anaphylactic reaction is a medical emergency, and prompt care is needed. If you have ever had a severe allergic reaction, your doctor may suggest that you carry an epinephrine syringe (such as EpiPen or Ana-Kit) designed for giving yourself a shot that will decrease the severity of the reaction. If you have had an allergic reaction to a drug, wear a medical identification bracelet that will tell health professionals about your allergy in case you cannot.

Prevention

• Avoid the substance that causes you to have allergy attacks if possible.

• Ask your doctor about allergy shots (immunotherapy). Allergy shots may help control some of the symptoms caused by allergies and asthma and may reduce your risk of having an anaphylactic reaction.

Home Treatment

If you can discover the source of your allergies, avoiding that substance may be the best treatment. Keep a record of your symptoms and the plants, animals, foods, or chemicals that seem to trigger them.

Here are some general tips for avoiding irritants:

• Avoid yard work (raking, mowing), which stirs up both pollen and mold. If you must do yard work, wear a mask and take an antihistamine beforehand.

• Avoid smoking and inhaling other people's smoke.

• Don't use aerosol sprays, perfumes, room deodorizers, cleaning products, and other substances that may trigger allergy symptoms.

If your symptoms are seasonal and seem to be related to pollen:

• Keep your house and car windows closed. Keep bedroom windows closed at night.

• Limit the time you spend outside when pollen counts are high. Dogs and other pets may bring large amounts of pollen into your house, so either leave them outside, or wash them frequently.

If your symptoms occur year-round and seem to be related to dust:

• Keep your bedroom and other places where you spend a lot of time as dust-free as possible.

• Avoid carpeting, upholstered furniture, and heavy draperies that collect dust. Vacuuming doesn't pick up house dust mites.

• Cover your mattress and box spring with dust-proof cases, and wipe them clean weekly. Avoid wool or down blankets and feather pillows. Wash all bedding in hot water once a week.

• Consider using an air conditioner or air purifier with a special HEPA filter. Rent one before buying to see if it helps.

If your symptoms occur year-round and are worse during damp weather, they may be related to mold or mildew:

• Keep your home well ventilated and dry. Keep the humidity below 50 percent. Use a dehumidifier during humid weather.

• Use an air conditioner, which removes mold spores from the air. Change or clean heating and cooling system filters regularly.

• Clean bathroom and kitchen surfaces often with bleach to reduce mold growth.

If you are allergic to a pet:

• Keep the animal outside, or at least out of your bedroom.

• Talk to your veterinarian about steps you can take to reduce your exposure to animal dander.

• If your symptoms are severe and your efforts to reduce your dander exposure do not help, the best solution may be to find a new home for the pet.

Antihistamines and decongestants may relieve some allergy symptoms. Use caution when taking these drugs. Your doctor may be able to prescribe an anti-histamine that does not make you sleepy. See pages 385 and 386.

 Call your doctor if allergy symptoms worsen over time and home treatment doesn't help. Your doctor may recommend stronger medication or allergy shots (immunotherapy).

For more information about allergies, including allergy shots, call Lung Line, a service of the National Jewish Medical and Research Center, at 1-800-222-LUNG (5864).

When to Call a Health Professional

Call 911 or other emergency services immediately if you develop signs of a severe allergic reaction (anaphylaxis). The following severe symptoms may occur soon after you take a drug, eat a certain food, or are stung by an insect:

MORE INFO **For more information, see the back cover.**

- Lightheadedness (feeling like you might pass out) or confusion

- Swelling around the lips, tongue, or face that is interfering with breathing or is getting worse

- Wheezing or difficulty breathing

Call a health professional:

- If your face, tongue, or lips are swollen, even if you are not having difficulty breathing and the swelling is not getting worse.

- If there is significant swelling around the site of an insect sting (for instance, an entire arm or leg is swollen).

- If you develop a skin rash, itching, a feeling of warmth, or hives.

Asthma

Asthma is a condition that causes long-term inflammation of the airways that lead to the lungs. The inflammation makes the airways overreact to certain triggers, such as cold air or particles in the air. When this reaction occurs, the muscles surrounding the bronchial tubes that carry air into the lungs go into spasm, the mucous lining of the lungs swells, and secretions build up in the lungs, suddenly making breathing difficult.

During an asthma episode (asthma attack), you may make a wheezing or whistling sound when you breathe. You will probably cough a great deal, and you may spit up mucus. Sometimes a chronic dry cough, especially at night or early in the morning, is the only symptom of mild asthma.

Many things can trigger asthma, including allergens such as dust and dust mites, pollen, cockroaches, and animal dander. Viral respiratory infections, such as colds, are common triggers of asthma. Other triggers include exercise, cold air, cigarette or wood smoke, chemical vapors, pain relievers (especially aspirin), food preservatives and dyes, and emotional stress.

 Most people can control asthma by avoiding triggers that cause attacks and using medications to treat chronic inflammation in their airways. Severe attacks can usually be treated with inhaled or injected medications. Asthma attacks are rarely fatal if they are treated promptly and appropriately.

Prevention

There is no way to prevent asthma. However, you may be able to prevent asthma symptoms or limit their severity by taking medications to treat inflammation in your airways and avoiding or limiting your exposure to things that trigger asthma symptoms.

- Review the home treatment for allergies on page 133.

Asthma Action Plan

An asthma action plan is a written plan that tells you how to manage your asthma symptoms at home. It helps take the guesswork out of treating your asthma. The plan will outline the medication you will take for your asthma symptoms and when to take it, depending on the zone you are in (green, yellow, or red). In order to determine what zone you are in, you will have to know how to use a peak flow meter to measure your ability to exhale. The plan may also tell you when to talk to your health professional about your asthma symptoms.

The asthma action plan zones include:

• Green zone plan: Routine care to keep asthma symptoms from starting.

• Yellow zone plan: How to stop asthma symptoms and keep an asthma episode (attack) from getting worse. This may involve taking other medications in addition to the ones you usually take to control your asthma.

• Red zone plan: What to do for a severe asthma episode. This is a medical emergency.

• Control cockroaches. Do not leave food or garbage in open containers. Use poison bait and traps to kill cockroaches. Avoid chemical sprays, which can trigger an asthma attack.

• Avoid smoke of all kinds. If you smoke cigarettes, stop. See page 18 for tips on quitting. Avoid places where other people may be smoking. Stay away from wood-burning stoves.

• Avoid irritants in the air. Stay indoors when the air pollution or pollen count is high. Try to avoid strong odors, fumes, and perfume.

• Avoid breathing cold air. In cold weather, breathe through your nose, and cover your nose and mouth with a scarf or a cold-weather mask.

• Aspirin, ibuprofen, and similar pain medications can cause severe asthma attacks in some people. Discuss the use of these medications with your doctor, and use them with caution. If these medications bother you, don't use them. Try acetaminophen instead.

• Do not use nonprescription cold and cough medications unless your doctor tells you to do so.

• Stress may be a factor in triggering asthma attacks. Practice the relaxation exercises on page 344.

• Reduce your risk of colds and flu by washing your hands often and getting a flu shot each year.

• If you use a humidifier, clean it thoroughly once a week.

• Build up the strength of your lungs and airways:

  - Get regular exercise. Swimming or water aerobics may be good choices because you are less likely to have an asthma attack when you breathe moist air. If vigorous exercise triggers asthma attacks, talk with your doctor. Adjusting your medication and your exercise routine may help.

- Practice roll breathing as described on page 344.

Home Treatment

Once an asthma attack begins, prompt home treatment can provide relief.

• Learn to use a metered-dose inhaler. Inhalers help get the right amount of medication to your airways. A device called a spacer is now recommended for use with an inhaler. Ask your doctor or pharmacist to watch you use your inhaler and spacer to make sure you are doing it right. With practice, most people can use an inhaler and spacer correctly.

• Drink extra fluids to thin the mucus in your bronchial tubes. Try to drink at least 2 quarts of water per day.

• Be confident that your home treatment will control the severity of the attack.

• Keep a diary outlining your asthma attacks. After you've had an attack, write down what triggered it, what helped end it, and any concerns you have about your asthma action plan. Take your diary when you see your doctor for your regular checkups. Ask questions you may have about your plan or medication.

To get more information about managing asthma, contact the National Asthma Center at 1-800-222-5864, or your local chapter of the American Lung Association.

When to Call a Health Professional

Always follow your asthma action plan if you have one. **Call 911 or other emergency services** if you are having severe asthma symptoms and:

• You are having severe difficulty breathing.

• Your medications have not helped after 20 minutes.

Call a health professional:

• If you have symptoms that may indicate heart problems, such as chest pain or shortness of breath. See Chest Pain on page 140.

• If you are having a severe asthma attack, even if your medications have relieved some symptoms.

• If your asthma symptoms don't get better after you follow your asthma action plan.

• If you have a fever or are coughing up yellow, dark brown, or bloody mucus.

• If acute asthma symptoms (wheezing, coughing, difficulty breathing) have happened for the first time.

• To discuss exactly what to do when an attack begins. Once you understand and have confidence in your asthma medication, you can often handle mild attacks without professional help.

- If you begin to use your asthma medication more often than usual. This may be a sign that your asthma is getting worse.

- If you or the people who live with you have not been educated about immediate treatment for asthma attacks.

- If the medication required to treat an asthma attack is not available.

- To talk about adjusting your medication. Your doctor needs your feedback to figure out the best medicine and the right dosage for you.

- To assess allergies, which may worsen asthma attacks.

- To get a referral to a support group. Talking with others who have asthma can give you information and boost your confidence in dealing with prevention and treatment.

Bronchitis

Bronchitis is an inflammation and irritation of the airways that lead to the lungs. Viruses are the usual cause of bronchitis, but it can also be caused by bacteria or by exposure to cigarette smoke or air pollution. The inflammation that develops in acute bronchitis is not permanent. It goes away when the infection or irritation goes away.

Symptoms of bronchitis usually begin 3 to 4 days after an upper respiratory infection, such as a cold, goes away. Symptoms often include a dry cough that may become productive (produce sputum), mild fever, fatigue, discomfort or tightness in the chest, and wheezing.

Having bronchitis and another lung disease, such as asthma, may increase your risk for pneumonia.

 Frequent lung infections, especially in a person who smokes, may lead to the development of chronic bronchitis. Tobacco smokers are also at high risk for developing emphysema. Chronic bronchitis, emphysema, and other lung conditions are known as chronic obstructive pulmonary disease (COPD). See page 145.

Prevention

Bronchitis usually cannot be prevented, but you can improve your body's ability to fight infection.

- Give proper home care to minor respiratory problems such as colds and flu. See pages 141 and 147.

- Stop smoking. People who smoke or who are around smokers have more frequent bouts of bronchitis.

- Avoid polluted air and don't exercise outdoors when the ozone concentration is high. (Daily ozone level reports usually appear in your local newspaper.)

Home Treatment

Most cases of bronchitis can be managed with home treatment. Here's what you can do at home to prevent complications and feel better.

- Drink 8 to 12 glasses of water per day. Liquids help thin the mucus in the lungs so it can be coughed out.

- Get some extra rest. Let your energy go to healing.

- Take aspirin, ibuprofen, or acetaminophen to relieve fever and body aches. Avoid aspirin if you have asthma.

- Use a nonprescription cough suppressant that contains dextromethorphan to help quiet a dry, hacking cough so you can sleep. Avoid cough preparations that contain more than one active ingredient. See Cough Preparations on page 385.

- Breathe moist air from a humidifier, hot shower, or a sink filled with hot water. The heat and moisture will thin mucus so it can be coughed out.

- If you have classic flu symptoms, you may want to contact your doctor about taking antiviral medications. Otherwise, try home treatment and reassess your symptoms in 48 hours. See Influenza (Flu) on page 147.

- If you have chronic bronchitis, try roll breathing (page 344) every day if it seems to help.

When to Call a Health Professional

- If you develop signs of a bacterial infection. See Viral or Bacterial? on page 150.

- If you are in frail health and coughing causes you to become weak or exhausted.

- If you are in frail health and have a fever of 100° or higher that lasts longer than 1 day.

- If you have a fever higher than 101° with shaking chills and a productive cough.

- If a fever higher than 103° does not come down after 2 hours of home treatment.

- If you feel significant chest-wall pain (pain in the muscles of the chest) when you cough or breathe.

- If you are unable to drink enough fluids to avoid becoming dehydrated or if you are unable to eat.

- If you are an older adult or have a chronic illness, especially a lung problem.

- If the person who is sick has a change in mental status (even a minor change in a person who is very old or in frail health), or if the person seems delirious. See Delirium on page 195.

Chest Pain

Call 911 or other emergency services immediately if you think you may be having a heart attack. Symptoms of a heart attack include squeezing or crushing chest pain that feels like someone is sitting on your chest. The pain or discomfort may increase in intensity or occur with any of the following symptoms:

- Pain spreading to your back, shoulder, neck, jaw or teeth, arm, or wrist

- Sweating

- Shortness of breath

- Dizziness or fainting

- Nausea or vomiting

- Unusual weakness

- Rapid and irregular heartbeat

- Sense of doom

Call your doctor if you have continuous chest discomfort or pain and there is no obvious cause.

If the person who is having heart attack symptoms loses consciousness, follow the Rescue Breathing and CPR guidelines on page 37.

Chest pain is a key warning sign of a heart attack (see page 53), but chest pain may also be caused by other problems.

If chest pain increases when you press your finger on the painful site, or if you can pinpoint the spot that hurts, it is probably **chest-wall pain**, which may be caused by strained muscles or ligaments in the chest wall or by a broken rib. An

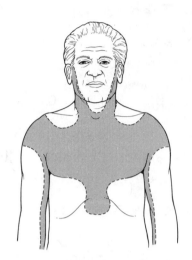

Chest pain caused by a heart attack can spread up the neck, into the jaw, down one or both arms, into the upper abdomen, or to the shoulders or upper back.

inflammation of the cartilage in the chest wall (called **costochondritis**) can also cause chest-wall pain. Chest-wall pain usually lasts only a few days. Aspirin or ibuprofen may help.

Chest pain caused by **pleurisy** (inflammation of the membrane that surrounds the lungs) or **pneumonia** (see page 151) will get worse when you take a deep breath or cough. An **ulcer** (see page 89) can cause chest pain, usually below the breastbone, that is worse when your stomach is empty. **Gallstones** (see page 77) may cause pain in the right side of the chest or around the shoulder blade. The pain may worsen after a meal or in the middle of the night. **Heartburn** (see page 78) can also cause chest pain. **Shingles** (see page 246) may cause a sharp, burning, or tingling pain that feels like a tight band around one side of the chest.

A shooting pain that lasts a few seconds, or a quick pain at the end of a deep breath, is usually not a cause for concern.

Home Treatment

For chest-wall pain caused by strained muscles and ligaments or a broken rib:

• Take pain relievers such as aspirin, acetaminophen, or ibuprofen. Applying products such as Ben-Gay or Icy-Hot to sore muscles may also help.

• Use an ice pack to help relieve pain the first few days after an injury.

• After applying ice during the first 72 hours (or until the swelling has gone down), apply a hot water bottle, warm towel, or heating pad to help relieve pain. Use heat that is no warmer than bath water or the low setting on a heating pad. To prevent burns, do not go to sleep with a heating pad turned on.

• Avoid any activity that strains the chest area. As your pain gets better, slowly return to your normal activities.

When to Call a Health Professional

Call 911 or other emergency services immediately if symptoms of a heart attack are present (see page 53).

If a doctor has diagnosed the cause of your chest pain and prescribed a home treatment plan, follow it. **Call 911 or other emergency services** if the pain worsens and may be caused by a heart problem, or if you develop any of the heart attack symptoms listed on page 53.

Call a health professional if minor chest pain occurs without the symptoms of a heart attack and any of the following apply:

• You have a history of heart disease or blood clots in the lungs.

• Chest pain is constant, nagging, and not relieved by rest.

• Chest pain occurs with symptoms of pneumonia. See page 151.

• Chest pain lasts longer than 2 days without improvement.

Colds

The common cold is brought to you by any one of 200 viruses. The symptoms of a cold include runny nose, red eyes, sneezing, sore throat, dry cough, headache, and general body aches. There is a gradual 1- or 2-day onset. As a cold progresses, the nasal mucus may thicken. This is the stage just before a cold dries up. A cold usually lasts a week or two. Colds occur throughout the year but are most common in late winter and early spring.

Using a mouthwash will not prevent a cold, and antibiotics will not cure a cold. There is no cure for the common cold. If you catch a cold, treat the symptoms.

Sometimes a cold will lead to a bacterial infection (see page 150), such as bronchitis or pneumonia. Good home treatment of colds can help prevent complications.

Prevention

• Eat well and get plenty of sleep and exercise to keep up your resistance.

• Try to avoid people who have colds.

• Keep your hands away from your nose, eyes, and mouth, but cover your mouth when you cough or sneeze.

• Wash your hands often, particularly when you are around people who have colds.

• Humidify your bedrooms or your whole house if possible.

• Don't smoke.

Home Treatment

Home treatment for a cold will help relieve symptoms and prevent complications.

• Get extra rest. Slow down just a little from your usual routine. It isn't necessary to stay home in bed, but take care not to expose others to your cold.

• Drink plenty of liquids. Hot water, herbal tea, or chicken soup will help relieve congestion.

• Take aspirin, ibuprofen, or acetaminophen to relieve aches. Avoid aspirin if you have asthma.

• Humidify your bedroom and take hot showers to relieve nasal stuffiness.

• Check the back of your throat for postnasal drip. If you see streaks of mucus, gargle with warm water to prevent a sore throat.

• Use disposable tissues, not handkerchiefs, to reduce the spread of the cold virus to others. If your nose is red and raw from rubbing it with tissues, put a dab of petroleum jelly on the sore area.

• Avoid cold remedies that contain a combination of drugs to treat many different symptoms. Treat each symptom separately. Take a decongestant for stuffiness and a cough medicine for a cough. See the home treatment for coughs on page 143.

• If you have high blood pressure or heart disease, do not take oral decongestants unless your doctor advises you to do so. Some decongestants can also be harmful to people with thyroid disease, glaucoma, urinary problems, an enlarged prostate, or diabetes. See page 385.

• Do not use nasal decongestant sprays for more than 3 days in a row. Continued use may lead to a "rebound" effect, causing the mucous membranes to become more swollen than they were before you used the spray. See page 384 to learn how to make nose drops at home.

• Avoid antihistamines. They are not an effective treatment for colds.

• If you have classic flu symptoms, you may want to contact your doctor about taking antiviral medications. Otherwise, try home treatment and reassess your symptoms in 48 hours. See Influenza (Flu) on page 147.

When to Call a Health Professional

- If you develop signs of a bacterial infection (see Viral or Bacterial? on page 150).

- If you develop facial pain, fever, and other signs of sinusitis (see page 152).

- If the person who is sick has a change in mental status (even a minor change in a person who is very old or in frail health), or if the person seems delirious. See Delirium on page 195.

Coughs

Coughing is the body's way of removing foreign material or mucus from the lungs. Coughs have distinctive traits you can learn to recognize.

Productive coughs produce phlegm or mucus (sputum) that comes up from the lungs. This kind of cough generally should not be suppressed. It is needed to clear mucus from the lungs.

Nonproductive coughs are dry coughs that do not produce sputum. A dry, hacking cough may develop toward the end of a cold or after exposure to an irritant, such as dust or smoke. Dry coughs that follow viral illnesses may last up to several weeks and often get worse at night. A dry cough can also be a side effect of certain medications.

A chronic dry cough, especially at night or early in the morning, may be the only symptom of mild asthma. It may also be an early sign of heart failure. See page 162.

Chronic coughs are often caused by the backflow (reflux) of stomach acid into the lungs and throat. If you suspect that problems with stomach acid reflux may be causing your cough, see Heartburn on page 78.

Prevention

- Don't smoke. See page 18 for tips on quitting. Avoid other people's smoke. A dry, hacking "smoker's cough" means that your lungs are constantly irritated.

- Drink 8 to 10 glasses of water every day. You are drinking enough if you are urinating more often than usual.

- Avoid exposure to dust, smoke, and other irritants, or wear an appropriate mask to protect yourself from the irritant.

Home Treatment

- Drink lots of water. Water helps loosen phlegm and soothe an irritated throat. Also try drinking hot tea or hot water with honey or lemon juice in it.

- Cough drops can soothe an irritated throat. Expensive, medicine-flavored cough drops are not any better than inexpensive, candy-flavored ones or hard candy.

Tuberculosis

Tuberculosis is a contagious disease caused by bacteria that usually infect the lungs (pulmonary TB). When a person who has pulmonary TB coughs, sneezes, or laughs, TB-causing bacteria are released into the air where other people can inhale them. This is how TB is spread. People with weak immune systems are particularly prone to TB.

Most people who are exposed to TB never develop symptoms because their immune systems are able to stop the disease. People who develop symptoms of TB, such as persistent cough, weight loss, fatigue, night sweats, and fever, need drug treatment to stop the disease from progressing and to reduce the risk of spreading TB to others. Treatment, which consists of several medications, may last from 6 months to 2 years.

People who have weak immune systems, abuse alcohol and drugs, or have a chronic lung disease called silicosis are at high risk for developing progressive TB, which can damage the lungs or spread to other parts of the body.

To prevent TB infection, avoid close contact with people who have TB if possible. If you live with someone who has TB, ask your doctor what you can do to protect yourself from TB infection. Also ask whether you need to be tested for TB.

- Elevate your head with extra pillows at night to ease a dry cough.

- Avoid cold remedies that combine drugs to treat many symptoms. It is generally better to treat each symptom separately. See Cough Preparations on page 385.

- Use cough suppressants wisely. Coughing is useful because it brings up mucus from the lungs and helps prevent bacterial infections. People with asthma and other lung diseases need to cough. If you have a dry, hacking cough that does not bring anything up, ask your health professional about an effective cough suppressant medication.

- Do not take anyone else's prescription cough medication.

When to Call a Health Professional

- If you develop signs of a bacterial infection (see Viral or Bacterial? on page 150).

- If a cough causes a person who is in frail health to become weak or exhausted.

- If a cough lasts longer than 2 weeks.

Emphysema

Emphysema is a chronic lung disease caused by repeated irritation or infection of the lung tissues. Emphysema almost always occurs in people who have been heavy smokers for a long time. Over time, the air sacs (alveoli) in the lungs become permanently damaged and can no longer add oxygen to the blood or remove carbon dioxide.

The primary symptom of emphysema is shortness of breath, especially on exertion, that worsens over time. Other symptoms can include fatigue, difficulty sleeping, weight loss, frequent colds and bronchitis, and wheezing. A mild productive cough (see page 143) may also be present. By the time symptoms develop, significant lung damage has already occurred.

Together with chronic bronchitis (see page 138), emphysema contributes to the condition known as **chronic obstructive pulmonary disease** (COPD).

 Emphysema and COPD must be diagnosed by a health professional. There is no cure, but early diagnosis and proper treatment will help you lead a more normal life.

Prevention

• Don't smoke, and avoid other people's smoke. The major cause of COPD and emphysema is cigarette smoking. For tips on quitting smoking, see page 18.

• Make sure your home and work areas are well ventilated, and wear a filtering mask to reduce your exposure to lung irritants.

Home Treatment

Self-care for emphysema and COPD focuses primarily on keeping your airways clear.

• If you smoke, quit. See page 18. Even though you cannot reverse lung damage caused by smoking, quitting now will prevent further damage.

• Take your prescribed medications as directed by your doctor.

• Drink at least 6 to 8 glasses of water and other fluids each day to keep mucus thin.

• Do roll breathing (page 344) every day if it helps your breathing.

• Exercise. General fitness can help you improve your lung function.

• Avoid exposure to colds or flu. Get a flu shot every year (see page 22).

• Make sure your pneumococcal vaccine is current (see page 25).

When to Call a Health Professional

• If you have been diagnosed with emphysema and you have any of the following symptoms:

  - Shortness of breath or wheezing that is rapidly getting worse.

- A cough that becomes more frequent or deeper, especially if it starts to bring up green, yellow, or rust-colored sputum.

- Coughing up blood.

- Increased swelling in your legs or abdomen.

- Fever higher than 100°.

- Severe chest pain.

- Flulike symptoms.

• If you have symptoms that may be caused by emphysema, such as chronic shortness of breath or a chronic cough, but your symptoms have not been evaluated by a doctor.

• If you are a smoker and you want help quitting. See page 18.

Fever

A fever is a high body temperature. It is a symptom, not a disease. A fever is one way the body fights illness. A temperature of up to 102° can help the body respond to infection. The height of a fever may not be related to the severity of an illness. This is especially true as a person ages, because with age the body loses some of its ability to produce a fever. An 80-year-old person with pneumonia who has a fever of 100° may be just as sick as a 24-year-old person with pneumonia who has a fever of 105°.

Older adults may develop symptoms that normally accompany fever even when they do not have a fever. These symptoms include headache, dizziness, restlessness, confusion, delusions, and paranoia. Such symptoms may indicate an infection even if fever is not present. Fevers are more likely to cause delirium (see page 195) or disorientation in older adults than in younger people.

Temperatures below normal (especially below 94°) may indicate a severe infection, a thyroid problem (see page 181), or hypothermia (see page 55).

A high fever can place increased strain on your heart. For people who have heart disease, a high fever can sometimes trigger heart failure.

Home Treatment

• Drink 8 to 12 glasses of water a day. You are drinking enough if you are urinating more often than usual.

• Watch for signs of dehydration. See page 73.

• Take and record your temperature every 2 hours and whenever your symptoms change.

• Take acetaminophen, aspirin, or ibuprofen to lower the fever.

• Take a sponge bath with lukewarm water if the fever is causing discomfort.

• Dress lightly.

• Eat light, easily digested foods, such as soup.

• If you have classic flu symptoms, you may want to contact your doctor about taking antiviral medications. Otherwise, try home treatment and reassess your symptoms in 48 hours. See Influenza (Flu) on page 147.

When to Call a Health Professional

• If a fever higher than 100° lasts longer than 1 day in a person who is in frail health.

• If a fever higher than 103° does not come down after 2 hours of home treatment.

• If you have a persistent fever. Many viral illnesses cause fevers of 102° or higher for short periods of time (up to 12 to 24 hours). Call a doctor if the fever stays high. For example:

 - 102° to 103° for 1 full day

 - 101° to 102° for 2 full days

 - 100° to 101° for 3 full days

• If your body temperature rises to 103° or higher, all sweating stops, and the skin becomes hot, dry, and flushed. These are symptoms of heat stroke. See page 54.

• If a fever occurs with other signs of a bacterial infection (see page 150).

• If the person who is sick has a change in mental status (even a minor change in a person who is very old or in frail health), or if the person seems delirious. See Delirium on page 195.

• If fever occurs with any of the following symptoms:

 - Very stiff neck and headache (see Encephalitis and Meningitis on page 189).

 - Shortness of breath and cough (see Bronchitis on page 138 and Pneumonia on page 151).

 - Pain above the eyes or the cheekbones (see Sinusitis on page 152).

 - Pain or burning when urinating (see Urinary Tract Infections on page 94).

 - Abdominal pain, nausea, and vomiting (see Stomach Flu and Food Poisoning on page 88).

 - Increased pain, redness, or tenderness around a skin wound, such as a cut or scrape (see Signs of a Wound Infection on page 59).

• If you develop a fever after you start taking a new medication.

Influenza (Flu)

Influenza, or flu, is a viral illness that commonly occurs in the winter and affects many people in a season. Flu is not the same as the common cold—the symptoms of flu are usually more severe and come on quite suddenly. Symptoms include fever (101° to 104°), shaking chills, body aches, muscle pain, headache, pain when you move your eyes, fatigue, weakness, and runny nose. Symptoms may last up to 10 days. Most other viral illnesses have milder symptoms that don't last as long.

Older adults who are in frail health or who have a chronic disease, especially lung diseases like asthma or emphysema, are at high risk of complications of influenza, such as bronchitis or pneumonia. Sinus or ear infections are other possible complications.

Prevention

- Get a flu shot each autumn if you are over 50; if you have a chronic illness, such as asthma, heart disease, or diabetes; if you are a health care worker; or if you live or work in a nursing home. See page 22 for more information about flu shots.

- Stop smoking to lower your risk of complications from the flu. See page 18 for tips.

- Keep up your resistance to infection by eating a healthy diet, getting plenty of rest, and exercising regularly.

- Avoid exposure to the virus. Wash your hands often, and keep your hands away from your nose, eyes, and mouth.

If you do get the flu, your doctor can prescribe an antiviral medication that may reduce the severity and duration of your symptoms. The medication is most effective if you start taking it within 48 hours after you start having flu symptoms.

Home Treatment

- Get plenty of rest.

- Drink extra fluids to replace those lost from fever, to ease a scratchy throat, and to keep the nasal mucus thin. Plain water, hot tea with lemon, fruit juice, and soup are all good choices.

- Take acetaminophen, aspirin, or ibuprofen to relieve fever, headache, and muscle aches. Avoid aspirin if you have asthma.

When to Call a Health Professional

When trying to decide if you need to see a health professional, consider the likelihood that you have the flu versus the possibility of a bacterial infection. If it is the flu season and many people in your community have similar symptoms, it is likely that you have the flu.

Call a health professional:

- Within the first 48 hours of flu symptoms developing if you are considering taking an antiviral medication to reduce the severity and duration of your illness. Medication is recommended for older adults and people with chronic health problems.

- If you develop signs of a bacterial infection. See Viral or Bacterial? on page 150.

- If you seem to get better, then get worse again.

- If the person who is sick has a change in mental status (even a minor change in a person who is very old or in frail health), or if the person seems delirious. See Delirium on page 195.

Laryngitis and Hoarseness

Laryngitis is an infection or irritation of the voice box (larynx). The most common cause is a viral infection such as a cold. Other causes include allergies; excessive talking, singing, or yelling; cigarette smoke; and the backflow (reflux) of stomach acid into the throat. Heavy drinking or smoking can lead to chronic laryngitis.

Symptoms of laryngitis include hoarseness or loss of voice, the urge to clear your throat, fever, tiredness, throat pain, and a cough.

Prevention

To prevent hoarseness, give your vocal cords a rest. As soon as you feel minor throat pain, try to talk less. Don't shout or whisper.

Home Treatment

- Your voice box will usually heal in 5 to 10 days. Medication does little to speed recovery.

- If hoarseness is caused by a cold, treat the cold (see page 141). Hoarseness may last up to 1 week after a cold goes away.

- Rest your voice. Talk as little as possible. Don't shout or whisper, and avoid clearing your throat.

- Stop smoking and avoid other people's smoke. See page 18 for tips on quitting.

- Humidify your bedrooms, or the whole house if possible. Try standing in the steam from a hot shower.

- Drink 8 to 12 glasses of water a day. You are drinking enough if you are urinating more often than usual.

- Gargle frequently with warm salt water (1 teaspoon of salt in 8 ounces of water), or drink weak tea or hot water with honey or lemon in it.

- If you think that problems with stomach acid reflux may be contributing to your laryngitis, see Heartburn on page 78.

When to Call a Health Professional

- If you develop signs of a bacterial infection. See Viral or Bacterial? on page 150.

- If hoarseness persists for 3 to 4 weeks.

Viral or Bacterial?

Viral infections

- Usually involve different parts of the body: sore throat, runny nose, headache, muscle aches. In the digestive system, viruses cause nausea, vomiting, or diarrhea.

- Typically include colds, flu, and stomach flu.

- Cannot be cured by antibiotics.

Bacterial infections

- Sometimes follow viral infections.

- Usually affect one area of the body: sinuses, lungs, an ear.

- Can be cured by antibiotics.

Call a health professional if you develop symptoms of a bacterial infection. These symptoms include:

- Fever of 103° or higher that does not go down after 2 hours of home treatment.

- Fever higher than 101° with shaking chills and productive cough (brings up sputum).

- Fever that persists despite home treatment. Many viral illnesses cause fevers of 102° or higher for short periods of time (12 to 24 hours). Call a doctor if the fever stays high:

  - 102° to 103° for 1 full day

  - 101° to 102° for 2 full days

  - 100° to 101° for 3 full days

- Labored, shallow, rapid breathing with shortness of breath.

- Sputum that is yellow, green, rust-colored, or bloody and occurs with other symptoms (fever, productive cough, fatigue) that are getting worse. Sputum that is coughed up from the lungs is more significant than mucus that has drained down the back of the throat (postnasal drip).

- Nasal discharge that changes from clear to colored (yellow or green) during the course of a cold (5 to 7 days) and occurs with other symptoms, such as sinus pain or fever.

- Nasal discharge that is colored from the time a cold starts and lasts longer than 7 to 10 days.

- Cough that lingers more than 7 to 10 days after other symptoms have cleared, especially if it is productive (brings up sputum). A dry, hacking cough may last several weeks after a viral illness such as a cold.

Pneumonia

Pneumonia is an infection or inflammation that affects the lungs. It is usually caused by bacteria, but viruses and other organisms can cause it as well. Pneumonia sometimes follows a viral upper respiratory infection, such as a cold or bronchitis. However, in a person who is very old or in frail health, pneumonia may develop even if the person hasn't been sick. A person who has bacterial pneumonia is usually very sick. Symptoms may include:

- A productive cough with yellow, green, rust-colored, or bloody sputum (mucus coughed up from the lungs).

- Fever and shaking chills.

- Sweating and flushed appearance.

- Rapid, shallow breathing.

- Chest-wall pain that is often made worse by coughing or taking a deep breath.

- Rapid heartbeat.

- Fatigue that is worse than you would expect from a cold.

- Mental status changes (confusion, disorientation).

Pneumonia can be a serious problem for older adults, especially those who have chronic diseases such as diabetes, heart disease, AIDS, or emphysema. The pneumococcal vaccine and good home care for colds and flu can help reduce the risk of getting pneumonia.

Prevention

- Get a pneumococcal vaccination if you are over 65, or if you are younger than 65 and have a chronic disease such as heart, lung, or kidney disease, diabetes, or cancer. See Pneumococcal Infection on page 25.

- Keep up your resistance to infection by eating a healthy diet, getting plenty of rest, and exercising regularly.

Home Treatment

Call a health professional if you suspect you have pneumonia. If pneumonia is diagnosed:

- Take the entire course of all prescribed medications.

- Drink 8 to 12 glasses of water a day. You are drinking enough if you are urinating more often than usual. Extra fluids help thin the mucus in the lungs.

- Get lots of rest. Don't try to rush your recovery.

- Take acetaminophen or aspirin to reduce fever and make you feel more comfortable. Avoid aspirin if you have asthma.

When to Call a Health Professional

- If you develop symptoms of pneumonia.

- If your breathing becomes rapid or labored during any respiratory illness.

- If you have new chest pain that gets worse whenever you take a deep breath.

Sinusitis

Sinusitis is an inflammation or infection of the mucous membranes that line the sinuses and nasal passages. The sinuses are hollow spaces in the head. Sinusitis causes the sinuses to become blocked, leading to pain and pressure in the face.

Sinusitis most often follows a cold and may also be associated with allergies, an infected tooth (dental abscess), or air pollution. The key symptom of sinusitis is pain over the cheekbones and upper teeth, in the forehead over the eyebrows, or around and behind the eyes. There may also be headache, swelling around the eyes, fever, stuffy nose, coughing, or mucus draining down the back of the throat (postnasal drip). Sinus headaches may occur when you get up in the morning, and they may get worse in the afternoon or when you bend over.

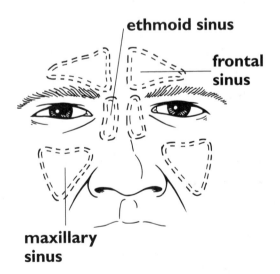

Sinusitis can cause pain in the cheekbones or forehead, or around the eyes.

If your symptoms are severe or continue for more than 10 to 14 days, you may need to take antibiotics. A sinus infection can lead to chronic sinusitis if it does not respond to home treatment or antibiotics, or if it is not treated at all.

Prevention

- Promptly treat nasal congestion caused by colds.

- Avoid cigarette, cigar, and pipe smoke in your home and workplace. Smoke irritates inflamed membranes in your nose and sinuses.

- If you have allergies, avoid the things that trigger your allergy attacks.

Home Treatment

Home treatment can often relieve early symptoms of sinusitis, such as facial pressure and stuffiness, and get your sinuses draining normally again so that you may not need antibiotic treatment.

- Drink extra fluids to keep mucus thin. Drink at least 8 to 10 glasses of water or juice per day.

- Apply moist heat (a warm towel or gel pack) to your face several times a day for 5 to 10 minutes at a time.

- Breathe warm, moist air from a steamy shower, a hot bath, or a sink filled with hot water.

- Increase the humidity in your home, especially in the bedrooms. Avoid cold, dry air.

• Take an oral decongestant, use a decongestant nasal spray, or use a mucus-thinning agent (see page 384). Do not use a nasal spray for more than 3 days in a row. Avoid products that contain antihistamines unless your symptoms may also be related to allergies.

• Take aspirin, acetaminophen, or ibuprofen to relieve facial pain and headache. Avoid aspirin if you have asthma.

• Check the back of your throat for post-nasal drip. If you see streaks of mucus, gargle with warm water to prevent a sore throat.

• Blow your nose gently. Do not close one nostril when blowing your nose.

• Salt water (saline) irrigation helps wash mucus and bacteria out of the nasal passages. Use nonprescription saline nose drops or a homemade solution (see page 384):

  - Use a bulb syringe and gently squirt the solution into your nose, or snuff the solution from the palm of your hand, one nostril at a time.

  - The salt water should go in through your nose and come out your mouth.

  - Blow your nose gently afterward. Repeat the salt water wash 2 to 4 times a day.

When to Call a Health Professional

• If cold symptoms last longer than 10 to 14 days or worsen after the first 7 days.

• If you have a severe headache that is different from a "normal" headache and is not relieved by acetaminophen, aspirin, or ibuprofen.

• If you have increased facial swelling, or if your vision changes or gets blurry.

• If you develop signs of a bacterial infection. See Viral or Bacterial? on page 150.

• If facial pain, especially in one sinus area or along the ridge between the nose and lower eyelid, persists after 2 days of home treatment. If you also have a fever and colored nasal discharge, call in 1 to 2 days.

• If sinusitis symptoms persist after you have taken a full course of antibiotics.

Sore Throat and Strep Throat

Most sore throats are caused by viruses and may occur with a cold or may follow a cold. A mild sore throat may be caused by dry air, smoking, air pollution, or yelling. People who have allergies or stuffy noses may breathe through their mouths while sleeping, which can cause a mild sore throat.

Strep throat is a sore throat caused by streptococcal bacteria. It is much more common in children than in older adults, but people of all ages can get it. You can get strep throat even if your tonsils have been removed.

In general, the more coldlike your symptoms are, the less likely it is that you have strep throat. Strep throat causes some or all of these symptoms:

• Sudden and severe sore throat

• Fever

• Swollen lymph nodes in the neck

• White or yellow coating on the tonsils

Strep throat is treated with antibiotics to prevent rheumatic fever. Antibiotics are effective in preventing rheumatic fever if they are started within 9 days of the onset of the sore throat.

A less common cause of sore throat is the backflow (reflux) of stomach acid into the throat. Although reflux is often associated with heartburn or an "acid" taste in the mouth, sometimes a sore throat is the only symptom. If you think stomach acid reflux may be causing your throat pain, see Heartburn on page 78.

Prevention

• Drink 8 to 12 glasses of water a day.

• Identify and avoid irritants that cause sore throat (such as smoke, fumes, or yelling). For tips on quitting smoking, see page 18.

• Avoid contact with people who have strep throat. If you have strep throat, stay home until 24 hours after starting antibiotics.

Home Treatment

Home care is usually all that is needed for viral sore throats. If you are taking antibiotics for strep throat, these tips will also help you feel better.

• Gargle with warm salt water (1 teaspoon of salt in 8 ounces of water). The salt reduces swelling and discomfort. If you have postnasal drip, gargle often to prevent more throat irritation.

• Drink more fluids to soothe your sore throat. Honey or lemon in hot water or in weak tea may help.

• Stop smoking, and avoid other people's smoke.

• Take acetaminophen, aspirin, or ibuprofen to relieve pain and reduce fever.

• Use nonprescription throat lozenges that contain a local anesthetic to soothe your throat, such as Sucrets Maximum Strength, Spec-T, or Tyrobenz. Regular cough drops or hard candy may also help.

When to Call a Health Professional

• If you develop any of the following symptoms:

  - Difficulty swallowing.

  - Excessive drooling caused by inability to swallow.

  - Labored or difficult breathing.

• If you develop a severe sore throat after being exposed to strep throat.

- If a sore throat occurs with 2 of these 3 symptoms of strep throat:

  - Fever.

  - White or yellow coating on the tonsils.

  - Swollen lymph nodes in the neck.

- If a rash occurs with sore throat. **Scarlet fever** is a rash that may occur when there is a strep throat infection. Like strep throat, scarlet fever is treated with antibiotics.

- If you cannot trace the cause of a sore throat to a cold, allergy, smoking, overuse of your voice, or other irritation.

- If a mild sore throat lasts longer than 2 weeks.

- If your throat is chronically sore and you have not had the problem evaluated by a health professional.

Snoring

Up to 50 percent of adults snore occasionally, and 25 percent of adults are habitual snorers. Snoring is caused by blockage of the airways in the back of the mouth and nose. These airways can be blocked for many reasons, such as excess neck tissue caused by being overweight or a stuffy nose caused by allergies or a cold. Some people who snore have sleep apnea. Sleep apnea is present when a person repeatedly stops breathing for 10 to 15 seconds or longer during sleep.

Snoring can disrupt a person's sleep patterns, so he or she may be sleepy and less alert during the day. A person's snoring can also disrupt the sleep of other family members or roommates. Here are some tips for people who snore:

- Exercise daily to maintain a healthy body weight and improve muscle tone. Avoid exercise within 2 hours of bedtime, because exercise may make it harder to fall asleep.

- Avoid heavy meals, alcohol, sleeping pills, and antihistamines before bedtime.

- Sleep on your side rather than your back. (Sew a pocket onto the back of your pajama top, and put a tennis ball inside the pocket. This will keep you from sleeping on your back.)

- Establish regular sleeping patterns. Go to bed at the same time every night, even on weekends.

- Let the person who doesn't snore fall asleep first.

 If snoring becomes a problem for you and affects your family life, see a health professional. An examination of the nose, mouth, and neck may be needed. Your doctor may also want to do a <u>sleep study</u> to see if sleep apnea is one of the reasons why you snore. Treatment will depend on what is causing you to snore.

Lung Cancer

Lung cancer kills more men and women than any other cancer does. It occurs most often in people over age 50 who smoked for many years. Lung cancer can develop when the lungs are damaged by repeatedly inhaling smoke (including secondhand smoke) or other harmful substances, including asbestos, radioactive dust, and radon.

Having a combination of risk factors, such as being a smoker who works with asbestos, greatly increases your risk of developing lung cancer.

Symptoms of lung cancer are similar to those of other chest and lung problems: chronic cough; shortness of breath; wheezing; hoarseness; repeated lung infections or pneumonia; pain in the chest wall, shoulders, or back; or coughing up pus-filled or bloody sputum. There may be no symptoms in the early stages. If you smoke, see your doctor about any chronic respiratory symptom.

If you've been diagnosed with lung cancer, see Winning Over Serious Illness on page 341.

If your heart has peace,
nothing can disturb you.
The Dalai Lama

8

Heart and Circulation Problems

Your heart and blood vessels make up your circulatory system, which supplies oxygen and nutrients to every cell in your body. A healthy circulatory system is the key to a physically robust life at any age, but especially as you get older. To a great extent, the health of your heart and blood vessels determines how far you can walk, how late you can dance, and how long you can garden.

The heart is a muscle with four hollow chambers. When it contracts, it pushes blood out through the arteries to the lungs, where the blood picks up oxygen. From the lungs, the oxygen-rich blood returns to the heart and is pumped to the rest of the body. Once the blood has delivered oxygen to the cells, it circulates through the veins back to the heart, where the whole process starts again.

Normally, the heart and blood vessels deliver a constant supply of oxygen and nutrients to the body. Therefore, if a problem develops in any part of the system, the whole body may be affected. Heart and circulatory diseases are the leading causes of death in adults. Read on for information about how to reduce your risk and manage these diseases.

Atherosclerosis

One of the most common problems to affect the circulatory system is atherosclerosis or "hardening of the arteries." Atherosclerosis is the buildup of cholesterol and calcium deposits (called plaques) inside the lining of the arteries. As plaques grow, the arteries become narrow. As a result, less blood is able to flow through the arteries, and less oxygen reaches the tissues that are supplied by those arteries.

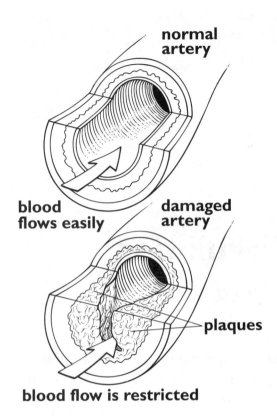

normal
artery

blood
flows easily

damaged
artery

plaques

blood flow is restricted

Atherosclerosis is the buildup of waxy deposits called plaques inside the arteries.

Atherosclerosis is the starting point for most heart and circulation problems:

- When atherosclerosis affects the arteries that supply blood to the heart muscle, it is called coronary artery disease (CAD). CAD may cause chest pain (angina), heart attack, heart failure, or other heart conditions. See Coronary Artery Disease on page 158.

- When atherosclerosis affects the arteries in the legs or other areas, it causes a circulation problem called peripheral vascular disease (PVD). See Peripheral Vascular Disease on page 169.

- When atherosclerosis affects blood vessels that supply the brain, it may cause transient ischemic attacks (TIAs) or strokes. See Stroke on page 63. Reduced blood flow to the brain caused by atherosclerosis can also cause multi-infarct dementia. See Dementia on page 196.

- When atherosclerosis affects the arteries that supply blood to the abdomen and pelvis, kidney or intestinal problems may result.

Other types of circulatory problems include high blood pressure, blood clots or inflammation in the veins (phlebitis), irregular heartbeats, and varicose veins. These problems may be related to atherosclerosis, but in some cases they are not.

Coronary Artery Disease

Coronary artery disease (CAD) is the most common type of heart disease. It develops when the coronary arteries, which supply blood to the heart muscle, become narrowed or blocked. This usually results from the buildup of fat and calcium deposits (called plaque) in the blood vessels, a process called "hardening of the arteries," or atherosclerosis (see page 157). When the coronary arteries are narrowed, less blood flows to the heart muscle. Decreased blood flow to the heart muscle can lead to one or more of the following problems.

Angina: Many people with CAD have no symptoms. Others may feel a pressure, heaviness, or tightness in the chest when they do things that make their heart work harder. This discomfort is called angina. The pain is signaling that the heart muscle needs more oxygen than can be delivered through the narrowed coronary arteries.

If you have had angina for a while, you may be able to predict almost exactly how much exertion will bring on your symptoms. Angina pain usually starts at a low level, then gradually increases over several minutes to a peak. Angina pain may spread to your abdomen, upper back, shoulders, neck, jaws, or arms. Angina pain that starts when you exert yourself will usually decrease when you stop the activity. This predictable type of discomfort is called **stable angina**. Your doctor may prescribe medications, such as nitroglycerin, for you to take when you have an episode of angina.

A change in your usual pattern of angina (**unstable angina**) may mean that blood flow to your heart has worsened. It is a warning sign that a heart attack may soon occur and needs immediate evaluation.

Chest pain is not always caused by angina or related to a heart problem. For more information about chest pain, see page 140.

Heart attack (myocardial infarction): If a blood clot forms in a narrowed coronary artery, the blood flow to a part of the heart may become completely blocked. This can cause a heart attack. During a heart attack, heart muscle cells die because blood, oxygen, and nutrients do not reach those cells. See Heart Attack on page 53.

Cardiomyopathy, irregular heartbeats, and heart failure: Over time, reduced blood flow to the heart may cause the heart muscle to weaken so that it is not able to pump effectively. This may result in other serious conditions such as irregular heartbeats (see page 167); heart failure (see page 162); or ischemic cardiomyopathy, in which the heart's chambers become enlarged and less effective.

Important risk factors for coronary artery disease include:

- Smoking.
- Being a man over age 45.
- Having a family history of early heart disease.
- Having uncontrolled high blood pressure, high cholesterol, or diabetes.

Other risk factors include not managing stress effectively, having an inactive lifestyle, being overweight, and having elevated levels of the amino acid homocysteine in your blood. If risk factors are identified early, it may be possible for you to prevent CAD by changing your lifestyle and taking medications to control high blood pressure, high cholesterol, and other conditions that increase your risk for CAD.

When blood flow to large areas of the heart muscle is restricted, other steps may need to be taken to restore blood flow to the heart. Angioplasty involves inserting a thin, flexible tube into a blocked coronary artery. A balloon at the end of the tube is inflated, and the pressure from the balloon presses the cholesterol and calcium deposits (plaques) that are blocking the artery against the artery wall. This makes it possible for more blood to flow through the artery. A small, expandable wire tube called a stent is often inserted into the artery to hold it open after the procedure. Coronary artery bypass surgery takes a blood vessel from another part of the body and uses it to detour (bypass) the blocked artery.

Whether you have angioplasty or bypass surgery depends on a number of factors, including how many blocked arteries you have, how badly the arteries are blocked, where the blockages are, other heart problems you may have, and your personal preferences.

 Getting all the facts and thinking about your own needs and values will help you make a wise decision about treatment for <u>coronary artery disease</u>. Regardless of which treatment you

choose, if you make lifestyle changes to control your risk factors, you can improve the quality of your life and, in all likelihood, have fewer future problems with your heart.

Prevention

A few risk factors for coronary artery disease, such as being a man over age 45 or having a history of early heart disease in your family, are outside your control. However, you can control many other risk factors for coronary artery disease, such as smoking, high blood pressure, and high cholesterol.

- Stop smoking. Smoking increases your risk of atherosclerosis. See page 18 for tips on quitting.

- Eat a healthy, low-fat diet. This can help lower your cholesterol levels and your weight. A very low-fat diet (less than 10 percent calories from fat) may even reduce the buildup of fat inside your blood vessels.

- Get regular aerobic exercise. Exercise helps to control your blood pressure and weight and helps to lower your cholesterol. For more information, read the Fitness chapter beginning on page 285.

- Manage stress and anger wisely. These emotions may increase your risk of having a heart attack. See Stress on page 342.

- Review the information about controlling high blood pressure on pages 165 to 167. Certain medications used to control high blood pressure may reduce your risk of heart attack.

- If you have diabetes, work with your doctor to keep your blood sugar levels within a safe range to help reduce your risk for heart disease. See the home treatment for diabetes on page 177.

- If you have elevated cholesterol levels, taking medications called statins may help prevent coronary artery disease and reduce your risk of heart attack.

- If you have elevated homocysteine levels, vitamins B_6 and B_{12} as well as folic acid may help lower homocysteine levels and reduce your risk of coronary artery disease. Eat a balanced diet that contains these nutrients, or talk to your doctor about taking supplements.

- If you are at increased risk for heart disease, talk to your doctor about whether you should take aspirin regularly to reduce your risk of heart attack.

Home Treatment

Coronary artery disease responds well to lifestyle changes and medications that reduce risk factors. If you stop smoking, maintain a healthy weight, exercise regularly, eat a healthy diet, and take prescribed medications as directed, you can reduce your risk of having a heart attack.

In some cases, you may be able to slow or reverse the process of atherosclerosis.

- Take your prescribed medications as directed. If your doctor has prescribed nitroglycerin to treat angina, be sure you understand when and how to use it and what to do if it doesn't seem to be working.

- If someone in your family has coronary artery disease, or has several risk factors for heart disease, take a cardiopulmonary resuscitation (CPR) course. CPR is a form of first aid for heart attacks, and it saves lives. See Breathing Emergencies on page 36.

- Follow the guidelines for quitting smoking, eating a low-fat diet, getting regular exercise, and managing stress that are provided in this book. Use the index to locate the topics about which you wish to learn more.

- Talk with your doctor about taking aspirin every day to reduce the risk of having a heart attack. Do not take aspirin regularly without first discussing it with your doctor.

- See Winning Over Serious Illness on page 341.

- Maintain a positive attitude. Learn all you can about heart disease and believe that you can manage it successfully. Studies show that a positive attitude helps people successfully recover from heart attacks.

When to Call a Health Professional

Call 911 or other emergency services immediately if you think you may be having a heart attack. Symptoms of a heart attack include chest pain that is squeezing or crushing, that feels like someone is sitting on your chest, or that occurs with any of the following symptoms:

- Sweating

- Shortness of breath

- Nausea or vomiting

- Pain that spreads from the chest to the abdomen, upper back, shoulder, neck, jaw, or arm

- Lightheadedness or dizziness

- Rapid or irregular heartbeat

- Signs of shock. See Shock on page 60.

- Angina that has been diagnosed by a doctor but has not gone away after using your treatment plan for angina

Do not try to drive yourself to the hospital. After calling 911, chew and swallow 1 adult aspirin (unless you are allergic to it).

If the person who is having heart attack symptoms loses consciousness, follow the Rescue Breathing and CPR guidelines outlined on page 37.

Quick action is vital when a person is having a heart attack. Medications that reduce the damage to the heart muscle are most effective when given within a few hours of the onset of symptoms.

Call your health professional:

- If you have new, more frequent, or severe episodes of chest pain or discomfort.

- If symptoms of angina do not respond to your prescribed treatment, or if the pattern of your angina changes (for example, if your symptoms begin to occur when you are at rest).

- If you develop minor chest pain without other symptoms of a heart attack and:

  - You have a history of heart disease or blood clots in your lungs.

  - Your chest pain is constant or nagging and is not relieved by rest.

- If pain or discomfort lasts longer than 30 minutes and there is no obvious cause, such as a pulled muscle or broken rib.

Heart Failure

Heart failure develops when the heart doesn't pump as much blood as the body needs. "Failure" doesn't mean that the heart has stopped pumping, but that it is failing to pump as effectively as it should.

Heart failure is most often caused by a problem with the left ventricle of the heart. The left ventricle is the lower left heart chamber that pumps blood out to the body. When the left ventricle cannot pump effectively, blood can back up inside the heart and lungs, leading to symptoms of heart failure.

Blood may also back up in the right ventricle of the heart. The right ventricle receives blood from the body and pumps it to the lungs, where oxygen enters the blood. When the right ventricle can't pump well, blood backs up in the body, causing fluid buildup in the abdomen, legs, ankles, and feet. Right-sided and left-sided heart failure can occur at the same time.

Symptoms of heart failure may include:

- Shortness of breath, especially when you are lying down. You may wake up coughing or wheezing and have a rapid heart rate and the feeling that you are being suffocated. These symptoms often improve when you sit or stand up.

- Difficulty breathing during routine activities that did not previously cause breathing problems.

- A dry, hacking cough, especially when you are lying down.

- Swelling caused by fluid buildup (edema), especially in the legs, ankles, and feet.

- Weight gain caused by fluid buildup. This may be sudden.

- Increased urination at night.

- Dizziness, fatigue, weakness, or fainting.

- Swelling and discomfort in the abdomen.

Heart failure is more likely to develop in people who have coronary artery disease or other types of heart disease. When the heart muscle has been damaged by long-term high blood pressure, coronary artery disease, injury (such as a heart attack), or infection, it may become harder for the heart to pump blood.

Heart failure is a chronic condition but can worsen suddenly in response to missed medication doses, a new heart attack, infection, alcohol use, a high-sodium meal, overexertion, or a low blood count. Sudden, or acute, heart failure is a medical emergency.

Prevention

The best way to prevent heart failure is to prevent atherosclerosis and coronary artery disease. See the prevention guidelines for coronary artery disease starting on page 160. Controlling high blood pressure (see page 165) and diabetes (see page 176) can also help.

Home Treatment

- Take your medications as directed. Not taking your pills regularly can make your symptoms worse. See page 379 for some suggestions on how to keep track of your pills.

- Limit the amount of salt in your diet. When you have heart failure, your body retains salt and water, which can lead to fluid buildup and swelling. See page 311.

- Your doctor may recommend that you limit the amount of liquid you drink each day. If so, keep track of how much you drink. Remember that juice, coffee, tea, milk, soda, and foods that melt (such as ice cream) or contain a lot of liquid (such as soup) all count toward your daily fluid intake.

- If your doctor wants you to weigh yourself every day, do it at the same time each day (before breakfast is a good time). Call your doctor if you gain more than 2 to 3 pounds in less than 1 week. This may mean that fluid is building up in your body.

- If your symptoms are severe or you are having a bad episode, don't try to continue with your usual activities. Your body needs to rest. However, if you are resting in bed, avoid lying flat on your back. Prop yourself up with pillows or move to an armchair, and flex and shift your legs often. This will help keep fluid from building up in your abdomen and chest and making it hard for you to breathe. Get help with household chores if needed.

- Ask your doctor about using nonprescription medications. Some antacids and stool softeners contain sodium or ingredients that can interfere with your prescription medications.

- Protect yourself against respiratory infections. Get a flu shot each fall and the pneumococcal vaccine as needed. See pages 22 and 25.

When to Call a Health Professional

Call 911 or other emergency services immediately:

- If you have chest pain that is not relieved by rest or medications, especially if the pain is pressing or crushing and occurs with shortness of breath, sweating, nausea, or other symptoms of a heart attack. See Heart Attack on page 53.

- If you have symptoms of a stroke. See Stroke on page 63.

- If you have severe shortness of breath (trouble getting a breath even when resting).

- If any chest pain or discomfort lasts longer than 30 minutes and there is no obvious cause.

- If you have a sudden episode of a prolonged irregular heartbeat or a very rapid heartbeat associated with dizziness, nausea, or fainting.

- If you have a cough that produces foamy, pink mucus.

- If you have a sense of doom that is associated with other heart or lung symptoms.

Call a health professional:

- If you have difficulty breathing during routine activities or exercise that did not previously cause a problem.

- If you become short of breath when you lie down, or if you wake up at night with shortness of breath or a feeling that you are suffocating.

- If you have a dry, hacking cough, especially when you lie down.

- If you have new and significant swelling in your feet, ankles, or legs, or if swelling that is typical for you worsens significantly.

- If you have gained more than 2 to 3 pounds in less than a week.

- If you have heart failure and your symptoms get worse. In general, it's a good idea to call your doctor whenever your symptoms change suddenly.

High Blood Pressure

Blood pressure is a measurement of the force of blood against the walls of the arteries. Blood pressure readings include two numbers, for example, 130/80. The first number in the reading is called the systolic pressure. It is the force that blood exerts on the artery walls as the heart contracts. The second number in the reading is the diastolic pressure. It is the force that blood exerts on the artery walls between heartbeats, when the heart is at rest.

If your blood pressure readings are consistently above 140 systolic and 90 diastolic, you have high blood pressure (hypertension).

Despite what a lot of people think, high blood pressure usually does not cause headaches, dizziness, or lightheadedness. Often called the "silent killer," it usually has no symptoms. However, high blood pressure increases your risk for heart attack, stroke, and kidney or eye damage. Your risk of developing these problems increases as your blood pressure rises.

Risk factors for high blood pressure and its complications include:

- Smoking.

- Being overweight.

- Having a family history of high blood pressure.

- Being of African-American descent.

- Having an inactive lifestyle.

- Drinking too much alcohol.

- Having too much salt or not enough potassium, calcium, or magnesium in your diet.

- Using medications such as steroids, decongestants, and anti-inflammatory drugs on a regular basis.

 Treating your high blood pressure, especially if you have moderate or severe high blood pressure, decreases your risk for coronary artery disease, heart attack, heart failure, stroke, and kidney disease and reduces your risk of dying from these conditions. If your blood pressure readings are consistently 120 to 139 systolic (the first or upper number) or 80 to 89 diastolic (the second or lower number), you are considered prehypertensive. Whether you have high blood pressure or prehypertension, treatment begins with making lifestyle changes like those outlined in Prevention. Whether you need treatment with medications depends on the severity of your high blood pressure and whether you have other health problems or conditions, such as heart failure or diabetes.

Prevention

Changes in your lifestyle can help prevent or lower high blood pressure.

- Maintain a healthy weight. This is especially important if you tend to put on weight around the waist rather than in the hips and thighs. (Weight gain around the waist is a risk factor for heart disease.) Losing even 10 pounds can help you lower your blood pressure.

- Exercise regularly. Thirty to 45 minutes of brisk walking 3 to 5 times a week will help you lower your blood pressure (and may also help you lose weight).

- Stop using tobacco products. Tobacco use increases your risk for heart attack and stroke. See page 18 for tips to help you quit.

- Drink alcohol only in moderation.

- Use salt moderately. Too much salt in the diet can be a problem for some people who have high blood pressure and are also salt-sensitive.

- Make sure you get enough potassium, calcium, and magnesium in your diet. Eating plenty of fruits (such as bananas and oranges), vegetables, legumes, whole grains, and low-fat dairy products will ensure that you get enough of these minerals.

- Reduce the saturated fat in your diet. Saturated fat is found in animal products (milk, cheese, and meat). Limiting these foods will help you lose weight and also lower your risk for coronary artery disease. See page 158.

- If your doctor recommends it, follow the Dietary Approaches to Stop Hypertension—or DASH—diet, which is described on page 314.

- Learn how to check your blood pressure at home. See page 377.

Home Treatment

- Follow the prevention tips listed earlier even more closely if you already have high blood pressure or if you are prehypertensive (120 to 139 systolic or 80 to 89 diastolic).

- Take any prescribed blood pressure medications exactly as directed, and see your doctor at least once a year. These medications help control high blood pressure but do not cure it. If you stop taking them, your blood pressure may go back up.

- If you are taking blood pressure medication, talk to your doctor before taking decongestants or anti-inflammatory drugs, because they can raise your blood pressure.

When to Call a Health Professional

• Call immediately if you have high blood pressure and:

- You develop chest pain or discomfort.

- Your blood pressure rises suddenly.

- Your blood pressure is 180/110 or higher.

- You have a sudden, severe headache.

• Call if your blood pressure is higher than 140/90 on two or more occasions (taken at home or in a community screening program). If one blood pressure reading is high, have another taken by a health professional to verify the first reading.

• Call if you develop uncomfortable or disturbing side effects from any medication you take for high blood pressure.

Irregular Heartbeat

Normally the heart beats in a regular rhythm and at a rate that is just right for the work the body is doing at any moment. Abnormal changes in heartbeats, called **arrhythmias**, occur when the heart beats too fast, too slow, or with an irregular rhythm. A change in your heart's rhythm may feel like a skipped beat, a strong and throbbing beat (palpitation), a flip-flop beat, or a fluttering in your chest.

Smoking heavily, drinking too much alcohol or caffeinated beverages (coffee, tea, or soda), or taking stimulants such as diet pills or decongestants may cause your heart to skip a beat. Your heartbeat can change when you are under stress or having pain. Your heart may beat faster when you have an illness or a fever. Hard physical exercise usually increases the heart rate, which can also cause heartbeat changes.

Many heartbeat changes are minor and do not require medical treatment. Others, such as atrial fibrillation, can be more serious because they may increase your risk for blood clots and strokes. Some skipped heartbeats may start in the lower heart chambers (ventricular arrhythmias) and can be life-threatening. If you have heart disease, heart failure, or a history of heart attack, pay close attention to changes in your usual heart rhythm or rate.

When you have a change in your heart rhythm or rate, you may also have other symptoms, such as chest pain, shortness of breath, lightheadedness, confusion, weakness, or fainting. When fainting occurs because of an irregular heartbeat, it is called cardiac syncope. Heartbeat changes with these other symptoms can be a sign of a serious heart problem.

 Your doctor may prescribe medications to help regulate your heartbeat or reduce your risk for blood clots, depending on the cause of your <u>arrhythmia</u>. If your risk for serious complications cannot be controlled with medications, you may need surgery. In this case, doctors will destroy your heart's natural pacemaker and implant an artificial pacemaker in your chest wall to regulate your heartbeat.

Prevention

• Prevent fatigue by getting plenty of sleep and rest. If you become overtired, your heartbeat changes may be more severe or occur more often.

• Cut back on or eliminate caffeine, including coffee, tea, colas, and chocolate. Some nonprescription medications, particularly headache remedies, contain caffeine. Caffeine increases your heart rate and can increase irregular heart rhythms.

• Cut back on or eliminate alcohol and tobacco, which contain substances that increase your heart rate.

• Stop using nonprescription medications (such as cough and cold remedies, nose drops, or allergy relief medications that contain phenylpropanolamine, pseudoephedrine, epinephrine, or ephedrine) that increase your heart rate. Ask your doctor or pharmacist for alternatives.

• If stress affects your heart rhythm or rate, try relaxation exercises and deep breathing techniques. See page 344. A healthy exercise program can also help reduce stress.

Home Treatment

• Take deep breaths and try to relax. This may slow a racing heart.

• If you start to feel lightheaded (like you might pass out), lie down to avoid injuries that might result if you pass out and fall down.

• Keep a record of the date and time; your pulse; your activities when the irregular heartbeat happened; how long the irregular beats lasted; how many "skipped" beats there were; and any other symptoms.

• Follow the prevention guidelines.

When to Call a Health Professional

Call 911 or other emergency services immediately:

• If a rapid or irregular heartbeat occurs with squeezing or crushing chest pain or other symptoms of a heart attack. See page 53.

• If you have signs of a stroke. See page 63.

• If you have an irregular heartbeat and faint or come close to fainting.

Call a health professional:

• If you suddenly experience a very rapid (more than 100 beats per minute) or very slow (less than 50 to 60 beats per minute) heartbeat without obvious cause.

- If you have repeated spells of light-headedness over a few days. Also see Dizziness and Vertigo on page 216.

- If your heart seems to beat irregularly all the time.

- If you think a prescription medication may be causing your irregular heartbeats.

- If you develop new shortness of breath that gets worse with exercise.

Peripheral Vascular Disease

If atherosclerosis (see page 157) develops in the arteries that supply blood to the legs, abdomen, pelvis, or arms, it is called peripheral vascular disease (PVD). The arteries in the legs are affected most often. As the artery is narrowed by atherosclerosis, the leg muscles don't get enough blood.

The main symptom of PVD in the leg is tightness or a squeezing pain in the calf, thigh, or buttock that occurs during exercise, such as walking up a steep hill or a flight of stairs. The pain usually occurs every time you do the same amount of exercise and is relieved by rest. This pain is called intermittent claudication. As PVD worsens, toe, foot, or leg pain may occur when you are resting.

Other signs of PVD include numbness, tingling, or cold skin on the feet or legs, loss of hair on the feet or legs, and irregular toenail growth. Your feet may become pale or blue-black in color. Minor skin injuries, especially on your feet, may turn into large sores that are slow to heal or that become infected easily. In severe cases, foot infections may lead to gangrene, and amputation of your foot or leg may be necessary.

If you have symptoms that you think may be caused by PVD, tell your doctor. If you have PVD, it is likely that you have atherosclerosis in other arteries, such as those that supply blood to your heart or brain. Detecting and treating atherosclerosis in these arteries is important in helping to prevent heart attack and stroke.

 The initial approach to treating peripheral vascular disease is to make lifestyle changes that may prevent or delay the progression of the disease. Treating high blood pressure, controlling high blood sugar levels caused by diabetes, lowering high cholesterol levels, and quitting smoking are all important lifestyle changes you can make.

Medications can also help control PVD risk factors and symptoms. Cholesterol-lowering medications can be used to help reduce the buildup of plaque in the arteries. Other medications may help improve symptoms of leg pain and prevent blood clots from suddenly forming and blocking a blood vessel. If you have severe PVD, you may need angioplasty to open clogged blood vessels or bypass surgery to redirect blood flow to your legs through healthy blood vessels.

Prevention

The best way to prevent peripheral vascular disease is to prevent atherosclerosis. See the prevention guidelines for coronary artery disease starting on page 160.

Home Treatment

Once peripheral vascular disease has been diagnosed, the following home treatment may be useful.

- Quit smoking. Smoking increases your risk for serious health problems related to peripheral vascular disease and makes atherosclerosis worse.

- Become more physically active. Start a walking program (with your doctor's approval). Each day, walk until the pain starts; then rest until it goes away before continuing. Try to walk a little farther each day before resting. Don't try to walk through the pain. The goal is to increase the amount of time you can exercise before the pain starts.

- Take steps to lower your cholesterol levels and blood pressure. If you have diabetes, keep your blood sugar levels within a safe range.

- Take good care of your feet. When your circulation is impaired, even minor injuries can lead to serious infections. See the foot care guidelines in the Diabetes topic on page 176.

- Don't wear shoes that are too tight or that rub your feet. Don't wear socks or stockings that leave elastic band marks on your legs.

When to Call a Health Professional

- If unexplained pain occurs deep in the leg or calf, especially if the leg is also swollen. See Thrombophlebitis on page 170.

- If you suddenly develop pain, cold, or numbness in the lower part of your leg.

- If the skin of one or both of your legs is pale or blue-black.

- If you develop leg pain whenever you walk a certain distance, and the pain goes away when you rest.

- If you have unexplained toe or foot pain when you are resting.

Thrombophlebitis

Thrombophlebitis occurs when a blood clot forms in a vein and the vein becomes inflamed. Thrombophlebitis can occur in any vein, but it is most common in the lower leg veins. A clot may form either in a vein just under the surface of the skin (superficial thrombophlebitis) or in a vein deep in the leg.

Symptoms of superficial thrombophlebitis include pain, tenderness, warmth, and redness along a leg vein. Clots in these veins rarely cause serious problems because they do not travel through the bloodstream.

Symptoms of thrombophlebitis in a deep leg vein include swelling and pain in one leg or a noticeable new difference in the size of one leg. You may also have pain when you walk or flex your foot upward. Deep vein thrombophlebitis is a serious condition because the clot may break loose, travel through the bloodstream to a lung, and cause a **pulmonary embolism**. A pulmonary embolism is a life-threatening situation. Symptoms may include chest pain, shortness of breath, or coughing up blood.

Your risk for thrombophlebitis is increased:

- If you have had surgery, especially if the surgery involved your lower abdomen or legs.

- If you are inactive for long periods of time, such as sitting during a long plane or car ride.

- If you have any major trauma to your legs, such as a broken leg.

- If you have a condition (such as heart disease or cancer) or take a medication (such as estrogen) that increases the likelihood that you will form blood clots.

Superficial thrombophlebitis is often treated with rest and anti-inflammatory medications. Deep vein thrombophlebitis usually requires hospitalization and medical treatment to avoid complications.

Cold Hands and Feet

Many older adults have cold hands and feet. Most often, this is due to reduced blood flow to the hands and feet, which can be caused by inactivity, cold weather, or circulation problems. The following may help:

- Avoid caffeine and nicotine, which can restrict blood flow to your skin.

- Keep indoor temperatures at 65° or higher.

- Wear layers of warm clothing. Wear cotton-blend or wool socks.

- Wear a hat. You lose more heat from your head than from any other part of your body.

- Wear mittens instead of gloves. Mittens are better than gloves for keeping fingers warm.

- Move around. Walking briskly or whirling your arms around like a windmill will get your blood moving and warm you up.

A low level of thyroid hormone may cause cold intolerance (see page 181). Raynaud's phenomenon is a blood vessel disorder that causes your fingers to turn white and feel cold and numb, usually when they are exposed to cold or even cool temperatures. As an attack ends, your fingers may become blue and red and swollen, tingle, and throb with pain. If these symptoms occur often, call your doctor.

Prevention

- Exercise your lower leg muscles to improve circulation. Try this exercise: Point your toes up toward your head so you stretch your calf muscles; then relax. Repeat. This exercise is especially important to do when you are sitting for long periods of time, for example, on long driving trips or airplane flights.

- Get out of bed as soon as possible after you have been ill or had surgery. If you cannot get out of bed, do the leg exercise described previously every hour to keep the blood moving through your legs.

- Quit smoking. This is especially important if you are taking any medications that contain estrogen, such as hormone therapy after menopause.

- Wear elastic stockings. Elastic stockings may help keep the blood from pooling in your lower legs. However, if the elastic stockings do not fit correctly, they can slow blood flow even more and do more harm than good. Ask your doctor or a pharmacist to help you select elastic stockings that fit correctly.

Home Treatment

Superficial thrombophlebitis may be treated at home once it has been diagnosed. If you suspect that you have deep vein thrombophlebitis, call your doctor immediately. Do not rub or massage the painful leg because doing so may cause the clot to come loose and travel through your bloodstream.

- Follow the prevention guidelines.

- Rest with your legs elevated, but be sure to continue your regular activities too. Avoid sitting or standing for long periods of time.

- Take aspirin or another anti-inflammatory medication as your doctor recommends.

- Apply warm, moist compresses to the painful area.

When to Call a Health Professional

Call 911 or emergency services immediately:

- If you have a sudden onset of shortness of breath or chest pain. Chest pain caused by a blood clot in the lung often gets worse when you take a deep breath.

- If you are coughing up blood.

Call your doctor:

- If you have swelling, warmth, or tenderness in the soft tissues of your leg.

- If you have leg pain that gets worse when you stand or walk. This is especially important if there is also swelling or redness in your leg.

Varicose Veins

Varicose veins are twisted, enlarged veins near the surface of the skin. They are most common in the legs and ankles.

Varicose veins develop when the vein walls become weak and stretched and can no longer help move blood against the force of gravity back to the heart. Blood pools in the legs, increasing pressure on the veins and causing them to swell. Varicose veins are more common in people who are overweight or who have to stand for long periods of time. Some women may develop them for the first time during pregnancy. They also run in families.

Varicose veins often cause no symptoms. You may feel aching or fatigue in your legs, especially at the end of the day. You may have minor swelling in your feet and ankles and feel itching over the vein. The blue color of the veins may be visible through your skin.

If varicose veins are more serious, your leg may swell and the skin over the enlarged veins may become stretched and thin. The thin skin can become dry and itchy and may break open easily and bleed heavily. Open sores may form that are slow to heal. The skin on your ankles and lower legs may look brownish because of the pooled blood in your legs.

Some people also have tiny red or blue varicose veins on the surface of the skin. These are often called **spider veins**, because they may resemble a spider's web. Spider veins usually do not cause symptoms.

 In most cases, varicose veins do not require treatment. Home treatment may help slow their progression, relieve symptoms, and prevent complications. Other treatments such as sclerotherapy or surgery may be helpful if your varicose veins are bothersome.

Home Treatment

• Wear supportive elastic stockings (full-length, not knee-highs). For mild symptoms, regular support panty hose may work. For more bothersome symptoms, buy compression stockings at a pharmacy or medical supply store. Your doctor can give you a prescription.

• Avoid tight clothing that limits circulation, such as tight belts, knee-high stockings that leave red marks around your legs, or pants that are tight in the waist and thighs. Tight clothing cuts off circulation and can worsen varicose veins.

• Elevate your legs on a footstool when you are sitting. Avoid crossing your legs at the knee when sitting. Put your feet flat on the floor, or cross your legs at the ankles. At the end of the day, lie down and prop your legs above heart level.

- Don't sit or stand for long periods of time. Get up and walk around often, or sit down and elevate your legs. Contracting the muscles in your legs helps move blood back toward your heart.

- Get regular exercise, such as walking, bicycling, dancing, or swimming. Working your leg muscles helps keep blood from pooling in the legs.

- Maintain a healthy body weight.

When to Call a Health Professional

- If your leg suddenly becomes swollen and painful. You may have a clot in a deep vein, which can be serious and may need prompt attention. See Thrombophlebitis on page 170.

- If the skin over a varicose vein bleeds heavily on its own or after an injury, elevate your leg and apply direct pressure to stop the bleeding. See Stopping Severe Bleeding on page 44. If you are unable to slow or stop the bleeding with direct pressure, call your doctor.

- If you develop an open sore on your leg or foot.

- If a tender lump appears on your leg with no apparent cause (you have not bumped or bruised your leg).

"Yes, I am an old enemy of the human race,
but I am not that unbeatable once my name is said,"
spoke the Pale Stranger.
From a Native American story about diabetes
by John McLeod

9

Diabetes and Thyroid Problems

Your endocrine system is your body's control system. The glands that make up the endocrine system include the pituitary, thyroid and parathyroids, pancreas, adrenals, and the ovaries or testes. Each gland releases special hormones—chemical messengers that travel to other parts of your body and help your body's organs do their jobs.

This chapter focuses on two common endocrine disorders: diabetes and thyroid problems. Successful management of diabetes starts with regular exercise and a healthy diet. In most cases, medications are needed to help control diabetes. Most thyroid problems respond well to medications. By following good health practices and getting early detection screening, you can help your endocrine system function at its best.

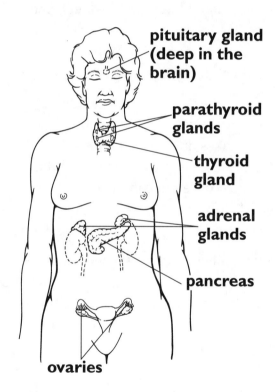

pituitary gland (deep in the brain)

parathyroid glands

thyroid gland

adrenal glands

pancreas

ovaries

Endocrine system (women). In men, the endocrine system includes the testes.

Diabetes

During digestion, the starches and sugars in food are converted to glucose, a sugar that your body uses for energy. The pancreas produces a hormone called insulin that helps glucose enter the body's cells. If the pancreas does not produce enough insulin or the body does not use insulin properly, glucose cannot get into the cells, and too much glucose stays in the blood. This is what happens when a person has diabetes. Over a long period of time, high blood glucose levels may damage blood vessels and nerves and increase a person's risk for problems that can affect the eyes, heart, kidneys, legs, and feet.

Type 1 diabetes occurs when the pancreas makes little or no insulin. Type 1 diabetes usually develops in childhood or adolescence but can develop at any age. People with type 1 diabetes must give themselves insulin shots every day.

Type 2 diabetes occurs when the pancreas cannot make enough insulin to meet the body's needs or when the body does not use insulin properly. Many people who have type 2 diabetes are able to control their blood glucose levels by managing their weight, exercising regularly, eating a healthy diet, and frequently testing their blood glucose levels. Some people may need to take oral medications or give themselves insulin shots to keep their blood glucose levels within a safe range.

Risk factors for type 2 diabetes include:

- Having a family history of type 2 diabetes.
- Being age 45 or over.
- Being overweight (20 percent or more over your healthy weight) or having a large percentage of body fat in the abdominal area.
- Having a physically inactive lifestyle.
- Having high blood pressure (above 140/90).
- Having an HDL cholesterol level below 40 or triglycerides above 250.
- Being of African-American, Hispanic, Asian, Pacific Island, or Native American descent.
- Having a history of diabetes during pregnancy (gestational diabetes) or having given birth to a baby over 9 pounds.
- Having prediabetes (blood sugar levels above normal, but not as high as diabetic levels).

The symptoms of diabetes vary from person to person and are common to many conditions. You may believe that your symptoms are caused by an illness or aging, not diabetes. Symptoms include:

- Dry mouth and increased thirst.
- Frequent urination (especially at night).
- Increased appetite.
- Unexplained weight loss.
- Weakness, tiredness, and dizziness.

• Frequent skin infections and slow-healing wounds.

• Recurrent vaginal infections.

• Blurry vision.

• Tingling or numbness in the hands or feet.

Your doctor needs to do a blood test to accurately diagnose diabetes.

Complications of Diabetes

Complications of diabetes are caused by the prolonged exposure of the body to high blood glucose levels. Some people develop complications early in the course of the disease; others develop them later. A person who develops complications of diabetes may have only one problem or several. By carefully controlling your blood glucose levels early in the course of the disease and practicing other healthy habits, you may reduce your risk of the following complications of diabetes:

• Heart disease and problems with circulation in the feet and legs (peripheral vascular disease)

• High blood pressure

• Stroke

• Nerve damage (neuropathy), which can decrease or completely block the movement of nerve impulses or messages through organs, limbs, and other parts of the body

• Impaired ability to fight infection and heal wounds

• Foot ulcers and other foot problems

• Joint and connective tissue disease

• Kidney disease (nephropathy)

• Eye disease (retinopathy) and other eye problems

• Gum disease

Prevention

At this time, there is no known way to prevent type 1 diabetes.

The risk for developing type 2 diabetes runs in families and increases with age. However, even if you have a history of type 2 diabetes in your family, you may be able to delay or prevent its onset by maintaining a healthy body weight and exercising regularly. If you are at risk for type 2 diabetes, talk to your doctor about taking metformin to reduce your likelihood of developing diabetes.

Home Treatment

Self-care for both type 1 and type 2 diabetes includes the following:

• **Take your medications as prescribed.** If your doctor has prescribed insulin or other medications to keep your blood glucose level within a safe range, take them as directed. If you improve your diet and exercise regularly, you may need less medicine. Check with your doctor before making any changes in your medication dosing schedule.

Diabetic Emergencies

	Low Blood Glucose (Hypoglycemia)	High Blood Glucose (Hyperglycemia)
Who can be affected?	Those who inject insulin or take certain oral hypoglycemic medications	Any person who has diabetes
How does it occur?	Rapidly, over minutes or hours	Gradually, over hours or days
Blood glucose range?	Less than 60 mg/dL*	More than 200 mg/dL*
Symptoms?	Fatigue, shakiness Headache Hunger Cold, clammy skin; sweating Sudden double vision or blurred vision Pounding heart, confusion, irritability; person may appear drunk Loss of consciousness	Frequent urination Intense thirst Dry skin Blurred vision Signs of ketoacidosis: rapid breathing with fruity-smelling breath Loss of consciousness
What to do?	If the person loses consciousness, **call 911 or other emergency services**. For other symptoms, have the person eat or drink something that contains sugar. If symptoms don't improve, call the doctor immediately.	If there are signs of ketoacidosis, call the doctor immediately. If the person loses consciousness, **call 911 or other emergency services**.

If you are unsure about the cause of the diabetic emergency in a person who uses medication, put something that contains sugar under the person's tongue (glucose gel, candy, honey or sugar dissolved in water, fruit juice, or a soft drink with sugar). Do not give an unconscious person anything to eat or drink. If you have been taught how to give glucagon to a person who is having a diabetic emergency, do so. Always make sure the glucagon kit has not expired.

May vary for individual people. If you have diabetes, ask your doctor what your safe blood glucose range is.

- **Eat a healthy diet.** A proper diet can help keep your blood glucose levels within a safe range. If you have type 2 diabetes, a good diet will also help you control your weight and help your body use insulin better. By improving your diet you may reduce your need for pills or insulin injections. See the Nutrition chapter starting on page 301 for basic guidelines on healthy food choices. In general, a person with diabetes needs to:

  - Eat less fat.

  - Eat more high-fiber foods such as whole-grain breads, vegetables, and fruit.

  - Use less salt.

  - Limit alcohol intake to no more than 1 to 2 drinks per day.

  - Avoid eating a lot of food at one meal, because eating too much at once overloads the blood with glucose. A person with diabetes should spread his or her calories over 4 to 6 meals.

- **Exercise regularly.** Regular aerobic exercise can help you keep your blood glucose level within a normal range, control your weight, and reduce your risk for heart disease. Before starting an exercise program, talk with your doctor. You will need to learn how exercise affects your blood glucose levels. Exercise tends to reduce blood glucose because the body can take more glucose into the cells and use it. (However, some people may have a rise in blood glucose during, or after, exercise.) If you take medicine to control your blood glucose levels, carry some type of carbohydrate, such as a granola bar, with you when you exercise. Learn the symptoms of low blood glucose (see page 178). Check back with your doctor whenever you increase your level of exercise. Your medication may need to be adjusted.

- **Check your blood glucose levels as often as your doctor has recommended.** Your doctor will probably tell you to measure your blood glucose levels at different times of the day. Keep a record of those measurements. It will help you and your doctor understand how your body reacts to different foods and to exercise, so you can decide on a treatment plan that will help keep your blood glucose level within a safe range. Keeping a daily record of the following things may make it easier for you to keep your blood sugar level within a safe range:

  - What you eat and when you eat it.

  - What kind of exercise you get and how long you do it.

  - How tired or energetic you feel.

  - What symptoms you have when your blood sugar is high or low (so that you can learn to recognize these states).

- **Talk to your doctor about taking a low-dose aspirin every day.** This may help prevent heart attack, stroke, and other large blood vessel disease.

- **Take care of your feet.** Diabetes can damage nerves and reduce blood flow to your feet. You may lose feeling in your feet, which can make it hard to notice when you have a small cut or injury. Small cuts, sores, and ingrown toenails can take longer to heal and may become infected. If you have a wound on your foot that won't heal or looks infected, see When to Call a Health Professional on page 181.

- Don't go barefoot, even indoors.

- Wash your feet daily with warm water and mild soap. Pay special attention to any cuts, cracking, or peeling between your toes or on the bottoms of your feet. Dry your feet well.

- Avoid putting strong chemicals, such as Epsom salts, iodine, and corn removers, on your feet. Do not do "bathroom surgery," such as trimming dead skin with nail scissors.

- Use a moisturizer to keep the skin on your feet soft. Do not put moisturizer between your toes.

- Cut and file your toenails straight across to avoid ingrown toenails.

- Break in new shoes slowly to avoid blisters.

- Have your doctor check your feet during each visit.

• **Stop smoking.** Smoking contributes to blood vessel damage that can lead to heart disease and circulation problems.

• **Have regular medical checkups.** Talk to your doctor about how often you need them. Diabetes requires lifelong care.

• **Have an eye exam every year.** Eye changes caused by diabetes often have no symptoms until they are quite advanced. Diabetic retinopathy is one form of diabetic eye disease that can cause blindness. Early detection and treatment of diabetic retinopathy may slow its progress and save your sight.

• **Join a support group.** Diabetes support groups can add a lot to your home treatment. These groups include supportive health professionals and people who have diabetes. Support groups are often offered at no charge and are excellent sources for the information you will need to help you manage your diabetes. Your local hospital may have information about diabetes support groups and other educational programs available in your community.

• **Wear medical identification at all times.** In an emergency, medical identification lets people know you have diabetes so they can give you appropriate care. Medical identification bracelets and necklaces are available at most pharmacies.

 Believe that you can live a healthy life with diabetes. Controlling diabetes requires making significant, long-term lifestyle changes that may seem overwhelming at first. However, if you adopt a "take charge" attitude about your health and focus on making one change at a time, you are more likely to be successful. Work with your doctor to develop a treatment plan that fits your needs.

MORE INFO ™ **For more information, see the back cover.**

The National Diabetes Information Clearinghouse is a good resource for more information about diabetes management. Contact them at 1 Information Way, Bethesda, MD 20892-3560.

When to Call a Health Professional

Call 911 or other emergency services if you develop signs of extreme high or low blood glucose (see page 178).

Call your health professional:

- If you develop signs of ketoacidosis (rapid breathing, fruity-smelling breath). See page 178.

- If signs of very low blood glucose do not go away after you eat or drink something that contains sugar or give yourself a glucagon shot. (Make sure your glucagon kit has not expired.)

- If there are signs of major changes in your normal blood glucose levels. Such signs include:

  - Unexplained changes in the results of your home blood glucose tests.

  - Changes in your mental functioning, such as confusion, drowsiness, or agitation.

- If you are sick for longer than 2 days (unless it is a mild illness, like a cold) or:

  - You have been vomiting or have had diarrhea for more than 6 hours.

  - You believe symptoms, such as extreme thirst and weakness, are caused by high blood glucose.

  - Your blood glucose levels are consistently greater than 250 mg/dL.

- If you notice any symptoms of long-term complications of diabetes, including:

  - Burning pain, numbness, or swelling in your feet or hands.

  - Dizziness or weakness when you sit up or stand up suddenly.

  - Vision problems, such as seeing flashing lights; large, floating red or black spots; or things that look like floating hair or spider webs.

  - A wound that won't heal or that looks infected. See Signs of a Wound Infection on page 59.

- If you suspect that you have diabetes but have not been diagnosed. See symptoms on pages 176 to 177.

Thyroid Problems

The thyroid is a butterfly-shaped gland that wraps around the windpipe. It functions as a kind of "throttle" for the body, regulating your metabolism. As the thyroid gland releases more hormones, the body runs faster. As thyroid hormone levels decrease, the body slows down. The pituitary gland in the brain controls the thyroid and usually keeps the level of thyroid hormones fairly constant. The pituitary gland is in turn controlled by the hypothalamus, another area of the brain.

Thyroid problems are common among older people. However, the symptoms may develop so slowly that they go unnoticed, or you may dismiss them as part of "normal aging."

 Thyroid hormone tests can detect changes in the amount of thyroid hormone in your body, even before you have noticed symptoms. If you have a family history of thyroid problems or have been exposed to radiation, either at work or as part of medical treatment, ask your doctor whether you need a thyroid test.

The thyroid gland can cause problems in two ways: by producing too much thyroid hormone or by producing too little of it. Symptoms of too much thyroid hormone, or **hyperthyroidism**, include:

- Weight loss with or without loss of appetite.

- Increased discomfort in warm temperatures.

- Soft stools or diarrhea.

- Itchy, irritated, and puffy eyes.

- Hair loss.

- Rapid , pounding, or irregular heart rhythm.

- Shortness of breath, even when resting.

- Night sweats.

- Difficulty sleeping.

- Chronic fatigue and lack of energy.

- Progressive muscle weakness, especially in the large muscles of the legs.

- Difficulty concentrating, mood swings, or nervousness.

- An enlarged thyroid gland, or goiter, which looks like a swollen area in the throat.

These symptoms are often confused with those caused by other diseases. Graves' disease, the most common cause of hyperthyroidism, occurs when the immune system makes the thyroid gland overactive. When drug treatment for hyperthyroidism is complete, thyroid function may return to normal. However, some people require radioactive iodine treatment to destroy part of the thyroid gland in order to cure hyperthyroidism. In rare cases, surgery to remove part or all of the thyroid gland may be necessary.

Symptoms of too little thyroid hormone, or **hypothyroidism**, include:

- Chronic fatigue, sluggishness, and weakness.

- Memory loss, difficulty concentrating, or depression.

- Inability to tolerate cold temperatures.

- Dry skin, brittle nails, and dry, coarse hair; hair loss.

- Constipation.

- Unexplained weight gain.

- Slowed heartbeat and reflexes.

- An enlarged thyroid gland, or goiter.

- Swelling of the arms, hands, legs, and feet, and facial puffiness, particularly around the eyes.

- Hoarseness.

Treatment of hypothyroidism is quite simple. Your doctor can prescribe a medication that acts like natural thyroid hormone in your body. You will probably have to take the medication for the rest of your life. You will need regular blood tests (usually once a year) to make sure your medication does not need to be adjusted.

Home Treatment

If you have a prescription for daily thyroid medications, take them every day.

When to Call a Health Professional

- If a person with **hyperthyroidism** develops any of the following symptoms:

  - Fever.

  - Extreme weakness or fatigue.

  - Rapid or irregular heartbeat.

  - Heavy sweating or inability to tolerate warm temperatures.

  - Restlessness, agitation, or delirium.

  - Abnormally high or low blood pressure.

  - Unexpected weight loss.

- If the following symptoms develop and persist, especially in a person who has been diagnosed with **hypothyroidism**:

  - Extreme intolerance of cold temperatures.

  - Weakness and fatigue.

  - Dry skin, brittle nails, or hair loss.

  - Constipation.

  - Memory problems, depression, or difficulty concentrating.

- If you suspect that you have a thyroid function problem.

- If you have a family history of thyroid problems or a history of radiation exposure, especially in the head or neck area.

*I'm very brave generally,
only today I happen to have a headache.*
Tweedledum in "Alice in Wonderland"

10

Headaches

Headaches are one of the most common health complaints. Some possible causes of headaches include muscle tension, eyestrain, arthritis, infections, allergies, injuries, hunger, changes in the flow of blood in the vessels of the head, and exposure to chemicals.

Most headaches are caused by tension and respond well to prevention and home treatment. See Tension Headaches on page 189. If a headache is caused by a serious illness, other symptoms may be present, such as vomiting, dizziness, a stiff neck, or changes in vision. A sudden, severe headache that is very different from any you have had before, or a change in the usual pattern of your headaches, is a cause for concern. See Headache Emergencies on page 187.

Headaches that routinely develop during or after physical exertion, sexual activity, coughing, or sneezing may be a sign of a more serious illness and should be discussed with a health professional.

Migraine Headaches

Migraine headaches are severe, usually one-sided headaches that often occur with nausea, vomiting, and extreme sensitivity to light or sound. People often describe migraine headaches as throbbing or piercing. The pain may range from mild to terribly severe.

Although migraine headaches are usually one-sided, there may be pain on both sides of the head. In some people, the pain may switch sides each time they have a migraine.

Migraine headaches sometimes occur with an aura, a group of symptoms that usually develop 5 to 30 minutes before a migraine begins. Visual disturbances, such as flashing lights, distortion in the size or shape of objects, or blind or dark spots in your field of vision, are the most common symptoms of an aura. An aura may also include symptoms that affect

185

Possible Headache Causes

If headache occurs:	Possible causes include:
Suddenly and is severe	Stroke, p. 63. Call a health professional immediately.
On awakening	Tension Headaches, p. 189; Migraine Headaches, p. 185; Allergies, p. 131; Sinusitis, p. 152; Neck Pain, p. 106; Sleep apnea, p. 333; TM Disorder, p. 232. May also be caused by low humidity.
With severe eye pain or vision disturbances	Temporal arteritis (p. 191) or closed-angle glaucoma (p. 209). Call a health professional immediately.
In jaw muscles or in both temples (may occur on awakening)	Tension Headaches, p. 189; TM Disorder, p. 232.
Each afternoon or evening; after hours of desk work; following a stressful event; with sore neck and shoulders	Tension Headaches, p. 189; Neck Pain, p. 106.
On one side of the head with visual disturbances or runny nose	Migraine Headaches, p. 185; Cluster Headaches, p. 190; Trigeminal neuralgia, p. 191.
After a blow to the head	Head Injuries, p. 51.
After exposure to chemicals (paint, varnish, insect spray, cigarette smoke)	Chemical headache. Get into fresh air. Drink water to flush poisons.
With fever, runny nose, or sore throat	Flu, p. 147; Sore Throat, p. 153; Colds, p. 141; Sinusitis, p. 152.
With fever, stiff neck, nausea, and vomiting	Encephalitis and Meningitis, p. 189.
With runny nose, watery eyes, and sneezing	Allergies, p. 131; Cluster Headaches, p. 190.
With fever and pain in the cheekbones or over the eyes	Sinusitis, p. 152.
On mornings when you drink less caffeine than usual	Caffeine withdrawal headache, p. 190.
After you start taking a new medication	Drug allergy. Call your doctor.

the nervous system, such as numbness or tingling in the face or arm, strange smells or strange sounds, or weakness on one side of your body. Some people have more vague symptoms, such as hunger, excessive thirst, or changes in mood or energy level, that appear 1 to 2 days before the headache develops.

The frequency of migraine attacks varies from person to person. Some people may have only a few migraines in their lifetime, while others have a migraine every few weeks or months. Migraine headaches usually last for 4 to 24 hours. Some migraine sufferers have attacks that last up to 3 days.

Migraines are more common in women than in men and are often associated with a woman's menstrual periods. The frequency of migraines may increase or decrease during pregnancy or at menopause. Hormone replacement therapy may make migraines worse.

People rarely start getting migraines after age 40. However, if you had migraine headaches before age 40, you may continue to get them after age 40, and they may continue to occur well into old age, especially in men. In general, however, migraines become less frequent and less severe as you age. Tell your doctor about any new and different headaches you develop.

Headache Emergencies

Call your doctor now if you have:

- A very sudden "thunderclap" headache.

- A sudden, severe headache unlike any you have had before.

- Headache with a stiff neck, fever, nausea, vomiting, drowsiness, or confusion.

- A sudden, severe headache and a stiff neck that develops soon after the headache starts.

- A different, severe headache that occurs with strenuous physical activity or sexual activity.

- Headache with weakness, paralysis, numbness, visual disturbances, slurred speech, confusion, or behavior changes.

- Headaches following a recent fall or blow to the head. See page 51 for information about head injuries.

- Headache with severe eye pain.

Prevention

- Keep a diary of your headache symptoms. See Tracking Your Headaches on page 188. Once you know what events, foods, medications, or activities bring on your headaches, you may be able to prevent or limit their recurrence.

- Do what you can to manage stress. See Stress on page 342 for tips.

Home Treatment

- At the first sign of a headache, try to go to a quiet, dark place to relax. Sleeping can relieve migraines.

- Some people find that taking a pain reliever such as aspirin, acetaminophen, or ibuprofen at the first sign of a headache brings relief. However, frequent use of pain relievers can cause rebound headaches, which are headaches that return as the effects of the pain relievers wear off.

- Apply a cold pack to the painful area, or put a cool cloth on your forehead. Do not apply heat, since it may make a migraine worse.

- Have someone gently massage your neck and shoulder muscles, or give yourself a massage.

- Practice a relaxation technique such as progressive muscle relaxation or roll breathing. See pages 344 and 345.

- If a doctor has prescribed medication for your migraines, take the recommended dose at the first sign that a migraine is starting.

When to Call a Health Professional

- If you suspect that your headaches are migraines.

- If your headaches are becoming more frequent or more severe.

- Also see Headache Emergencies on page 187.

Tracking Your Headaches

If you have recurring headaches, keep a record of your symptoms. This record will help your doctor if medical evaluation is needed. Write down:

1. The date and time each headache starts and stops.

2. Any factors that seem to trigger the headache, such as food, smoke, bright light, stress, or activity.

3. The location and nature of the pain: throbbing, aching, stabbing, dull.

4. The severity of the pain.

5. Other physical symptoms, such as nausea, vomiting, visual disturbances, or sensitivity to light or noise.

6. If you are a woman, note any association between headaches and your menstrual cycle or use of hormone replacement therapy.

 Professional diagnosis and treatment, combined with your self-care, can help decrease the impact of migraines on your life. Discuss relaxation and biofeedback techniques with your doctor. They help many people prevent migraines. If non-drug treatments are not effective, there are many new prescription drugs available that can reduce the severity of migraines or eliminate migraines altogether.

Encephalitis and Meningitis

Encephalitis is an inflammation of the brain that may occur following a viral infection such as the flu. Mosquitoes and ticks spread encephalitis in some parts of the world, including the United States.

Meningitis is a viral or bacterial infection that causes inflammation in the tissues that surround the brain and spinal cord. It may follow an infection, such as an ear or sinus infection, or a viral or bacterial illness.

Encephalitis and meningitis are serious illnesses with similar symptoms. Call a health professional immediately if you develop the following symptoms, especially after a viral illness or after you have been bitten by mosquitoes:

- Severe headache with stiff neck, fever, nausea, and vomiting

- Drowsiness, lack of energy, confusion, memory problems, or unusual behavior

Tension Headaches

Most headaches are tension headaches, which become more frequent and severe during times of emotional or physical stress. Having arthritis in your neck, a previous neck injury, or a habit of clenching your jaw muscles can also cause tension headaches.

A tension headache may cause pain or a pressure sensation all over your head or a feeling like there is a tight band around your head. Your head may feel like it is in a vise. Some people feel a dull, pressing, burning sensation above their eyes. The tightness and pain may also affect the muscles in your jaws, face, neck, shoulders, and upper back. You can rarely pinpoint the center or source of the pain.

Prevention

- Reduce emotional stress. Take time to relax before and after you do activities that have caused headaches in the past. Try the progressive muscle relaxation or roll breathing techniques on pages 344 and 345.

- Reduce physical stress. When sitting at a desk, change positions often, and stretch for 30 seconds each hour. Make a conscious effort to relax your jaw, neck, shoulder, and upper back muscles.

- Evaluate your neck and shoulder posture at work or at home, and make adjustments if needed. See Neck Pain on page 106.

- Exercise daily. Regular exercise can help relieve tension and stress.

- If muscle tension seems to be related to teeth clenching, try a relaxation technique. See page 344.

- Treat yourself to a massage. Some people find regular massages very helpful in relieving tension. See page 354.

- Limit your caffeine intake to 1 to 2 caffeinated beverages per day. People who consume a lot of caffeine often develop a headache several hours after they have their last caffeinated beverage or may wake with a headache that can be relieved by drinking a caffeinated beverage. Cut down slowly to avoid caffeine-withdrawal headaches.

Home Treatment

- Stop whatever you are doing, and sit quietly for a moment. Close your eyes, and inhale and exhale slowly. Try to relax your head and neck muscles.

- Take a stretch break or try a relaxation technique. See page 344.

- Gently and firmly massage your neck muscles. See the neck exercises on page 107.

- Use a heating pad, a hot water bottle, or warm water from a shower to apply heat to the painful area.

- Lie down in a dark room with a cool cloth on your forehead.

- Taking aspirin, acetaminophen, or ibuprofen often helps relieve a tension headache. However, using non-prescription or prescription headache medications too often may make headaches more frequent or severe when the medication wears off.

Cluster Headaches

Cluster headaches are sudden, very severe, sharp, stabbing headaches that occur on one side of the head, usually in the temple or behind the eye. They are much more common in men than in women.

During a cluster headache, the eye and nostril on the affected side may be runny, and the eye may also be red. The pain often begins at night and may last from a few minutes to a few hours.

Cluster headaches occur in periods of time called cluster periods, which may last days or months and then disappear for months or even years. During a cluster period, a person may have headaches several times a day. To prevent headaches during a cluster period, avoid alcohol and tobacco products, maintain a regular sleep schedule, and try to reduce your overall stress level.

See your doctor if you think you have cluster headaches or if you have persistent, severe headaches with no apparent cause. Also see Headache Emergencies on page 187.

When to Call a Health Professional

- If a headache is very severe and cannot be relieved with home treatment. This could be a sign of a serious health problem, such as a stroke, and may require immediate treatment.

- If a headache occurs with fever of 103° or higher (100° in a person who is very old or in frail health) and no other symptoms.

- If unexplained headaches continue to occur more than 3 times a week.

- If headaches become more frequent and severe.

- If headaches occur during or after physical exertion, sexual activity, coughing, or sneezing.

- If headaches awaken you from a sound sleep or are worse first thing in the morning.

- If you need help discovering or eliminating the source of your tension headaches.

- If your headaches last for long periods of time and significantly affect your quality of life or your ability to do daily activities.

Also see Headache Emergencies on page 187.

Other Causes of Head or Facial Pain

Headaches are not the only causes of head and facial pain. Other causes include sinus infections (page 152), shingles (page 246), and temporomandibular disorder (page 232).

Temporal arteritis is an inflammation of the artery in the temple. It also may affect a nerve in the eye and can cause vision problems or blindness if it is not treated promptly. Temporal arteritis most commonly affects people over age 50. Call your doctor immediately if you have a new or different headache in one or both temples, especially if you have any vision loss.

Trigeminal neuralgia (tic douloureux) is a painful condition caused by pressure on the trigeminal nerve, which is located in front of the ear. Symptoms include attacks of stabbing or electric shocklike pain on one side of the face, usually around the mouth, upper jaw, and the side of the nose. The pain may occur for no apparent reason, or it may occur when the side of the face or the mouth is touched or when the face is exposed to extreme heat or cold. The pain usually lasts for just a few seconds or minutes.

Medications or, in some cases, surgery may be used to control the pain of trigeminal neuralgia. Progressive muscle relaxation may help relieve the pain and anxiety caused by the condition. See page 345.

If the brain was simple enough for us to understand it,
we would be too simple to understand it.
Ken Hill

11

Nervous System Problems

It's a myth that getting old means getting senile. Most people retain their mental vitality as they age, though some changes do occur. (For more information about memory changes with aging, see Memory Loss on page 331.) A number of conditions can affect mental functioning, including medication side effects, depression, infections, or heavy alcohol intake. Treating such conditions sometimes clears up the problem with mental functioning. Other illnesses, such as Alzheimer's disease, may cause a progressive decline in mental functioning that cannot be reversed or cured.

This chapter provides some basic information about conditions that affect the nervous system: delirium, dementia, Alzheimer's disease, Parkinson's disease, and tremor. Some of these illnesses respond well to treatment. Some, like dementia and Alzheimer's disease, can be managed but not cured.

This chapter will help you better understand some common nervous system problems that can occur as you get older, so that you can seek care for yourself or someone else if serious symptoms develop.

Alzheimer's Disease

Alzheimer's disease is a condition that damages parts of the brain involved in memory, intelligence, judgment, language, and behavior. It is the most common cause of mental decline (dementia) in older adults. Alzheimer's disease usually starts with mild memory loss and progresses over a few years to severe mental and functional problems and, eventually, death. There is currently no cure for Alzheimer's disease, but there are medications that may temporarily improve some of the thinking and memory problems that it causes.

Alzheimer's disease usually develops very slowly. If confusion and other changes in mental abilities come on suddenly, the problem may be delirium. See page 195. During the first few years, the only symptoms of Alzheimer's disease may be memory loss for recent events and occasional disorientation or confusion.

It may be difficult to distinguish the earliest symptoms of Alzheimer's disease from normal changes in the speed of memory recall that may occur with aging. However, the memory changes associated with Alzheimer's disease are very different from typical age-related memory changes.

Normal forgetfulness:

• Forgetting parts of an experience

• Forgetting where the car is parked

• Forgetting events from the distant past

• Forgetting names, remembering them later

Memory loss caused by Alzheimer's disease:

• Forgetting an entire experience

• Forgetting how to drive the car

• Forgetting recent events

• Forgetting ever having known a person

There are no definitive tests to identify the early stages of Alzheimer's disease. Alzheimer's disease is diagnosed only after other causes of dementia have been ruled out.

As Alzheimer's disease progresses, memory loss worsens and language skills and judgment become impaired. During the later stages of the disease, a person may have difficulty doing routine activities such as bathing, dressing, and eating. In the final stage of the disease, a person may become completely dependent upon others for assistance with everyday activities.

Prevention

Medical science is getting closer to finding the cause of Alzheimer's disease. However, at this time, prevention guidelines are limited. Do your best to stay physically healthy and mentally active.

Recent research suggests that some common drugs may lower the risk of Alzheimer's disease or delay its onset. These drugs include vitamin E and nonsteroidal anti-inflammatory drugs (NSAIDs) such as aspirin or ibuprofen. More research on the possible preventive use of these medications is needed before they can be recommended. None of these substances have been proven to prevent Alzheimer's disease.

Home Treatment

Most people with Alzheimer's disease are cared for at home by family and friends. The home treatment guidelines for Alzheimer's disease are the same as those for dementia on page 199.

For more information, contact the Alzheimer's Association, 919 N. Michigan Ave., Suite 1100, Chicago, IL 60611-1676, 1-800-272-3900.

Being a caregiver for someone with Alzheimer's is not easy, no matter how much you know about the disease and how committed you are to taking care of the person. As the disease progresses, caring for the person at home usually becomes more and more difficult. The decision to place your family member in a nursing home or other facility can be a very difficult one, but sometimes nursing home placement is the best thing to do.

 Getting all the facts and thinking about your own needs and values, as well as those of the person you are caring for, will help you make a wise decision about whether to place your loved one in a nursing home.

When to Call a Health Professional

- If symptoms such as a shortened attention span, memory problems, or seeing or hearing things that aren't really there (hallucinations) develop suddenly over hours to days. See Delirium on page 195.

- If a person who has Alzheimer's disease has a sudden, significant change in behavior, or if symptoms suddenly become worse. See Delirium on page 195.

- If symptoms such as a shortened attention span, memory problems, or false beliefs (delusions) develop gradually over a few weeks or months.

- If memory loss and other symptoms begin to interfere with work, hobbies, or friendships, or could result in injury or harm.

- If you need help caring for a person with Alzheimer's disease.

Delirium

Delirium is a sudden change in a person's mental functioning that leads to confusion and unusual behavior. It is a sign that a health problem is becoming more serious.

Unlike dementia (see page 196), which comes on slowly over several months, symptoms of delirium usually develop over the course of a few hours to a few days. Symptoms of delirium may include:

- Disorganized thinking, disorientation, and confusion, all of which may cause the person's speech to ramble or make no sense. The person may see or hear things that aren't really there (hallucinations) or imagine people or things to be what they are not (illusions).

- An unusually short attention span; the person may be easily distracted or have difficulty shifting his or her attention to something new.

- A disrupted sleep-wake cycle, which may cause daytime sleepiness and nighttime wakefulness.

- Fluctuations between periods when the person is very active and when he or she is very sleepy or hard to keep awake.

- Agitation and, in some cases, violent behavior.

- Seizures.

Symptoms of delirium may come and go. A person may be alert and coherent one minute, confused and drowsy the next. Delirium requires immediate medical attention so that the underlying cause can be detected and treated.

Many things can cause delirium, including:

- Certain medications, taking too large a dose of a medication, or sudden withdrawal of certain medications.

- Having an infection, such as pneumonia, flu, a urinary tract infection, meningitis, or encephalitis.

- Going through a major change in your daily routine, such as being ill and having to stay in the hospital.

- Drinking a lot of alcohol or sudden withdrawal from regular use of alcohol.

- Worsening of a chronic disease such as emphysema, heart disease, diabetes, or a thyroid disorder.

If a person can recover from the underlying condition that is causing delirium, the symptoms of delirium will usually go away.

When to Call a Health Professional

Call 911 or other emergency services if a person has had a sudden change in mental functioning and you suspect that he or she is delirious.

You can give the health professionals who respond to your call information that may help reveal the cause of delirium. Tell them:

- Whether the person has a chronic disease, such as diabetes, heart disease, lung disease, or anemia.

- What prescription and nonprescription medications the person has taken, and the doses.

- Whether the person has a fever or has been ill or hospitalized recently.

- If the person has been drinking alcohol, and how much.

- If the person recently suffered an injury.

Dementia

Dementia is a term used to describe a condition of persistent and progressive mental decline. Dementia involves memory, problem solving, learning, and other mental functions. The mental changes associated with dementia usually come on slowly over months. Little change is noticed day to day, although many people with dementia seem better or worse at different times of the day. Over time, the mental impairment becomes severe enough to interfere with daily activities.

> ## What About Ginkgo Biloba?
>
> Ginkgo extract, from the leaves of the *Ginkgo biloba* tree, has been used for thousands of years in traditional Chinese medicine. Although the benefits of ginkgo are not clearly understood, it has been used to treat a variety of health conditions, such as blood clots, Raynaud's phenomenon, and peripheral vascular disease; dementia; memory and concentration problems; and anxiety, stress, and other mood problems.
>
> Be sure to tell your doctor if you are taking ginkgo. Ginkgo appears to be safe and has few side effects. However, it is not recommended for people who are taking extremely high doses of vitamin E or medications that thin the blood (anticoagulants), such as warfarin or aspirin. This is because ginkgo also thins the blood and may reduce the blood's ability to clot. The combined effect of the medications may be harmful.

The general symptoms of dementia include:

- Short-term memory loss (more than just an occasional forgetting of appointments, names, or where things were put). A person may remember events from 20 years ago but may not remember what happened 2 hours ago.

- Inability to complete everyday tasks, such as making soup from a can.

- Confusion.

- Impaired judgment, such as walking into traffic.

- Getting lost in familiar places.

- Suspicion of others (paranoia); strange behavior.

If confusion and other changes in mental abilities come on suddenly, the problem may be delirium, not dementia. See Delirium on page 195.

There are more than 100 separate health conditions that can cause or mimic dementia. For some causes of dementia, such as Alzheimer's disease, no effective treatment is currently available. However, in some cases, if the underlying problem can be successfully managed, dementia symptoms may be reversible. Depression, for example, is a common problem in older adults, and its symptoms are often confused with signs of dementia. Treatment for depression is often effective in reversing dementia-like symptoms.

In about 20 percent of cases, dementia is caused by repeated strokes or blockages of blood vessels in the brain. This is called **multi-infarct dementia** or vascular dementia. People with untreated diabetes or high blood pressure are at increased risk for multi-infarct dementia. The symptoms vary depending on which area of the brain is affected. Unlike Alzheimer's disease, which develops and worsens slowly, multi-infarct dementia usually develops suddenly and gets worse in distinct phases. Symptoms develop in stages, with some improvement between major declines in functioning. The prevention tips for Stroke (see page 64) may help prevent this type of dementia or slow its progress.

Other common causes of dementia include:

- Parkinson's disease (see page 201), especially in its later stages.

- Hypothyroidism (see page 181).

- Deficiency in vitamin B_1 (thiamine), vitamin B_{12}, or folic acid.

- Reactions to medications.

- Long-term, heavy alcohol intake.

- Chronic infections of the brain.

Early Symptoms of Dementia

Early symptoms of mental impairment can include the following:

Personality changes

- A usually social person becomes withdrawn.

- A person has unusual or wild mood swings.

Behavior changes

- A normally tidy person becomes messy.

- A person stops previous routines for no obvious reason.

Skill changes

- Loss of skill in balancing a checkbook

- Loss of skill in shaving or putting on makeup

- Loss of skill in cooking a favorite recipe

- Inability to find previously familiar places

- Increasing and repeated confusion about times and dates

- Increasing forgetfulness about where items are kept

Don't be overly concerned about minor changes in these areas. However, if the changes are major, unexplained, and causing increasing trouble or getting worse, they can be clues that a more significant problem is developing. A review of the causes of dementia on pages 196 to 198 may help you identify or rule out possible problems. Call a health professional if you suspect dementia.

Distinguishing Between Delirium and Dementia

Delirium and dementia are different. Delirium comes on quickly, over a few hours to days. Dementia develops gradually, often over several months. See pages 195 and 196 for help in understanding the differences between delirium and dementia. People with dementia are more likely to become delirious when they have an acute illness like a cold or the flu. Delirium is a medical emergency. If you suspect that the problem is delirium, call a doctor immediately.

Caring for a Person With Dementia

Most people who have dementia or Alzheimer's disease are cared for at home by relatives and friends.

• Discuss important matters like a will, a living will, and a power of attorney early in the course of the disease when the person's judgment is clearer. See page 362.

• Arrange for respite care. Your need for rest will increase as your loved one's dementia worsens. Taking regular breaks from caregiving will help give you the stamina you need to care for the person as long as possible. Family and friends can help, but explore other options too. See page 372.

• Recognize when placement in a residential care or nursing home becomes appropriate. When home care can no longer be provided safely or without harm to others, consider placement away from home. Ask if the staff is particularly knowledgeable about dementia. Some facilities have special units designed for people who have dementia.

Home Treatment

If you suspect that a person has dementia, it is important that he or she be evaluated by a doctor to rule out any underlying causes that might be treatable. After a diagnosis is made, the following guidelines can be helpful no matter what the cause of the dementia.

• Let the person make decisions about activities, food, clothing, and other choices for as long as he or she is able. However, keep the number of options limited to avoid confusion.

• Reinforce and support the person's efforts to remain independent, even if tasks take more time or aren't done perfectly. When the person needs help, offer it gently and discreetly to protect the person's self-esteem.

• Provide visual cues to time and place: clocks, a current monthly calendar with upcoming holidays highlighted, pictures of the place where the person is living and scenes from the current season.

• Simplify the person's daily routine by establishing regular times for meals, baths, and activities.

• Label often-used rooms and objects.

• Be aware that the person may become more confused and agitated in the early evening. Don't plan complicated activities for that time.

• Create a safe but interesting living environment. See the safety tips starting on page 26 and the prevention guidelines for falls on page 48; add the following:

  - Use locks on doors and cupboards. Lock away knives, scissors, medications, cleaning supplies, and other dangerous objects and substances.

  - If the person may wander outside and become lost, lock all doors that lead outside and use alarms to alert you if the person opens an outside door. Get a medical ID bracelet for the person so you can be contacted if the person is found wandering outside.

- Don't argue with the person if he or she becomes agitated. Offer reassurance, and try to distract the person or focus the person's attention on something else.

- Review all the person's medications and their dosages with a doctor or pharmacist.

- Provide well-balanced meals and healthy snacks. If the person cannot use utensils, prepare foods that can be eaten with the fingers. Allow plenty of time for the person to eat his or her meals.

- Review the home treatment tips for depression (page 326). Depression often occurs with dementia.

- Also see Caregiver Secrets starting on page 367.

When to Call a Health Professional

- If mental impairment has come on suddenly. See Delirium on page 195.

- If a person's symptoms cause you to suspect dementia.

- If a person with dementia becomes uncontrollably hostile or agitated.

- If you want a referral to a gerontologist or neurologist. These doctors have special training to identify causes of dementia. Some causes of dementia are reversible, and many symptoms can be effectively managed.

Tremor

Tremor is an involuntary shaking movement that is repeated over and over. Although it may affect any part of the body, tremor most often affects the hands and head. Occasionally the feet or torso may also shake.

Essential tremor, which sometimes runs in families, is one of the most common types of tremor. It causes shaking that is most noticeable when you are doing something like lifting a cup or pointing at an object. The shaking does not occur when you are not moving. The tremor may also affect your voice. Medication can help reduce the shaking. Brain surgery can be helpful in some cases.

Tremors can also be caused by conditions or medications that affect the nervous system, including Parkinson's disease (page 201), liver failure, alcoholism, mercury or arsenic poisoning, lithium, and certain antidepressants.

If you notice a tremor, observe it carefully and note what seems to make it better or worse before calling your health professional. If a cause is discovered, the disease will be treated rather than the tremor.

Home Treatment

- Stress reduction can sometimes help reduce tremor. See Stress on page 342.

- Add a little weight to your hand by wearing a heavy bracelet or watch or holding something in your hand. This may reduce some tremors and restore more control to your hands.

- Drink beverages from half-filled cups or glasses, and use a straw.

- Get enough rest and sleep. Fatigue often makes a tremor worse.

When to Call a Health Professional

- If you suddenly develop a tremor or if an existing tremor becomes worse.

- If tremor interferes with your ability to do daily activities or keeps you from taking part in social events.

- If you suspect that tremor may be a side effect of a medication.

Parkinson's Disease

Parkinson's disease occurs when brain cells that produce dopamine, a chemical needed to control muscle movements, break down. Parkinson's disease seldom affects people younger than 50. Symptoms of Parkinson's disease come on slowly and gradually worsen over time. They may include:

- Tremor or shaking, often in a hand, arm, or leg.

- Stiff muscles.

- Slow, limited movement.

- Balance problems, stooped posture, and a shuffling walk.

- A loss of expression in the face.

- Speech changes, such as loss of volume or a flat tone to the voice, or difficulty starting to speak.

 No treatment can halt or reverse the breakdown of nerve cells that causes Parkinson's disease. Medications can relieve some symptoms, and regular exercise can help a person maintain flexibility, strength, and endurance. Some people may benefit from surgery or a procedure called deep brain stimulation.

For more information, contact the American Parkinson Disease Association at 1-800-223-2732 or the National Parkinson Foundation, Inc. at 1-800-327-4545.

You can observe a lot just by watching.
Yogi Berra (naturally)

12

Eye and Vision Problems

This chapter includes information about eye problems that are common with aging and that can impair your vision, such as cataracts, glaucoma, and retinal disorders. These conditions usually require medical treatment. You will also find information about eyelid problems, dry eyes, excessive tearing, and floaters and flashes—annoying problems that respond well to self-care and usually do not affect your vision.

By age 50, most people have become aware of changes in their vision. Typical changes include:

- A gradual decline in the ability to see small print or focus on close objects (presbyopia).

- A decrease in the sharpness of vision.

- The need for more light for reading, driving, sewing, and other activities.

- Some trouble distinguishing subtle color differences; blue may appear gray, for example.

The information in this chapter will help you adjust to normal vision changes and know what symptoms may indicate a serious problem.

Eye Emergencies

If you have any of the following symptoms, call your eye doctor immediately:

- Severe pain in your eye.

- Sudden onset of new vision disturbances, such as floaters or flashes of light, partial blindness, or a shadow across part of your field of vision.

These symptoms may indicate a serious eye problem that could lead to blindness if not treated. Immediate medical care may help save your sight.

Eye Problems

Symptoms	Possible Causes
Sudden, severe pain in eye, blurred vision, or a reddened eyeball	Call a health professional immediately! Possible closed-angle glaucoma, p. 209.
Sudden onset of vision changes such as flashes of light, partial blindness, or shadow across part of visual field	Call a health professional immediately! Possible retinal detachment, p. 212.
Gradual onset of cloudy, filmy, or fuzzy vision; difficulty seeing close objects	Presbyopia, p. 211; Cataracts, p. 205.
Tunnel vision (gradual loss of side or peripheral vision)	Glaucoma, p. 209.
Halos around lights	Cataracts, p. 205; Glaucoma, p. 209.
Distorted vision, dark spot in center of vision; straight lines appear wavy	Macular Degeneration, p. 212.
Red spot on white of eye	Blood in the Eye, p. 205.
Excessive discharge from eye; red, swollen eyelids; sandy feeling in eyes	Eye Infections, p. 207.
Dry, scratchy eyes	Dry Eyes, p. 207.
Red, irritated, scaly eyelids	Eyelid Problems, p. 209.
Drooping eyelids; excess tearing	Eyelid Problems, p. 209.
Pimple or swelling on eyelid	Styes, p. 214.
Object or chemical in eye	Objects in the Eye, p. 58; Burns, p. 40.

Vision Protection Tips

Protect your sight throughout your life by following these general guidelines:

• Avoid overexposure to sunlight to reduce the risk of cataracts (page 205). Wear sunglasses that screen out ultraviolet (UV) rays.

• Wear goggles or protective glasses when handling chemicals, operating power tools, or playing racket sports.

• Get periodic eye exams. If you have diabetes, a diagnosed vision disorder (such as glaucoma, cataracts, or macular degeneration), or a family history of eye disorders, have your eyes checked according to the schedule your eye doctor recommends.

• Keep your blood pressure under control. High blood pressure can damage the blood vessels that supply blood to your eyes. See High Blood Pressure on page 165.

• If you have diabetes, follow the home treatment guidelines on page 177. People with diabetes are at risk for a vision problem called diabetic retinopathy.

Blood in the Eye

Blood vessels in the clear membrane (conjunctiva) that covers the white of the eye sometimes break, causing red spots or specks to form on the eye. This is called a subconjunctival hemorrhage, and it may be caused by coughing, sneezing, or a blow to the eye. The blood in your eye may look alarming, especially if the spot is large. However, it is usually not a cause for concern and will clear up on its own in 2 to 3 weeks.

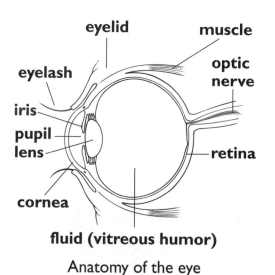

eyelid

muscle

optic nerve

eyelash

iris

pupil

lens

retina

cornea

fluid (vitreous humor)

Anatomy of the eye

When to Call a Health Professional

• If there is blood in the colored part of your eye (iris).

• If you have blood in the white of your eye and any of the following problems:
  - Pain in the eye.
  - Sensitivity to light.
  - Vision changes.

• If blood covers more than one-fourth of the white of your eye.

• If the bleeding started following a blow to the eye.

• If you have blood in the white of your eye and you are taking blood thinners (anticoagulants).

Cataracts

A cataract is a painless, cloudy area in the lens of the eye. A cataract blocks the passage of light through the lens to the nerve layer (retina) at the back of the eye, and it may cause vision problems.

Cataracts are very common in older adults and can result from normal age-related changes in the lens. They can also occur after an eye injury, as a result of eye disease, as a side effect of certain medications, or as a result of medical conditions such as diabetes.

Symptoms of cataracts include cloudy, fuzzy, or filmy vision; decreased night vision; problems with glare; and double vision. You may see spots or halos around lights. Your eyeglasses prescription may change frequently.

 Without treatment, some cataracts can become larger or denser over time, making your vision problems worse. However, cataracts do not always need to be removed. The vision loss that results from cataracts often develops slowly and may never become severe. Many people with cataracts get along very well with the help of eyeglasses, contact lenses, and other vision aids and are able to avoid or delay surgery. The decision whether to have cataract surgery often depends on how much cataracts are interfering with a person's ability to do daily activities.

Prevention

There is no proven way to prevent cataracts. However, certain health habits may help slow cataract development. These include:

- Not smoking.
- Wearing a hat or sunglasses when you are in the sun and avoiding sunlamps and tanning booths.
- Eating a diet rich in vitamins C and E.
- Limiting your alcohol intake.
- Avoiding the use of steroid medications when possible.
- Keeping high blood pressure and diabetes under control.

Home Treatment

Home treatment will not cure cataracts, but it may help you avoid or delay surgery. There are many things you can do to make the gradual changes in your vision easier to live with.

- Reposition room lights and use window shades to prevent glare on TV and computer screens.
- Use table or floor lamps for close reading and other fine work.
- Put more lights or use higher-watt bulbs over steps and in hallways.
- Use contrasts in color and brightness to make things easier to find at home. For example, if you have light-colored walls, use dark switch plates to mark the location of switches. Use colored, high-contrast labels to "color code" medications, spices, stove dials, and other items.
- Keep your eyeglasses prescription current. Update your prescription before considering surgery.
- Try reading large-print books and newspapers. Also, bank checks, medication labels, and other items are often available in large print. Magnifying glasses may help you read some things, but only if the type is very clear. Magnified blurry print will be larger but will still be blurry.

For more information about cataracts and other vision problems, contact The Lighthouse, 111 East 59th Street, New York, NY 10017, 1-800-829-0500.

When to Call a Health Professional

• If you have severe eye pain.

• If you have a change in your vision, such as vision loss, double vision, or blurred vision.

• If your eyeglasses prescription changes frequently.

• If daytime glare is a problem.

• If you have difficulty driving at night because of glare from oncoming headlights.

• If vision problems are affecting your ability to do daily activities.

Dry Eyes

Eyes that don't have enough moisture in them may feel dry, hot, sandy, or gritty. Low humidity, smoke, the natural aging process, and certain medications (diuretics, antihistamines, decongestants, antidepressants) can cause dry eyes.

Home Treatment

• Give your eyes a rest. While reading, watching television, or using a computer, take frequent breaks and close your eyes. If you can, blink your eyes more often.

• Avoid smoke and other irritants when possible.

• Try a nonprescription artificial tear solution, such as Akwa Tears, Duratears, or HypoTears. Do not use eyedrops for reducing redness (such as Visine) to treat dry eyes.

When to Call a Health Professional

Call a health professional if your eyes are persistently dry and artificial tears do not help. Excessive dryness can damage your eyes.

Eye Infections

Conjunctivitis, or pinkeye, is an inflammation of the membrane (conjunctiva) that lines the eyelids and the surface of the eyes. Bacteria and viruses (which can be very contagious), allergies, dry air, and irritants in the air such as smoke, fumes, or chemicals can cause pinkeye.

The symptoms of pinkeye may include red, itching, burning eyes; red, swollen eyelids; lots of tears; a sandy feeling in the eyes; and sensitivity to light. There may be a colored discharge that causes your eyelids to stick together during sleep.

Prevention

• Do not share towels, linens, pillows, handkerchiefs, eye makeup, eye medication, or contact lens equipment or solutions.

• Wash your hands before and after treating pinkeye in your own eyes or someone else's eyes.

- To prevent irritation, wear eye protection when your eyes might be exposed to wind, heat, or cold.

- Wear safety glasses when working with chemicals.

Home Treatment

Although most cases of pinkeye will clear up in 5 to 7 days with treatment, viral pinkeye can last many weeks. Pinkeye caused by allergies or pollution will last as long as you are exposed to the irritating substance. Good home care will speed healing and ease the discomfort.

- Don't wear contact lenses or eye makeup until the inflammation is gone. If pinkeye was caused by an infection, throw away your old eye makeup and buy new products. Clean your contact lenses and your lens case thoroughly before you start wearing your contacts again, or use a new pair of disposable lenses.

- Apply cold or warm compresses several times a day to relieve discomfort.

- Gently wipe the edge of the eyelid with moist cotton or a clean, wet washcloth to remove encrusted matter. Wipe from the inside (next to your nose) to the outside, and use a clean surface with each wipe.

- If eyedrops are prescribed, insert them as follows: Pull your lower lid down with two fingers to create a little pouch. Put the drops there. Close your eye for 30 to 60 seconds to let the drops move around.

- Be sure the dropper is clean. If the dropper touches your eye, eyelid, or eyelashes, don't put it back in the medication bottle. Throw it away and replace it.

- Make sure any nonprescription medicine you use is ophthalmic (for eyes), not otic (for ears).

- Wash your hands thoroughly after treating pinkeye.

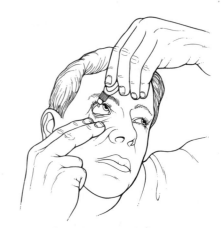

Inserting eyedrops

When to Call a Health Professional

- If you have pain in your eye (not an irritated, scratchy feeling), blurring, or loss of vision that is not cleared even momentarily by blinking.

- If you have drainage from one or both eyes.

- If your eye is painfully sensitive to light.

- If your symptoms last more than a few days.

- If your symptoms do not start to improve within 48 hours after you start using an antibiotic medication to treat an eye infection.

- If you wear contact lenses and you have had pinkeye more than once.

Eyelid Problems

One of the most common eye problems in older adults is a skin condition called **blepharitis**. Symptoms include redness, irritation, and scaly skin at the edges of the eyelids. The scales may be dry or greasy. Eyelashes may fall out as well. The cause of blepharitis is not known, but it is more common in people who have dandruff, skin allergies, or eczema and in those who often have styes. The problem is often chronic.

Another common age-related eye change is drooping eyelids. Drooping is the result of reduced muscle tone in the muscles that control the eyelids. If your lower eyelids droop low enough (**ectropion**), they may no longer be able to protect your eyes, and your eyes may become dry and irritated. If your upper eyelids droop low enough (**ptosis**), they may interfere with your vision.

Drooping eyelids can prevent tears from draining normally, so tears may run down your cheeks. Excessive tearing can also be a sign of increased sensitivity to light or wind, an eye infection, or a blocked tear duct. If your eyes tear when they are exposed to bright light or wind, wear protective glasses.

Home Treatment

To treat blepharitis at home, wash your eyelids, eyebrows, and hair daily with baby shampoo. To wash your eyelids, put a few drops of shampoo in a cup of water, dip a cotton ball, cotton swab, or washcloth in the solution, and gently wipe your eyelids. Rinse well with clear water.

When to Call a Health Professional

- Blepharitis often requires antibiotic treatment. Call a health professional:

  - If your eye is painful.

  - If your eyelids are bleeding.

  - If the problem is not improving after 1 week of home treatment.

- If your eyelids suddenly start to droop.

- If drooping eyelids interfere with your vision.

- If your eyes are dry and irritated, or if your eyelids do not close completely when you sleep.

- If your eyelashes start to rub on your eyeball.

Glaucoma

Glaucoma causes damage to the optic nerve that results in the loss of eyesight. The optic nerve, which is located at the back of the eye, carries signals from the eye to the brain. The brain translates those signals into images that you see. In a person with glaucoma, increased pressure inside the eye may be part of the reason why the optic nerve becomes damaged. The pressure increase is caused by the buildup of fluid inside the eye.

There are two types of glaucoma that can occur in adults:

- **Open-angle glaucoma**, the most common form of glaucoma, is usually painless and can develop gradually over several years without being detected. Both eyes can be affected at the same time. However, one eye may be affected more than the other. Open-angle glaucoma often affects side (peripheral) vision first. By the time you notice a change in your vision, the damage is permanent.

- **Closed-angle glaucoma** comes on suddenly and can lead to permanent eye damage in a matter of hours. Symptoms of closed-angle glaucoma include severe eye pain, blurred vision, redness in the eye, and possibly nausea and vomiting. Call a health professional immediately if you develop these symptoms.

Untreated glaucoma is a leading cause of blindness in older adults. African Americans, people who have high pressure in their eyes (intraocular pressure), and those who have a family history of glaucoma are at increased risk for developing glaucoma.

Prevention

 Regular eye exams, including glaucoma tests, will help detect glaucoma before it affects your eyesight. Talk to your doctor about how often you should be tested for glaucoma. If there is a history of glaucoma in your family or you have other risk factors for glaucoma, talk with your health professional about having more frequent eye exams. If you are at increased risk for glaucoma, you need to have regular eye exams by an eye specialist (ophthalmologist).

Home Treatment

If you have been diagnosed with glaucoma, use your prescribed medications exactly as directed.

When to Call a Health Professional

Call 911 or other emergency services immediately:

- If your vision in one eye suddenly becomes severely blurred.

- If there is severe pain in the affected eye.

- If the affected eye is red.

- If you see colored halos around lights.

- If you have nausea or vomiting in addition to the above symptoms.

Call a health professional:

- If you have noticed blind spots in your side (peripheral) vision in one or both eyes.

• If you have noticed that over time you are having more difficulty seeing.

• If you have a family history of open-angle glaucoma and you have not had an eye exam in more than a year.

PRK and LASIK

PRK and LASIK are two different surgical procedures that can correct vision problems such as nearsightedness, farsightedness, and astigmatism. For each procedure, a surgeon uses laser instruments to reshape the cornea (the clear tissue that covers the iris and pupil) in a way that allows improved vision. These procedures take only a few minutes to complete. If both eyes need correction, they can be treated at the same time.

People who wore glasses or contact lenses before having corrective surgery may still need to wear them after the surgery, especially when light is dim and at night (usually the prescription is not as strong). A person may see halos around lights for up to 6 months after having corrective eye surgery.

PRK and LASIK cannot restore vision loss caused by cataracts or macular degeneration; nor can they prevent these age-related eye changes from happening. PRK and LASIK are not appropriate if you have glaucoma.

Floaters and Flashes

Floaters are spots, specks, and lines that float across your field of vision. They are caused by stray cells or strands of tissue that float in the vitreous humor, the gel-like substance that fills your eyeball. Floaters can be annoying but are not usually serious. However, if you notice a sudden increase in the number of floaters you see, if floaters occur with flashes of light, or if you notice a persistent shadow across part of your field of vision, call your eye doctor or family doctor. These may be signs of retinal detachment. See page 212.

Presbyopia

Presbyopia is a condition that affects almost everyone sometime after age 40. As the eyes age, the lenses become less flexible, which makes it harder for them to focus on close objects or small print. You may find that you have to hold objects at arm's length to see them clearly. (People with presbyopia sometimes say that they don't need glasses; they just need longer arms.)

Home Treatment

Glasses or contact lenses can usually give you clear vision again. If you already wear glasses, you may need bifocals, which will allow you to see objects that are close up and those that are far away. Nonprescription reading glasses may be appropriate for some people.

When to Call a Health Professional

Presbyopia usually develops gradually, over months to years. If your vision changes more quickly, over just a few weeks, call your doctor. This may be an early symptom of another condition, such as diabetes.

Retinal Disorders

The retina is a thin membrane made up of nerve cells that lines the back of the eyeball. The nerve cells in the retina detect light and send signals to the brain about what the eye sees. Problems with the retina can lead to impaired vision or blindness.

Torn or Detached Retina

Retinal detachment occurs when the retina becomes separated from the wall of the eye. Once the retina becomes detached, it stops working properly. This causes vision loss in the affected area of the retina. Although retinal detachment may occur at any age, older people, those who are nearsighted, and those with a family history of retinal detachments are at higher risk. Most retinal detachments are caused by age-related changes in the gel-like substance (vitreous) that fills the eye. A blow to the head or eye may also cause the retina to detach. Symptoms of a retinal tear or detachment may include seeing floaters or flashes of light or seeing a new shadow or "curtain" across part of your field of vision.

Many retinal tears do not require treatment. Tears that occur with symptoms, such as floaters or flashes of light, are more likely to require surgical treatment to prevent retinal detachment and vision loss.

Treatment for retinal detachment always involves surgery. In most cases, good vision can be restored if surgery is done soon after retinal detachment occurs.

Macular Degeneration

Macular degeneration is an eye disease that destroys central vision by damaging the macula. The macula is the part of the retina that provides clear, sharp central vision that you use to focus on what's in front of you. Macular degeneration may occur in one or both eyes. Signs of the disease may range from dim or fuzzy vision to a blank or dark spot in the center of your visual field. Straight lines (such as in the Amsler grid on page 213) may appear wavy, and colors may appear faded or dim.

As the condition progresses, central vision is lost. Peripheral (side) vision is not affected, and many people function well despite the loss of central vision, although walking, reading, driving, and other activities that require central vision are much more difficult.

Smoking increases your risk for macular degeneration. There is some evidence that eating plenty of dark, leafy green vegetables, such as spinach and collard greens, may reduce your risk for macular degeneration.

Laser surgery may prevent or delay further loss of vision in one type of macular degeneration if the condition is detected early.

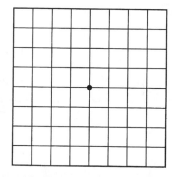

Amsler grid: Cover one eye and look at the grid above. Repeat with the other eye covered. If the lines around the center dot look wavy or distorted, you may have a macular problem.

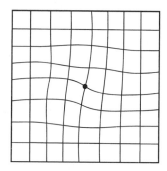

This is how the first grid might look to someone who has macular degeneration.

Diabetic Retinopathy

Diabetic retinopathy develops when the blood vessels that supply blood to the retina are damaged by diabetes. It often has no symptoms until it is quite advanced. If it is not treated, diabetic retinopathy can lead to blindness. Regular eye exams can detect this problem early, when it can be more successfully treated. Keeping your blood sugar levels in a safe range is important to help reduce your risk for retinal changes. See Diabetes on page 176.

When to Call a Health Professional

Call a health professional immediately if you have a sudden onset of vision disturbances, such as floaters and flashes of light, partial blindness, or dark spots in your field of vision.

Call your doctor:

- If straight lines appear wavy or curved, or the size or shape of objects begins to look different or distorted.

- If you often see new floaters or flashes of light.

If you are at high risk for macular degeneration or diabetic retinopathy, have eye exams according to the schedule recommended by your doctor and report any new changes in your vision as soon as possible.

Styes

A sty is a noncontagious infection of an eyelash follicle. It looks like a small, red bump, much like a pimple, either in the eyelid or on the edge of the lid. It comes to a head and breaks open after a few days.

Styes are very common and are not a serious problem. Most will go away on their own with home treatment and don't require removal.

Home Treatment

- Do not rub your eye, and do not squeeze or try to open the sty.

- Apply warm, moist compresses for 10 minutes, 3 to 6 times a day, until the sty comes to a point and drains.

- Do not wear eye makeup or contact lenses until the sty heals.

When to Call a Health Professional

- If the sty is very painful, grows larger quickly, or continues to drain.

- If the sty interferes with your vision.

- If the sty gets worse despite home treatment or doesn't heal within a week.

- If redness and swelling centered on the sty spread to your entire eyelid or eyeball.

The Eye Specialists

Ophthalmologists are medical doctors (MDs) or osteopathic doctors (DOs) who are trained and licensed to provide total eye care. They can prescribe corrective lenses, diagnose and treat eye disorders, and perform eye surgery.

Optometrists (ODs) perform eye examinations and prescribe corrective lenses. In some states, they are also licensed to diagnose and treat some types of eye problems.

Opticians make eyeglasses and fill prescriptions for corrective lenses.

13

Ear and Hearing Problems

The human ear is designed to channel and modify sound waves. Sound waves enter the ear and cause the eardrum to vibrate, setting in motion the tiny bones of the middle ear: the hammer, anvil, and stirrup. These bones magnify and transfer sounds to the structures of the inner ear: the cochlea and auditory nerve. The cochlea contains tiny hairs that convert sounds to nerve impulses, which are transmitted to the brain by the auditory nerve.

As people age, a number of changes within the ear can affect how well they hear. For example, the tiny hairs in the cochlea begin to break down and do not conduct sound vibrations as well as they once could. This breakdown is probably the result of lifelong exposure to noise.

It is impossible to undo noise damage, but there is still plenty you can do to get the most out of your hearing.

This chapter will tell you how to protect your hearing and what you can do to cope with hearing loss and other ear problems.

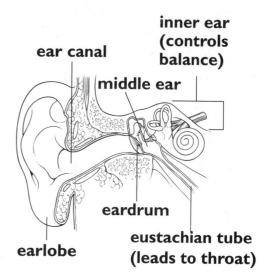

Infections can occur in the ear canal, middle ear, or inner ear. Dizziness can be caused by an inflammation of the middle or inner ear.

Ear Problems

Symptoms	Possible Causes
Ear pain and fever	Ear Infections, p. 219.
Ear pain while chewing; headache	TM Disorder, p. 232.
Feeling of fullness in the ear, with runny or stuffy nose, cough, fever	Colds, p. 141; Ear Infections, p. 219.
Hearing loss	Hearing Loss, p. 222; Earwax, p. 221.
Dizziness or lightheadedness; sensation that room is spinning around you; problems with balance	Dizziness and Vertigo, p. 216; Meniere's Disease, p. 217.
Ringing or noise in the ears	Tinnitus, p. 224.

Dizziness and Vertigo

Dizziness is a word that is often used to describe two different sensations: lightheadedness and vertigo. It is important to know exactly what you mean when you say, "I feel dizzy," because it can help you and your health professional narrow down the list of possible problems.

Lightheadedness is a feeling that you are about to pass out (faint). Although you may feel unsteady, there is no sensation of movement.

Lightheadedness usually goes away or improves when you lie down. If lightheadedness gets worse, it can lead to a fainting spell with nausea or vomiting.

Lightheadedness usually does not indicate a serious problem. It is common to feel lightheaded occasionally. Lightheadedness is often caused by a momentary drop in blood pressure and reduced blood flow to the head when you get up too quickly from a seated or lying position. This is called **orthostatic hypotension**. It may be caused by dehydration or medications such as water pills (diuretics), certain high blood pressure medications, and certain heart medications.

Lightheadedness is common when you have the flu, a cold, or allergies. Vomiting, diarrhea, and fever can cause dehydration and lightheadedness. Other common causes of lightheadedness include hyperventilation, stress, anxiety, drinking alcohol, or using illegal drugs. A more serious cause of lightheadedness is bleeding. If a person is bleeding internally, lightheadedness and fatigue may be the first noticeable symptoms of blood loss.

An uncommon cause of lightheadedness is an abnormality in your heart rhythm that reduces blood flow. This can cause recurrent spells of lightheadedness and can lead to a fainting spell (cardiac syncope). Unexplained fainting spells need to be evaluated by a health professional. See Fainting and Unconsciousness on page 46.

Vertigo is a sensation that your body or the world around you is spinning or moving when there is no actual movement. Vertigo is often related to inner ear problems. Severe vertigo can cause nausea and vomiting. Standing or walking may be impossible when you have severe vertigo.

The most common form of vertigo is triggered by changes in the position of your head, such as when you move your head from side to side or bend your head back to look up. This is called **benign positional vertigo**. Vertigo also may be caused by labyrinthitis, an inflammation or infection in the part of the inner ear that controls balance. Labyrinthitis is usually caused by a viral infection and sometimes follows a cold or the flu.

Other underlying problems that can contribute to vertigo are Meniere's disease (see page 217), multiple sclerosis, stroke, and, in rare cases, a brain tumor.

Meniere's Disease

Meniere's disease is a balance problem that is believed to be caused by a buildup of fluid in the inner ear. The symptoms include attacks of vertigo and unsteadiness, tinnitus, hearing loss in one ear, nausea, and vomiting. You may also have a feeling of fullness in your ear and be very sensitive to loud noises. The attacks can last for hours or days and occur as frequently as once a week or as seldom as once every few years.

If you have been diagnosed with Meniere's disease, these measures may help ease your symptoms:

• Avoid salt, caffeine, and alcohol.

• Stop smoking.

• Relax. Episodes of Meniere's disease can cause your stress level to increase, which can make your ear and balance problems worse. Ease stress by using relaxation techniques. See page 344.

 In some cases, medications that keep the body from retaining fluid (diuretics) may help make vertigo attacks less frequent. Medications like those used to treat motion sickness may make symptoms less severe when attacks do occur.

Home Treatment

Lightheadedness is usually not a cause for concern unless it is severe or persistent or occurs with other symptoms such as an irregular heartbeat or fainting. The greatest danger of lightheadedness or vertigo is the injuries that you might suffer if you fall.

- When you feel lightheaded, lie down for a minute or two. This will allow more blood to flow to your brain. After lying down, sit up slowly and remain sitting for 1 to 2 minutes before slowly standing up.

- If you have a cold or the flu, get extra rest and drink extra fluids to prevent dehydration, which can cause or increase lightheadedness.

- Do not drive, operate machinery, or put yourself in any other potentially dangerous situation while you are feeling lightheaded or having vertigo.

- When you are having vertigo, avoid lying flat on your back. Propping yourself up slightly may relieve the spinning sensation. Keep your eyes open.

When to Call a Health Professional

Call 911 or other emergency services immediately:

- If vertigo is accompanied by headache, confusion, loss of speech or sight, weakness in the arms or legs, or numbness in any part of the body. See Stroke on page 63.

- If lightheadedness occurs with squeezing or crushing chest pain or any other symptoms of a heart attack (see page 53).

- If someone who is feeling dizzy loses consciousness and you are unable to wake the person.

- If vertigo or loss of balance occurs with other signs of serious illness, such as headache with severe stiff neck, fever, irritability, confusion, or a seizure. (See Encephalitis and Meningitis on page 189.)

- If severe and persistent lightheadedness is accompanied by a sudden change in your normal heart rate.

Call a health professional:

- If lightheadedness or vertigo develops after an injury.

- If you have vertigo that is severe or that occurs with hearing loss.

- If you suspect your dizziness may be a side effect of a medication.

- If you experience vertigo that:

  - Occurs frequently and has not been diagnosed.

  - Lasts longer than 5 days.

  - Is significantly different from other episodes.

- If you have repeated spells of lightheadedness over a few days.

- If you feel lightheaded and your pulse rate is fewer than 50 or more than 150 beats per minute. See page 47 to learn how to take your pulse.

Ear Infections

Inflammation and infection can develop in the ear canal, causing what is known as otitis externa or swimmer's ear. These same problems can develop in the middle ear (see illustration on page 215). Middle ear infections are called otitis media.

Swimmer's ear often develops after water, sand, or other debris has gotten into the ear canal. Other causes of inflammation in the ear canal include a scratch from a cotton swab or other object; frequent use of cotton swabs deep in the ear canal; prolonged use of earplugs; soap or shampoo buildup; and chronic skin conditions.

Symptoms of swimmer's ear include pain, itching, and a feeling of fullness in the ear. The ear canal may be swollen. A more severe infection can cause increased pain, discharge from the ear, and possibly some hearing loss. The pain caused by ear canal inflammation gets worse when you chew, press on the "tag" in front of your ear, or wiggle your earlobe.

Middle ear infections are much more common in children, but they do occur in adults. They usually start when a cold causes the eustachian tube (which leads from the middle ear to the throat) to swell and close. When the eustachian tube is closed, air cannot reach the middle ear. This creates a vacuum that draws fluid into the middle ear. Bacteria or viruses then grow in the fluid, causing a middle ear infection. As your body fights the infection, pressure builds up in the middle ear, causing pain. If the ear infection is not treated, the pressure may continue to build until the eardrum ruptures.

Symptoms of a middle ear infection include ear pain, dizziness, ringing or a feeling of fullness in the ear, hearing loss, fever, headache, and runny nose. Drainage from the ear that is bloody or looks like pus may indicate a ruptured eardrum. Ear pain usually improves once an eardrum ruptures.

Bacterial ear infections are usually treated with antibiotics. Antibiotics stop bacterial growth, and by doing so they help relieve pressure and pain.

Prevention

To prevent ear infections:

- Keep your ears dry. After swimming or showering, shake your head to get water out of your ear canals. Gently dry your ears with the corner of a tissue or towel, or use a blow-dryer on its lowest setting, held several inches from your ear.

- Put a few drops of rubbing alcohol mixed with an equal amount of white vinegar in your ears after swimming or showering. Pull your ear up and back to let the liquid go deep into the ear canal; then tilt your head and let the liquid drain out. You can also use nonprescription drops, such as Star-Otic or Swim-Ear, to prevent swimmer's ear.

- Never use cotton swabs, hairpins, or any other objects to clean your ears. Avoid prolonged use of earplugs. Putting objects in your ears may plug the ears with wax. See Earwax on page 221.

- Avoid getting soap and shampoo in your ears. To remove dirt or sand that gets into the ear during swimming, direct a gentle stream of warm water from the shower or a bulb syringe into your ear; then tip your head to let the water drain out.

- Follow any instructions your health professional has given you to treat skin problems, such as eczema, psoriasis, or seborrhea, that may cause ear canal irritation.

- Stop smoking. Smoking irritates the mucous membranes that line the nose, sinuses, and lungs, and may contribute to inflammation or infection of the ear.

- Blow your nose gently to avoid forcing fluid into your eustachian tubes.

Home Treatment

For swimmer's ear:

- Using a bulb syringe, gently rinse the ear with equal parts vinegar and rubbing alcohol. Make sure the solution is at body temperature. Putting cool or hot fluids in the ear may cause dizziness. Bulb syringes are inexpensive and available at most pharmacies and drugstores.

- Avoid getting water in the ear until the irritation clears up. Cotton coated with petroleum jelly can be used as an earplug.

- If your ear is itchy, try nonprescription swimmer's eardrops (see Prevention) before and after getting your ears wet.

- To ease ear pain, use a warm washcloth or a heating pad set on low. (Never use a heating pad in bed; you could fall asleep and burn yourself.) There may be some drainage when the heat melts earwax. As long as the drainage does not contain pus or blood, it is not of concern.

For otitis media:

- Apply heat to the ear to ease pain. Use a warm washcloth or heating pad set on low.

- Take aspirin, ibuprofen, or acetaminophen to help relieve pain.

- Rest. Let your energy go to fighting the infection.

- Drink more clear liquids.

- If dizziness occurs, see page 216.

- If your eardrum ruptures, avoid getting water in your ear until the eardrum heals. This usually takes 3 to 4 weeks.

When to Call a Health Professional

• If ear pain is severe, or if any ear pain or itching lasts longer than 3 days. If hearing loss or a significant feeling of fullness in the ear persists after the pain is gone, call your doctor.

• If ear pain occurs with other signs of serious illness, such as a headache and severe stiff neck, fever, nausea, vomiting, confusion, or memory problems. See Encephalitis and Meningitis on page 189.

• If you suspect that your eardrum has ruptured or if there is drainage from your ear that looks like pus or contains blood.

• If your ear canal is swollen, red, and very painful.

• If there is redness or swelling around or behind your ear.

• If there is no improvement in your symptoms after you have taken antibiotics for 2 to 3 days.

Earwax

Earwax is a protective secretion that filters dust, repels water, and keeps the ears clean. Normally, earwax is semisolid, clears spontaneously from the ear canal, and does not cause problems.

Occasionally, earwax will build up, harden, and cause some hearing loss or discomfort. Poking at the wax with cotton swabs, fingers, or other objects will only push the wax deeper into your ear canal and pack it against your eardrum. When wax is tightly packed, professional help is needed to remove it.

In general, it is best to leave earwax alone. You can handle most earwax problems that do occur by avoiding cotton swabs and following the home treatment tips. You should be concerned only if the earwax causes ringing or a full feeling in your ear, some hearing loss, or vertigo.

Home Treatment

Home treatment is not appropriate if you suspect that the eardrum is ruptured or if there is drainage from the ear that looks like pus or contains blood.

To remove earwax safely:

• Soften and loosen the earwax with body temperature mineral oil. Place 2 drops of mineral oil in your ear twice a day for 1 or 2 days.

• Once the wax is loose and soft, all that is usually needed to remove the wax from the ear canal is the spray from a warm, gentle shower or a bulb ear syringe. With the affected ear down, direct the water into the ear, and then tip your head to let the earwax drain out. Bulb syringes are inexpensive and available at most pharmacies and drugstores.

• If the warm mineral oil and water do not work, use a nonprescription wax softener, such as Debrox or Murine, followed by gentle flushing with warm water from a bulb ear syringe, each night for 1 to 2 weeks. Make sure the solution is body temperature. Putting cool or hot fluids in the ear may cause dizziness.

When to Call a Health Professional

• If home treatment does not work and the wax buildup remains hard, dry, and compacted.

• If earwax is causing ringing in your ears, a full feeling in your ears, or hearing loss.

• If earwax buildup occurs with other problems such as nausea or difficulty with balance.

Hearing Loss

Hearing loss is one of the most common conditions that affects people over 50. Most hearing loss in adults is caused by damage to the inner ear resulting from exposure to loud noise, certain medications (including high doses of aspirin), or changes that come with age (presbycusis). People with these types of hearing loss may have trouble understanding other people's speech yet be very sensitive to loud sounds. They may also hear ringing, hissing, or clicking noises.

Caregiver Tips: Living With a Hearing-Impaired Person

• Speak to the person at a distance of 3 to 6 feet. Make sure that your face, mouth, and gestures can be seen clearly. Arrange furniture so everyone is completely visible.

• Avoid speaking directly into the person's ear. Visual clues will be missed.

• Speak slightly louder than normal, but do not shout. Speak slowly.

• Cut down on background noise. Turn down the television or radio. Ask for quiet sections in restaurants.

• If a particular phrase or word is misunderstood, find another way of saying it. Avoid repeating the same words over and over.

• If the subject is changed, tell the person, "We are talking about _____ now."

• Treat the hearing-impaired person with respect and consideration. Involve the person in discussions, especially those about him or her. Do what you can to ease feelings of isolation.

Hearing loss may also develop when something prevents sound from reaching the inner ear. The most common cause is packed earwax in the ear canal, which can be easily treated (see page 221). Infection, abnormal bone growth, and excess fluid in the middle or inner ear are other causes of this type of hearing loss.

When sound doesn't reach the inner ear, your own voice may sound loud while other voices sound muffled. You may also hear ringing in your ears (tinnitus).

Some hearing loss may be the result of decreased blood flow to the inner ear. If you have circulatory problems caused by heart disease, high blood pressure, high cholesterol, hypothyroidism, or diabetes, be sure to follow your care plan for keeping those conditions under control.

Stroke or head injury can damage the hearing centers in the brain, causing central deafness. This type of hearing loss is rare.

Hearing Aid Considerations

- Not all hearing loss can be corrected with hearing aids. Whether hearing aids will be useful depends on the underlying cause of your hearing loss.

- Hearing aids work by making all sounds, both soft and loud, louder. They do not restore normal hearing. Digitally programmable hearing aids may allow you to choose different settings depending on whether you are in a noisy or quiet place.

- It takes time and practice to get used to hearing aids; you may need to try more than one type to get the best results. Wear your hearing aids every day, and gradually accustom yourself to the way they work.

Prevention

- Avoid loud noise whenever possible, and wear earplugs or protective earmuffs when you are going to be exposed to loud noises. The noise generated by snowmobiles, lawnmowers, guns, power tools and appliances, high-volume music, and other sources can permanently damage your hearing.

- Never use cotton swabs, hairpins, or other objects to deeply clean your ears. They can damage the ear canal or eardrum. See Earwax on page 221.

- Ask your pharmacist whether the medications you are taking can affect your hearing. For example, the use of certain antibiotics, blood pressure medications, ibuprofen, or large doses of aspirin (8 to 12 tablets per day) is linked to hearing loss.

- Keep circulatory problems, such as heart disease, high blood pressure, and diabetes, under control. Some hearing loss may be the result of decreased blood flow to the inner ear.

Home Assessment

Age-related hearing loss often occurs so gradually that many people may not even realize they have a hearing loss. However, it is important to recognize hearing loss, whatever the cause. When undetected and untreated, hearing loss can contribute to depression, social isolation, and loss of independence, especially in older adults.

Here are three simple tests you can do to test your hearing.

The Clock Test

- Have a friend hold a ticking clock out of sight some distance from one side of your head.

- Have the person slowly move the clock closer to your ear. Tell the person when you first hear the clock ticking.

- Repeat the test for your other ear. For each ear, you should hear the ticking sound when the clock is about the same distance away.

- Test your friend's hearing in the same way to see if he or she can hear the clock from much farther away than you can. Be sure to ask a friend whose hearing is good!

The Radio Test

Have someone adjust the volume on a radio or television set so it is pleasing to that person. Can you hear it well, or do you have to strain to hear it?

The Telephone Test

When you talk on the telephone, switch the phone from ear to ear to hear if the sound is the same. Although hearing loss that is associated with aging usually affects both ears, it is possible for only one ear to be affected.

When to Call a Health Professional

- If hearing loss develops suddenly (within a matter of days or weeks).

- If you have hearing loss in one ear only.

- After age 50, hearing assessments are recommended periodically during regular doctor visits. Have exams more frequently if hearing problems exist.

- If you are thinking about wearing hearing aids. Make an appointment with an ear specialist (otolaryngologist) if:

  - You often ask people to repeat themselves or you have difficulty understanding words.

  - You have difficulty hearing when someone speaks in a whisper.

  - You cannot hear soft sounds, such as a dripping faucet, or high-pitched sounds.

  - You continuously hear a ringing or hissing background noise.

  - A hearing problem is interfering with your life.

The otolaryngologist can refer you to a hearing specialist (audiologist) or hearing aid dispenser if needed.

Tinnitus

Most people experience occasional ringing, roaring, hissing, buzzing, or tinkling in their ears. The sound usually lasts only a few minutes. If it becomes persistent, you may have tinnitus.

Tinnitus is often the result of damage to the nerves in the inner ear caused by prolonged exposure to loud noise. Other causes include excess earwax, fluid in the middle ear, ear infection, dental problems, head or ear injuries, and medications, especially antibiotics and large amounts of aspirin. Excessive alcohol or caffeine intake can also cause tinnitus or make existing tinnitus worse. In rare cases, tinnitus can be caused by a brain tumor.

Most intermittent tinnitus does not require medical treatment. However, if tinnitus is accompanied by other symptoms, becomes persistent, or starts to localize to one ear, a visit to a health professional usually is needed.

Often there is no cure for tinnitus, but your health professional can help you learn how to live with the problem.

Prevention

Follow the prevention tips on page 223.

Home Treatment

- Cut back on or eliminate alcohol and beverages containing caffeine.

- Limit your use of aspirin, ibuprofen, and naproxen sodium.

- If you think earwax may be the cause of tinnitus, see Earwax on page 221.

- Find emotional support. Tinnitus can be difficult to deal with. The American Tinnitus Association is a helpful support group. Write P.O. Box 5, Portland, OR 97207, or call 1-503-248-9985.

When to Call a Health Professional

- If tinnitus develops suddenly and affects only one ear.

- If you have new tinnitus with other symptoms such as significant hearing loss, vertigo (see page 216), loss of balance, nausea, or vomiting.

- If tinnitus develops after an injury to the head or ear.

- If tinnitus lasts longer than 2 weeks despite home treatment.

Help for Hearing Problems

- National Institute on Deafness and Other Communication Disorders (NIDCD)

  - 1-800-241-1044 (Voice)

  - 1-800-241-1055 (TTY)

- American Speech-Language-Hearing Association

  - 1-800-638-8255 (Voice)

- SHHH (Self Help for Hard of Hearing People, Inc.)

  - 1-301-657-2248 (Voice)

  - 1-301-657-2249 (TTY)

The Hearing Specialists

Otologists or **otolaryngologists** are medical doctors (MDs or DOs) who can diagnose and treat hearing disorders and perform surgery.

Audiologists are hearing specialists who are trained to identify, diagnose, and measure hearing problems and recommend the most appropriate method to treat hearing loss. Look for an audiologist who is licensed by the state or who is certified by the American Speech-Language-Hearing Association (the letters CCC-A will appear after the audiologist's name).

Hearing aid specialists or **dispensers** are licensed in nearly all states and may be certified by the National Board for Certification in Hearing Instrument Sciences (BC-HIS). They can fit you with hearing aids.

If you are considering buying hearing aids, first have an evaluation by a medical doctor and an audiologist to help determine what type of hearing loss you have and whether it can be treated in other ways.

Be true to your teeth or your teeth will be false to you.
Dental Proverb

14

Mouth and Dental Problems

Your teeth and gums will last a lifetime if you care for them properly. Understanding how your mouth and teeth may change as you age will help you keep your mouth healthy and your smile attractive. Possible changes include:

- A dryer mouth, which can alter your sense of taste and also increase your risk for tooth decay.

- Receding gums, which expose the roots of your teeth, making them more sensitive to temperature changes and prone to cavities. Decay may also occur around the edges of fillings.

- Loss of teeth, which can affect your ability to eat a healthy diet. Dentures and bridgework require special care. See page 229.

This chapter also covers irritations to your mouth that know no age limits, such as canker sores and cold sores.

Dental Problems

Dental disease is preventable. You can keep all of your teeth by practicing good home care and having regular professional checkups.

Plaque and Tooth Decay

Germs are always present in the mouth. When they are not removed by brushing and flossing, bacteria stick to the teeth and multiply into larger and larger colonies called plaque. Plaque appears as a sticky, colorless film on the teeth.

Plaque damages the teeth in two ways. First, food particles, especially refined sugars, stick to it. The plaque uses that food to grow more bacteria and to produce acid. Second, the plaque holds the acid against the surface of the teeth. If it isn't removed, the acid will eventually eat through the tooth enamel, causing tooth decay.

Mouth and Dental Problems

Symptoms	Possible Causes
Sores, white spots, or bleeding in mouth or on lips	Canker and Cold Sores, p. 234; Oral Cancer, p. 232.
Bleeding gums	Gum disease. See Plaque and Gum Disease, p. 228.
Toothache	See p. 230.
Bad breath	May be a sign of gum disease, a dental cavity, indigestion, or an upper respiratory infection.
Pain and stiffness in jaw (there may be noise in jaw), with headache	Temporomandibular Disorder, p. 232; Tension Headaches, p. 189.
Hoarseness or voice changes	Laryngitis and Hoarseness, p. 149.
Dry mouth	See p. 231; may be a reaction to a medication.

Tooth decay can occur anytime. However, tooth decay is more likely to happen in the first 30 minutes after you eat, when bacteria produce more acid.

Plaque and Gum Disease

Gum (periodontal) disease is the result of long-term infection of the gums, bone, and other tissues that surround and support the teeth. It is the primary cause of tooth loss in older adults. It is caused by plaque that grows above and below the gumline.

The early stage of gum disease, called **gingivitis**, is marked by red, swollen gums that bleed easily when you brush them or press on them with your finger. Because gingivitis usually does not cause pain, it often is not treated promptly.

As the disease progresses, the gums pull away from the teeth, leaving deep pockets where plaque can grow and do further damage. This stage of gum disease is called **periodontitis**. Eventually gum disease can damage the bones that support the teeth, and the teeth may become loose or fall out.

Denture Care

• Clean your dentures every day with a brush and a denture cleaner, such as Polident or Efferdent.

• Clean fixed bridges with a floss threader or special floss with a stiff threader section.

• Store dentures in lukewarm water or denture-cleansing liquid overnight. Don't let them dry out.

• Examine your gums daily before putting in your dentures. Let red, swollen gums heal before you wear your dentures again. If the redness does not go away in a few days, call your dentist. White patches on the inside of your cheeks could also indicate poorly fitting dentures.

• Give your mouth at least 6 hours of rest from your dentures every day. Your mouth heals more slowly as you age and needs time to recover from the friction of wearing dentures.

• Don't put up with dentures that are too big, click when you eat, or feel uncomfortable. Dentures take some time to get used to, but if they are still giving you trouble after the first few weeks, consult your dentist about a refitting.

• Have your dentures replaced about every 5 years. Dentures suffer from daily wear and tear and need to be replaced regularly.

About 75 to 80 percent of Americans have some form of gum disease. People who have dry mouth (see page 231), those with diabetes, and those who smoke or chew tobacco are at increased risk.

Occasional bleeding when you brush or floss your teeth is an early sign of gum disease. However, if you improve your daily dental care habits (see Prevention) and see your dentist regularly, your gums will eventually tighten up against your teeth and return to a normal pink color. Your dentist can remove plaque and mineral buildup (tartar) from your teeth and gums and may prescribe a special mouthwash that contains chlorhexidine, a drug that kills plaque and helps prevent gum disease.

Prevention

• Brush your teeth and gums at least twice a day, and floss once a day. Brush all surfaces of your teeth, including the inner surfaces (next to the tongue) and outer surfaces (next to the cheek).

• Use a toothbrush with soft bristles and a small head that allows you to reach all parts of your teeth and mouth. Replace your toothbrush every 3 to 4 months. Electric toothbrushes are also effective.

• Brush your tongue regularly. Use toothpaste, and brush vigorously. This will leave your breath sweeter and cleaner.

• Use a fluoride toothpaste. Fluoride is a mineral that strengthens tooth enamel and reduces the harmful effects of plaque.

• Snack on mozzarella cheese, peanuts, yogurt, milk, or sugar-free chewing gum. They help clear the mouth of harmful sugars and protect your teeth against plaque. Avoid high-sugar foods and drinks. Use a toothpick after eating a snack if you can't brush right away (but be careful not to cut your mouth or swallow the toothpick).

• Have your teeth checked and cleaned at least twice a year by a dentist or dental hygienist.

Home Treatment

• Follow the prevention guidelines.

• Call your dentist if you develop a toothache. Toothaches occur when the inside of your tooth (the dentin) is exposed to air. The pain of a toothache may go away temporarily, but the problem that is causing it will not. Take aspirin, ibuprofen, or acetaminophen for pain relief until you can see your dentist. Putting a cold pack on your jaw may also help. Some people find that applying oil of clove to the painful tooth relieves pain too.

When to Call a Dentist

• If you have loose teeth or your teeth have shifted or moved, creating spaces between your teeth.

• If you have pus or blood coming from your gums.

• If your gums have pulled away from your teeth.

• If you have bad breath that doesn't go away with proper dental care.

Get Hold of Your Toothbrush

If you have difficulty brushing your teeth because your hands are stiff, painful, or weak, consider these simple solutions:

• Enlarge the handle of your toothbrush by wrapping a sponge, an elastic bandage, or adhesive tape around it. Or push the handle through a rubber ball for a better grip.

• Lengthen the handle by taping Popsicle sticks or tongue depressors to it.

• Use an electric toothbrush.

You can also buy specially designed toothbrushes, toothpaste dispensers, and floss holders.

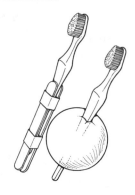

• If you have red, swollen gums or your gums are tender to the touch.

• If you have a toothache.

• If your gums bleed easily when brushed, or if blood from your gums appears on food you are eating (for example, an apple).

• If you have not seen a dentist in 6 months.

Dry Mouth

Many older adults have a dry mouth (xerostomia). Dry mouth can be caused by:

- Breathing through your mouth, especially when the air is dry.

- Having diabetes.

- Taking certain medications, particularly water pills (diuretics), antihistamines, and some antidepressants.

- Not drinking enough water throughout the day.

- Having gum disease.

- Getting radiation treatments to your head or neck.

Sjögren's syndrome is a condition that affects some older women. It causes dry mouth; itchy, burning eyes; and vaginal dryness. Sjögren's syndrome often accompanies autoimmune diseases such as rheumatoid arthritis or lupus.

Chronic lack of saliva can cause mouth problems such as tooth decay, bacterial infections, and bad breath.

Prevention

- Drink 2 quarts of water every day.

- Humidify your home, especially your bedroom.

- Breathe through your nose rather than through your mouth.

- Avoid antihistamines, which dry out the inside of your mouth.

Home Treatment

- Follow the prevention guidelines.

- Practice good dental care. Because lack of saliva increases your risk of tooth decay, regular brushing and flossing are very important to protect your teeth.

- Suck on sugarless candies or chew sugarless gum to increase saliva production.

- Add extra liquid to foods to make them easier to chew and swallow. Drink water with meals.

- Avoid caffeinated beverages, tobacco, and alcohol, all of which increase dryness in your mouth.

- Try saliva substitutes, such as Xerolube, which are available without a prescription.

When to Call a Health Professional

- If dry mouth is making it hard for you to swallow food.

- If dry mouth is accompanied by a persistently sore throat.

- If dry mouth causes denture discomfort.

- If you think dry mouth may be linked to medications you are taking.

Oral Cancer

Oral cancer may develop in any part of the mouth. Risk factors for oral cancer include smoking or chewing tobacco and excessive use of alcohol.

It is important to check regularly for symptoms of oral cancer. See When to Call a Health Professional for a list of symptoms.

Prevention

- Don't use tobacco in any form.
- Drink alcohol only in moderation.
- Get dental checkups twice a year so signs of oral cancer can be detected early.

When to Call a Health Professional

Call if one or more of the following symptoms last longer than 2 weeks without explanation:

- A sore in your mouth that bleeds easily and does not heal
- A lump or thickening in your cheek that you can feel with your tongue
- A white or red patch on your gums, tongue, or the lining of your mouth
- Sore throat or a feeling that something is caught in your throat
- Unexplained difficulty chewing or swallowing, or moving your jaw or tongue
- Numbness in your tongue or other areas of your mouth
- A swelling in your jaw that makes your dentures fit poorly or cause discomfort

Temporomandibular Disorder

The temporomandibular joint (TMJ) is located in front of the ear and connects the lower jawbone to the skull. Pain and discomfort in this joint and in the muscles of the jaw is called temporomandibular disorder (TM disorder).

The symptoms of TM disorder may include:

- Pain in one or both jaws when chewing or yawning.
- Painful clicking, popping, or grating in the jaw joint.
- Locking of the jaw in an open or closed position, or being unable to "open wide."
- Headache, neck pain, facial pain, or shoulder pain.

The most common cause of TM disorder is tension in the jaw, neck, or shoulder muscles. This can be brought on by stress or by habits such as clenching or grinding your teeth. TM disorder can also develop when there is a problem in the temporomandibular joint itself, such as arthritis or an injury resulting from a blow to the face or head.

Home treatment and non-surgical treatments can bring relief for most symptoms of <u>TM disorder</u>. Your doctor may recommend that you use a plastic mouth plate (splint), have physical therapy, or take prescription pain relievers to ease your symptoms. Surgery is rarely needed and may cause further problems.

Prevention

The key to preventing TM disorder is to reduce muscle tension in the jaw. You can do this by following these guidelines:

- Relax. If you have a lot of stress and anxiety in your life, try some relaxation techniques (see page 344).

- Don't bite your nails or cradle the telephone receiver between your shoulder and jaw.

- Stop chewing gum or tough foods at the first sign of pain or discomfort in your jaw muscles.

- Change your diet. Eat softer foods, and use both sides of your mouth to chew your food.

- Maintain good posture. Poor posture may disturb the natural alignment between your facial bones and muscles and cause pain.

- Get regular dental checkups.

Home Treatment

- Continue to follow the prevention tips.

- Avoid opening your mouth too wide.

- Rest your jaw, keeping your teeth apart and your lips closed. Keep your tongue on the roof of your mouth, not between your teeth.

- Put an ice pack on the painful area for 10 minutes, 3 times a day. Gently open and close your mouth while the ice pack is on your jaw. If your jaw muscle is swollen, apply ice 6 times a day.

- Take aspirin, ibuprofen, or acetaminophen to reduce swelling and pain.

- If there is no swelling, apply moist heat (no warmer than bath water) to your jaw muscle 3 times a day for 10 to 15 minutes. Gently open and close your mouth while you apply the heat. Alternate heat treatments with the ice pack treatments.

- Seek help if you are under severe stress or suffer from anxiety or depression. See Mental Health starting on page 317.

When to Call a Health Professional

- If you have severe pain.

- If TM disorder symptoms occur after you have injured your jaw.

- If your jaw locks in certain positions.

- If any jaw problem or pain lasts longer than 2 weeks without improvement.

- If you have noticed a change in the way your teeth fit together when you close your mouth.

Canker and Cold Sores

Canker sores are painful, open sores that form on the inside of the mouth. Possible causes of canker sores include injury to the inside of the mouth, infection, certain foods or medications, stress, a genetic tendency to get canker sores, and female hormones. The sores usually heal in 7 to 10 days. If they are very painful or numerous, see your doctor.

Cold sores (fever blisters) are small, red blisters that usually appear on the lip and outer edge of the mouth. They often weep a clear fluid and scab over after a few days.

Cold sores are caused by a herpes virus. Herpes viruses (chickenpox is another kind) stay in the body after the first infection. Later, something triggers the virus to become active again. Cold sores may appear after you've had a cold or fever, been exposed to the sun, experienced stressful times, or stretched your mouth during a dental appointment. Sometimes cold sores develop for no apparent reason.

Call a health professional:

• If sores develop after you start taking a new medication.

• If a sore does not heal after 14 days.

• If sores are very painful or come back often.

They aren't making mirrors like they used to.
Tallulah Bankhead

15

Skin, Hair, and Nail Problems

Your skin and nails are often where the first telltale signs of age begin to appear. As you age, your skin grows thinner, gets drier, becomes less elastic so wrinkles appear, and takes longer to heal when it is cut or bruised. These changes are more pronounced and come earlier in people whose skin has been repeatedly exposed to sun over the years.

Your nails may get drier and more brittle with age. They may also develop ridges. These changes are usually normal.

The good news is that while some of the skin problems that arise with age may be a nuisance, few are dangerous. Except for certain skin cancers that are not caught early, skin problems rarely cause death. Even though you can't slow down or prevent every change that occurs with age, good self-care can help you keep your skin, hair, and nails looking and feeling as healthy as ever.

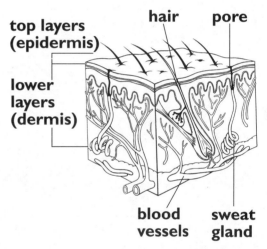

Skin protects your body from dirt and germs and helps you maintain a steady body temperature.

Blisters

Blisters are usually the result of persistent or repeated rubbing against the skin. Some illnesses, such as shingles, cause blisterlike rashes. See Shingles on page 246. Burns can also cause your skin to blister. See Burns on page 40.

235

Skin, Hair, and Nail Problems

Symptoms	Possible Causes
Raised, red, itchy welts or fluid-filled bumps after an insect bite or after taking a drug	Hives, p. 241; Bites and Stings, p. 32.
Red, painful, swollen bump under the skin	Boils, p. 237.
Red, flaky, itchy skin	Dry Skin, p. 239; Fungal Infections, p. 239; Rashes, p. 243.
Rash that develops after you wear new jewelry or clothing, eat a new food, take a new drug, or are exposed to poisonous plants	Rashes, p. 243; Allergies, p. 131.
Red, itchy, blistered rash	Poison ivy, oak, or sumac. See Rashes, p. 243.
Painful blisters in a band around one side of the body	Shingles, p. 246.
Change in the shape, size, or color of a mole, or persistently irritated mole; sore that does not heal	Skin Cancer, p. 247.
Cracked, blistered, itchy, peeling skin between the toes	Athlete's foot. See Fungal Infections, p. 239.
Red, itchy, weeping rash on the groin or thighs	Jock itch. See Fungal Infections, p. 239.
Flaky, silvery patches of skin, especially on the knees, elbows, or scalp	Psoriasis, p. 245.
Sandpapery skin rash with sore throat	Scarlet fever. See p. 155.
Reddish yellow, scaly patches on scalp, forehead, sides of nose, eyebrows, behind ears, center of chest	Seborrheic Dermatitis, p. 243.
Chafing rash between folds of skin in armpit or groin or under breasts	Intertrigo (Chafing), p. 243.
Fingernails or toenails that are thickened, discolored, or soft and crumbly	Fungal Infections, p. 239.
Red or dark spot on skin that does not turn white when you press on it and still looks discolored 30 minutes or more after you change position to take pressure off the area	Pressure Sores, p. 244.

Prevention

- Avoid shoes that are too tight or that rub on your feet.

- Wear gloves to protect your hands when doing heavy chores.

Home Treatment

- If a blister is small and closed, leave it alone. Apply a loose bandage to protect the blister from further rubbing. Avoid the activity or shoes that caused the blister to form.

- If a small blister is in a weight-bearing area, protect it with a doughnut-shaped moleskin pad. Leave the area over the blister open.

- If a blister is larger than 1 inch across, it is usually best to drain it. The following is a safe method:

  - Wash your hands before touching the blister.

  - Sterilize a needle with rubbing alcohol.

  - Gently puncture the blister at the edge.

  - Carefully drain the blister fluid by pressing it toward the hole you have made.

- Once you have opened a blister, or if it has torn open:

  - Wash the area with soap and water.

  - Do not remove the flap of skin covering a blister unless it is very dirty or torn, or if pus is forming

under the skin flap. Gently smooth the skin flap over the tender skin underneath.

  - Apply an antibiotic ointment and a sterile bandage. Do not use alcohol or iodine. They will delay healing.

  - Change the bandage once a day or anytime it gets wet to reduce the chance of infection.

  - Remove the bandage at night to let the area dry.

When to Call a Health Professional

- If blisters form often and you do not know the cause.

- If signs of infection develop. See Signs of a Wound Infection on page 59.

- If you have diabetes or peripheral vascular disease and blisters are forming on your hands, feet, or legs.

Boils

A boil is a red, swollen, painful bump under the skin, similar to an overgrown pimple. Boils are often caused by infected hair follicles. Bacteria from the infection form an abscess or pocket of pus. The abscess can become large and may be extremely painful.

Boils occur most often in areas where there is hair and chafing. The face, neck, armpits, breasts, groin, and buttocks are common sites.

Prevention

- Wash boil-prone areas often with soapy water. An antibacterial soap may help. Dry thoroughly.

- Avoid clothing that is too tight.

Calluses and Corns

Calluses and corns are areas of hard, thickened skin that form when skin is exposed to friction and pressure. Calluses are common on the soles of the feet, the heels, and the hands. Corns usually form on the toes, where shoes press and rub against bone.

You can prevent corns and calluses by avoiding shoes that pinch or cramp your toes or by using insoles to cushion your feet. If you cannot avoid wearing shoes that rub your feet, use moleskin pads for protection.

If a callus or corn becomes painful, soak the area in warm water, and rub the callus or corn with a towel or pumice stone. You may need to do this for several days until the thickened skin is gone. Nonprescription products for removing calluses and corns are also available. If a corn or callus breaks open or becomes sore, see your doctor.

Do not try to cut or burn off corns or calluses. If you have diabetes or peripheral vascular disease, talk with your doctor before attempting to remove troublesome corns or calluses.

Home Treatment

- Do not squeeze, scratch, drain, or open the boil. Squeezing can push the infection deeper into the skin. Scratching can spread the bacteria to other parts of the body.

- Wash yourself well with an antibacterial soap to keep the infection from spreading.

- Apply hot, wet washcloths to the boil for 20 to 30 minutes, 3 to 4 times a day. Do this as soon as you notice a boil. The heat and moisture can help bring the boil to a head, but it may take 5 to 7 days. Applying a hot water bottle or a waterproof heating pad over a damp towel also may help.

- Continue using warm compresses for 3 days after the boil opens. Apply a bandage to keep the draining material from spreading, and change the bandage daily.

When to Call a Health Professional

If it is needed, your doctor can drain the boil and treat the infection. Call your doctor:

- If the boil is on your face, near your spine, or in the anal area.

- If signs of worsening infection develop. See Signs of a Wound Infection on page 59.

- If any other lumps, particularly painful ones, develop near the infected area.

- If the pain limits your normal activities.

- If you have diabetes.

- If the boil is as large as a Ping-Pong ball.

- If the boil has not improved after 5 to 7 days of home treatment.

- If many boils develop over several months.

Dry Skin

As you age, your skin produces less of the natural oil that helps it retain moisture. Dry indoor air can cause your skin to become dry, as can excessive bathing in hot water.

Prevention

- Avoid showers. They strip the natural oil that helps the skin hold in moisture. Baths are much kinder to the skin than showers are.

- Use bath oils in the tub. (Be careful, because bath oil will make the tub slippery!)

- Use mild soaps, such as Dove or Cetaphil, especially under the arms and in the genital area.

- Use a moisturizing lotion immediately after your bath.

Home Treatment

- Follow the prevention guidelines above.

- For very dry hands, try this for a night: Apply a thin layer of petroleum jelly, and wear thin cotton gloves to bed. (Dry feet may benefit from similar treatment.)

- If dry, brittle nails are a problem, use lotion on your nails as well.

- Avoid scratching, which damages the skin. If itching is a problem, see Relief From Itching on page 240.

When to Call a Health Professional

- If you itch all over your body but there is no obvious cause or rash.

- If itching is so bad that you cannot sleep, and home treatment is not helping.

- If your skin is badly broken from scratching.

- If signs of infection develop. See Signs of a Wound Infection on page 59.

Fungal Infections

Fungal infections of the skin most commonly affect the feet, groin, scalp, or nails. Fungi grow best in warm, moist areas of the skin, such as between toes, in the groin, and in the area beneath the breasts.

Athlete's foot is the most common fungal skin infection. Symptoms include cracked, blistered, and peeling areas between the toes; redness and scaling on the soles of the feet; and itching. Athlete's foot often recurs and must be treated each time.

Jock itch causes severe itching and moistness on the skin of the groin and upper thighs. There are usually red, scaly, raised areas on the skin that weep or ooze pus or clear fluid.

Fungal infections of the **fingernails** and **toenails** cause discoloration, thickening, and often softening of the nails. These infections are difficult to treat and often cause permanent damage to the nails.

Relief From Itching

- Keep the itchy area well moisturized. Dry skin may make itching worse.

- Take an oatmeal bath to help relieve itching: Wrap 1 cup of oatmeal in a cotton cloth, and boil as you would to cook it. Use this as a sponge and bathe in tepid water without soap. Or try an Aveeno colloidal oatmeal bath.

- Apply calamine lotion to poison ivy or poison oak rashes.

- Try a nonprescription 1% hydrocortisone cream for small itchy areas. Use it very sparingly on the face or genitals. If itching is severe, your doctor may prescribe a stronger cream.

- Try a nonprescription oral antihistamine, such as Chlor-Trimeton or Benadryl.

- Cut your nails short or wear gloves at night to prevent scratching.

- Wear cotton or silk clothing. Avoid wool and acrylic fabrics next to your skin.

Prevention

- Keep your feet clean, cool, and dry. Dry well between your toes after swimming or bathing. Use antifungal powder to prevent infection or reinfection.

- Wear leather shoes or sandals that allow your feet to "breathe," and wear cotton socks to absorb sweat. Use powder on your feet and in your shoes. Give shoes 24 hours to dry between wearings.

- Wear thongs or shower sandals in public pools and showers.

- Keep your groin area clean and dry. Wash and dry well, especially after exercising, and apply talcum powder to absorb moisture. Wear cotton underclothes and avoid tight pants and panty hose.

- Don't share hats, combs, brushes, or towels.

Home Treatment

- Follow the prevention guidelines.

- For athlete's foot and jock itch, use a nonprescription antifungal powder or lotion, such as Lamisil, Micatin, or Lotrimin AF. Use the medication for 1 to 2 weeks after the symptoms clear up to keep the infection from recurring. Do not use hydrocortisone cream on a fungal infection.

When to Call a Health Professional

• If signs of infection are present. See Signs of a Wound Infection on page 59.

• If you have diabetes and develop athlete's foot. People with diabetes are at increased risk for infection and may need professional care.

• If home treatment fails to clear up athlete's foot or jock itch after 2 weeks.

• If you experience the sudden loss of patches of hair together with broken hairs, flaking, and inflammation of the scalp; or if several members of your household are experiencing hair loss.

 If a <u>fungal infection</u> does not improve after 2 weeks or clear up after 1 month despite home treatment, you may want to consider prescription medication. Discuss the options with your doctor.

Hives

Hives are raised, red, itchy, often fluid-filled patches of skin called wheals or welts that may appear and disappear at random. They range in size from less than ¼ inch to 3 inches across or larger, and they may last a few minutes or a few days.

A single hive commonly develops after an insect sting. Multiple hives often develop in response to a medication, food, or infection. Other possible causes of hives include plant allergies; inhaled allergens; allergy to natural rubber or latex; stress; cosmetics; exposure to heat, cold, or sunlight; or pressure of clothing. Often a cause cannot be found.

Prevention

• Avoid substances that cause you to break out in hives.

• If you know that outbreaks of hives are stress-related, do what you can to reduce stress in your life. See Stress on page 342.

Home Treatment

• Follow the prevention guidelines.

• Apply cool water compresses to help relieve itching. Also see Relief From Itching on page 240.

• Take an oral antihistamine, such as Benadryl or Chlor-Trimeton, to treat the hives and relieve itching. Once the hives have disappeared, decrease the dose of the medication slowly over 5 to 7 days.

When to Call a Health Professional

Call 911 or other emergency services if spreading hives occur with dizziness, wheezing, difficulty breathing, tightness in the chest, or swelling of the throat, tongue, lips, or face.

Call a health professional:

- If hives cover all or most of your body.

- If you develop hives soon after you start taking a new medication.

- If hives persist for 24 hours despite home treatment.

Ingrown Toenails

Ingrown toenails usually develop when an improperly trimmed toenail cuts into the skin at the edge of the nail or when you wear shoes that are too tight. Because the cut can easily become infected, prompt care is needed.

Prevention

- Cut toenails straight across and leave the nails a little longer at the corners so that the sharp ends don't cut into the skin.

- Wear roomy shoes, and keep your feet clean and dry.

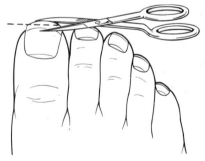

Cut toenails straight across.

Nail Care Tips for Caregivers

People with poor eyesight, joint stiffness, or tremor may have difficulty providing proper nail care for themselves. Present them with the gift of a foot bath, foot massage, and toenail and fingernail trim every few weeks.

Use care when trimming toenails and fingernails for a person who has diabetes or peripheral vascular disease. See pages 169 and 176.

Home Treatment

If you have diabetes or another condition that causes decreased blood circulation to your legs and feet, you may want to contact your doctor to make sure the home treatment tips that follow are appropriate for you.

- Soak your foot in warm water for 15 minutes to soften the skin around the nail.

- Wedge a small piece of wet cotton under the corner of the nail. This will cushion the nail and keep it from cutting the skin. Repeat daily until the nail has grown out and can be trimmed.

- Soaking your foot once or twice a day in warm water will help relieve swelling or tenderness while toenails grow out.

When to Call a Health Professional

- If signs of infection develop. See Signs of a Wound Infection on page 59.

- If you have diabetes or circulatory problems and develop an ingrown toenail.

Rashes

A rash—or dermatitis—is any irritation or inflammation of the skin. Rashes can be caused by infection, allergies, or heat, and sometimes by emotional stress. If you have a rash that developed after you were bitten by a tick, see Bites and Stings on page 32.

Poison ivy and other plant rashes are often red, blistered, and itchy and appear in lines where the plant's leaves brushed against the skin.

When you first get a rash, ask yourself the following questions to help determine its cause (also see page 236):

- Did a rash that affects a specific area of your body (localized rash) develop after you came in contact with anything new that could have irritated your skin: poison ivy, oak, or sumac; soaps, detergents, shampoos, perfumes, cosmetics, or lotions; jewelry or fabrics; new tools, appliances, latex gloves, or other objects? The location of the rash is often a clue to the cause.

- Have you eaten anything new that you may be allergic to?

- Are you taking any new medications, either prescription or nonprescription?

- Have you been unusually stressed or upset recently?

- Is there joint pain or fever with the rash?

- Is the rash spreading?

- Does the rash itch?

Seborrheic Dermatitis

Older adults are especially prone to a rash called seborrheic dermatitis. Small, scaly, reddish yellow patches develop in areas that are particularly oily: behind and in the ears, in the center of the chest, and on the scalp, forehead, eyebrows, and the sides of the nose.

This common problem is caused by overactive oil glands in the skin. Emotional stress, physical exertion, and certain medications can trigger flare-ups. Seborrheic dermatitis responds well to home treatment with dandruff shampoos and nonprescription hydrocortisone creams.

Intertrigo (Chafing)

Intertrigo is a chafing rash that occurs between skin folds. Common sites are the armpits, groin, inner thighs, anal region, and the area beneath the breasts. Moisture, warmth, and friction combine to cause chafing.

Weight loss and some of the home treatment tips that follow can clear up the problem. If the rash is not treated, bacterial or fungal infections may develop.

Pressure Sores

People who have difficulty changing positions while sitting in a chair or lying in bed may develop pressure sores. Pressure sores usually form on bony parts of the body, such as the elbows, heels, knees, buttocks, tailbone, and along the spine. The skin and underlying tissues in these areas are thinner than they are elsewhere on the body. When pressure from a bed or chair limits blood flow to one of these bony areas, the skin and underlying tissues start to break down, and a sore forms.

A pressure sore may first appear as a red or dark spot on the skin that does not turn white when you press on it. The spot will still look discolored 30 minutes or more after you have changed position to take pressure off the area. The area around the sore may feel warm. Over time the sore may deepen, looking like an open wound or a scabbed-over blister.

Pressure sores can become very deep and usually take a long time to heal. They are also prone to bacterial infections, which must be treated with antibiotics.

If you know someone who has difficulty moving by him- or herself, help the person change positions every 1 to 2 hours. Place pillows under bony areas when the person is sitting or lying down. Using a special mattress designed to redistribute the person's weight can also help. Make sure the person eats a nutritious diet, as this is important for maintaining healthy skin.

Check the person's skin daily for signs of pressure sores. Call your doctor immediately if you see signs of a pressure sore.

Prevention

- Avoid products that have caused rashes in the past, such as detergents, cosmetics, lotions, clothing, or jewelry.

- Use fragrance- and preservative-free or hypoallergenic detergents, lotions, and cosmetics if you have frequent rashes.

- If you are exposed to poison ivy, oak, or sumac, wash your skin with dish soap and plenty of water within 30 minutes to get the allergy-causing oil off your skin. This may help prevent or reduce the rash. Also wash your clothes, your dog, and anything else that may have come in contact with the plant.

Home Treatment

- Wash affected areas with water. Soap can be irritating. Pat dry thoroughly.

- Apply cold, wet compresses to reduce itching. Repeat frequently. Also see Relief From Itching on page 240.

- Keep cool and stay out of the sun.

• Leave the rash exposed to the air. Baby powder can help keep it dry. Avoid lotions and ointments until the rash heals. However, calamine lotion is helpful for plant rashes. Use it 3 to 4 times a day.

• Use hydrocortisone cream to provide temporary relief of itching. Use it very sparingly on the face and the genital area.

• Rashes on the feet or groin may be caused by a fungal infection. See Fungal Infections on page 239.

When to Call a Health Professional

• If signs of infection develop. See Signs of a Wound Infection on page 59.

• If you suspect a medication reaction caused the rash.

• If a rash occurs with fever and joint pain.

• If a rash occurs with sore throat. See When to Call a Health Professional in the Sore Throat and Strep Throat topic on page 154.

• If a rash appears and you aren't sure what is causing it.

• If a rash does not go away after 2 to 3 weeks of home treatment.

Psoriasis

Psoriasis is a chronic skin condition that causes raised red patches topped with silvery, scaling skin. The patches most commonly develop on the knees, elbows, scalp, and back. The fingernails, palms, and soles of the feet may also be affected. Psoriasis is not contagious.

The patches, called plaques, are made of dead skin cells that accumulate in thick layers. Normal skin cells are replaced every 28 days. In people who have psoriasis, skin cells are replaced every 3 to 6 days. Psoriasis can also cause a form of arthritis.

Small patches of psoriasis can often be treated with regular use of corticosteroid cream. Other products (lotions, gels, shampoos) may also be useful, although they may increase your skin's sensitivity to the sun. Exposing affected areas to the sun may also help. But be sure to limit the amount of time you spend in the sun, and protect unaffected skin by wearing sunscreen.

Stress may contribute to psoriasis. Stress reduction may help in some cases. See page 342.

Call your doctor if psoriasis covers much of your body or is very red. Extensive or severe cases often need professional care.

Shingles

Shingles (herpes zoster) is an infection caused by reactivation of the chickenpox virus years after the initial illness. After you get over chickenpox, the varicella virus moves to the roots of your spinal nerves and remains there in an inactive state. Later in life the virus may become active again at a time when you are under physical or emotional stress. The reactivated virus causes shingles.

Shingles can affect anyone who has had chickenpox. However, older adults and people with weakened immune systems are more likely to get shingles. Exposure to the shingles rash can cause chickenpox in a person who has not had chickenpox.

Once reactivated, the varicella virus follows the path of the spinal nerves where it was living in an inactive state and infects the skin supplied by those nerves. Since each spinal nerve supplies feeling to one side of the body in a bandlike pattern, the pain and rash of shingles develop in a bandlike pattern. This is the most typical feature of shingles.

The symptoms of shingles develop in stages. First, there is a tingling, burning, throbbing, or stabbing pain on one side of your body. The pain is usually worse when shingles affects your face or scalp. A rash of small blisters appears 2 to 3 days after the pain begins. The blisters scab over after a few days and drop off over the course of a few weeks.

About half of people over 60 who get shingles experience lingering pain called **post-herpetic neuralgia** in the affected nerve. The pain can last for months or even years.

Medication can help limit the pain and discomfort caused by shingles and reduce your risk of developing complications such as post-herpetic neuralgia if it is started within the first 2 to 3 days of the rash.

Prevention

- If you have never had chickenpox, avoid exposure to people who have shingles or chickenpox.

- Consider getting the chickenpox vaccine. It may prevent shingles if you have never had chickenpox. However, it will not prevent shingles if you already have had chickenpox.

- If you have had chickenpox, reduce your chance of getting shingles by maintaining a strong immune system through good nutrition, regular exercise, and healthy living.

Home Treatment

- Avoid picking and scratching blisters. If left alone, blisters will crust over and fall off naturally.

- Apply cool, moist compresses to the rash if you find that this eases discomfort. Calamine or a similar lotion may be applied after the wet compresses. Don't apply so much lotion that it cakes and is hard to remove.

- Applying cornstarch or baking soda to the sores may help dry them so they heal more quickly. After the sores have formed crusts, soaking them with water or Burow's solution (available at most pharmacies) can help clean away the crusts, decrease oozing, and dry and soothe your skin.

- If the rash becomes infected, it should be treated with an antibiotic cream or ointment prescribed by your doctor.

- Avoid contact with children, pregnant women, and other adults who have never had chickenpox until your shingles blisters have dried completely.

When to Call a Health Professional

- If you suspect you might have shingles. If medications are taken near the beginning of an outbreak, they can limit the pain and rash.

- If pain or blisters affect your eyes or eyelids, your forehead, or the tip of your nose; or if you notice changes in your vision.

- If you develop symptoms that indicate shingles may have affected your central nervous system. These symptoms include:

  - Headache and stiff neck.

  - Dizziness.

  - Weakness.

  - Hearing loss.

  - New changes in your thinking and reasoning abilities.

- If skin sores seem to be spreading to other parts of your body.

- If you develop pain in your face or inability to move one or more facial muscles.

- If the rash looks like it has become infected. See Signs of a Wound Infection on page 59.

- If the rash does not heal after 2 to 3 weeks.

Skin Cancer

Skin cancer is the most common type of cancer. Most skin cancer is caused by sun damage and develops on the face, neck, and arms, where sun exposure is greatest. People with light skin and blue eyes are most likely to develop skin cancer. Dark-skinned people have less risk, but they can still develop skin cancer.

Most skin cancers are nonmelanoma skin cancer, which includes basal cell and squamous cell carcinoma. Nonmelanoma skin cancer is rarely life-threatening. Melanoma is a more serious type of skin cancer. It may affect only the skin, or it may spread (metastasize) to other organs and bones. Melanoma can be life-threatening.

 Most nonmelanoma skin cancers are easy to treat if they are caught early. Early surgical removal of thin melanomas can cure the disease in many cases.

Skin cancers differ from noncancerous growths in the following ways:

- They tend to bleed more than non-cancerous growths do and are often open sores that do not heal.

- They tend to be slow-growing. However, malignant melanoma may appear suddenly and grow quickly.

Prevention

Most skin cancers can be prevented by avoiding excessive exposure to the sun. Unfortunately, sun damage from earlier years is often the cause of skin cancer later in life.

Home Treatment

Examine all areas of your skin with a mirror, or have someone else do it for you. Look for unusual moles, spots, bumps, or sores that won't heal. Pay special attention to areas that get a lot of sun exposure: hands, arms, chest, neck, face, ears, etc. Report any changes to your doctor.

When to Call a Health Professional

Call your doctor if you notice any unusual skin changes or growths, especially if they bleed and continue to change.

Asymmetrical shape

Border irregular

Color varied

Diameter larger than a pencil eraser

Watch for these "ABCD" mole changes.

If your moles do not change over time, there is little cause for concern. If you have a family history of malignant melanoma, let your doctor know, because you may be at higher risk for malignant melanoma. Call your doctor if you notice any of the following "ABCD" changes in a mole:

- **A**symmetrical shape: One half does not match the other half.

- **B**order irregularity: The edges are ragged, notched, or blurred.

- **C**olor not uniform: Watch for shades of red and black, or a red, white, and blue mottled appearance.

- **D**iameter: The mole is larger than a pencil eraser. (Harmless moles are usually smaller than this.)

Also call if you notice:

- Scaliness, oozing, bleeding, or spreading of color into surrounding skin.

- Appearance of a bump or nodule on the mole, or any change in the appearance of the mole.

- Itching, tenderness, or pain.

Skin Growths

Most bumps and lumps that occur as a person ages are harmless growths, spots, or skin tags that remain stable once they have appeared.

Seborrheic keratoses are flat, waxy-looking, noncancerous growths that appear on the scalp, face, neck, and trunk. They may look as if they could be easily "picked" off the skin. They are usually light brown when they first appear and may become darker over time.

Cherry angiomas, or ruby spots, are small, reddish purple spots most often found on the trunk and upper legs, but also on the face, neck, scalp, and arms. These harmless bumps are clusters of dilated blood vessels. They will bleed profusely if punctured. Cherry angiomas are increasingly common after age 40.

Skin tags are fleshy, taglike growths of skin that appear on the face, neck, chest, underarms, and groin.

Sebaceous gland growths are small, yellowish bumps that appear on the forehead and face.

Lumps Under the Skin

Most lumps under the skin are not cause for concern. Swollen lymph nodes often develop when the body fights minor infections caused by colds, insect bites, or small cuts. More serious infections may cause the nodes to become very large, firm, and tender.

A lump under the skin that is not related to a swollen lymph node may be a noncancerous growth, such as a lipoma, ganglion or sebaceous cyst, or thyroid nodule; a pocket of pus (abscess) resulting from an infection under the skin; an organ or blood vessel pushing against the skin; or, rarely, a cancerous lump. For information about breast lumps, see Breast Health on page 255.

There is no specific home treatment for swollen lymph nodes other than treating the infection that is causing the lymph nodes to swell.

See a health professional about any lump that concerns you, especially a breast lump; a testicular lump; a lump in your neck that interferes with your breathing; a lump that pulsates like a heartbeat in your abdomen or groin or behind your knee; a painful lump that does not get better after 2 weeks; or a new, hard, fixed lump that changes or grows over the course of several weeks.

Age Spots

Age spots are areas of skin that have changed color because of long-term exposure to sunlight. People used to think that the yellow, red, tan, or brown spots were a sign of liver ailments, hence the name "liver spots." However, the spots have nothing to do with your liver or any other organ except the skin.

Age spots are usually harmless. If you notice a spot that has become irritated or is changing in color, size, or shape, let your doctor know.

Solar or **actinic keratoses** are small red or yellow-brown patches caused by long-term exposure to sunlight. These patches have a crusted, scaly surface. They are considered to be precancerous. If protected from the sun, the patches may grow smaller and disappear. If sun exposure continues, they may eventually change into skin cancers.

Prevention

- Noncancerous growths, such as skin tags, sebaceous gland growths, and seborrheic keratoses, usually cannot be prevented.

- To help prevent actinic keratoses, always use a sunscreen that has a sun protection factor (SPF) of 30 or higher.

When to Call a Health Professional

- If any skin growth changes in size, shape, texture, or color.

- If any sore lasts 4 weeks or longer without healing.

- If a skin growth bleeds or breaks off.

- If a skin growth repeatedly becomes irritated when you shave or when clothing rubs on it.

- If signs of skin cancer develop. See Skin Cancer on page 247.

Sunburn

A sunburn is usually a first-degree burn that involves the outer surface of the skin. Sunburns are uncomfortable but usually can be treated at home unless they are extensive. Severe sunburns in older adults can be serious. Repeated sun exposure and sunburns increase your risk for skin cancer.

Prevention

If you are going to be in the sun for more than 15 minutes, take the following precautions:

- Wear light-colored, loose-fitting, long-sleeved clothes and a broad-brimmed hat to shade your face. Wear sunglasses that provide ultraviolet protection.

• Use a sunscreen that has a sun protection factor (SPF) of 30 or higher. Sunscreens labeled "broad spectrum" can protect the skin from the two types of harmful sun rays (UVA and UVB).

• Apply sunscreen at least 30 minutes before you will be exposed to the sun.

• Apply sunscreen to all the skin that will be exposed to the sun, including your nose, ears, neck, scalp, and lips. Sunscreen needs to be applied evenly over the skin.

• Reapply sunscreen every 2 to 3 hours while in the sun or more often if you are swimming or sweating a lot.

• Drink lots of water to stay hydrated and promote sweating. Sweating helps cool the skin.

• Avoid the sun between 10 a.m. and 4 p.m., when the burning rays are strongest.

Please note: You need a minimal amount of sunshine on your skin to produce vitamin D. Vitamin D and calcium are needed to strengthen bones and prevent osteoporosis. Sunscreens block vitamin D production, so if you use them all the time, you may want to consider boosting the amount of vitamin D in your diet. You can do this by drinking lots of milk fortified with vitamin D or by taking a low-dosage vitamin D supplement (no more than 1,000 IU per day).

Home Treatment

• Drink plenty of water and watch for signs of dehydration. See page 73. Also watch for signs of heat exhaustion. See page 54.

• Cool baths or compresses can be very soothing. Take acetaminophen or aspirin for pain.

• A mild fever and headache can accompany a sunburn. Lie down in a cool, quiet room to relieve headache.

• There is nothing you can do to prevent peeling; it is part of the healing process. Lotion can help relieve itching.

When to Call a Health Professional

• If you develop signs of heat stroke (red, hot, dry skin; confusion). See page 54.

• If symptoms of heat exhaustion (dizziness, nausea, headache) persist after you have cooled off.

• If there is severe blistering (over 50 percent of the affected body part) with fever or if you feel very ill.

• If you have a fever of 102° or higher.

Warts

Warts are skin growths that are caused by a virus. They can appear anywhere on the body. Warts are not dangerous, but they can be bothersome.

Little is known about warts. Most types are only slightly contagious. They can spread to other areas on the same person but rarely to other people. Genital and anal warts are exceptions: they are easily transmitted through sexual contact, and certain types increase a woman's risk for cervical cancer. See pages 259 and 279.

Plantar warts appear on the soles of the feet. Most of the wart lies under the skin surface and may make you feel like you are walking on a pebble.

Warts appear and disappear on their own. They may last a week, a month, or even years. Because warts seem to come and go for little reason, it's possible that they are sensitive to slight changes in the immune system. Although there is no scientific explanation for why it works, in some cases you can "think" warts away.

If it is necessary, your doctor can remove warts. Unfortunately, they often come back.

Home Treatment

- Try the least expensive method of treating warts first. You may save a trip to your doctor. If you find something that works for you, stick with it.

- If you have diabetes or peripheral vascular disease, talk to your health professional before trying home treatment to remove a wart.

- If the wart bleeds a little, cover it with a bandage and apply light pressure to stop the bleeding.

- If the wart is in the way, rub it with a pumice stone or a file, or apply a nonprescription product containing salicylic acid. If you have diabetes or peripheral vascular disease, do not irritate the wart or use salicylic acid on it without first discussing these treatments with a health professional.

- If treatment with salicylic acid causes the area to become tender, taking a 2- to 3-day break from treatment may help relieve pain.

- If you use a pumice stone or file, don't use these items for any other purpose or you may spread the wart-causing virus. Both the debris from the wart and the area of the pumice stone or file that touched the wart can be infectious. Wash your hands with soap after you touch the debris from the wart or the pumice stone or file.

- For plantar warts, apply a doughnut-shaped pad to cushion the wart and relieve pain. Before you go to bed, apply salicylic acid to the wart, and cover the wart with a bandage (or wear a sock). Wash the medication off in the morning.

- Don't cut or burn off a wart.

When to Call a Health Professional

- If the wart area looks infected after being irritated or after the wart is knocked off.

- If a plantar wart is painful when you walk, and foam pads do not help.

- If you have warts in the anal or genital area. See Sexually Transmitted Diseases on page 279.

- If a wart develops on your face and is a cosmetic concern.

 If a wart causes continual discomfort, or if warts are numerous enough to be a problem, they may need to be surgically removed. Talk with your doctor about the risks and benefits of <u>removing warts surgically</u>.

Hair Loss

Many people lose hair as they grow older. Such hair loss is natural and is largely the result of heredity. Balding poses no health risks other than sunburn, which you can prevent by wearing a hat and using sunscreen when outdoors. While men tend to lose hair from the hairline and crown of the head, women's hair becomes thinner all over.

 If you are thinking about medication (such as minoxidil) or surgical treatment for <u>hair loss</u>, make sure you understand the risks of treatment, how many treatments you will need, and how long the results will last.

Bald spots are not the same as baldness. Wearing tight braids or habitually tugging or twisting your hair may cause bald spots.

Ringworm is a fungal infection that causes scaly bald spots. See Fungal Infections on page 239. A condition called alopecia areata causes patchy hair loss that may require treatment with steroid medications.

Thinning hair can signal problems such as thyroid disease or lupus. Emotional or physical stress can cause short-term hair loss, as can changes in hormone levels during menopause.

Hair loss can also be caused or accelerated by a variety of medications, including some drugs for high blood pressure, high cholesterol, arthritis, ulcers, or cancer. If hair loss is sudden, or if it develops after you start taking a new medication, call your doctor.

The most creative force in the world is the
menopausal woman with zest.
Margaret Mead

16

Women's Health

This chapter focuses on health problems that are unique to women. If you are looking for general guidelines for making healthy lifestyle choices to prevent illness and injury, see Aging With Vitality starting on page 15. Specific tips for developing a fitness plan, eating a healthy diet, maintaining a healthy body weight, managing stress, and preventing sexually transmitted diseases are included in other chapters. Use the index to find the information you need.

Breast Health

A woman's risk for developing breast cancer increases as she ages, and the risk is significantly greater after age 50. The good news is that breast cancer can often be cured if it is detected early. There are three methods of early detection: mammography, clinical breast exam, and breast self-exam.

Mammography

A mammogram is a breast X-ray that can reveal breast tumors that are too small to be found by physical examination. The earlier breast cancer is detected, the more likely it is that the cancer can be successfully treated.

Studies have shown that mammograms save lives. In women over 50, mammograms reduce breast cancer death rates by up to one-third.

 The recommended schedule for women over 50 (more specifically, for women past menopause) is a mammogram every 1 to 2 years. Yearly <u>mammograms</u> are recommended for any woman who has had cancer in a breast or has a family history of breast cancer. Don't put it off. You can get information about where to get a mammogram from your doctor or a local hospital or chapter of the American Cancer Society.

Breast Self-Exam

The breast self-exam is a simple technique to help you learn what is normal for you and become aware of any changes. It takes a little practice to learn. At your regular checkup, ask your doctor to show or remind you how to examine your breasts.

If you want to do breast self-exams, a good time is a few days after your period ends, when your breasts are less likely to be swollen or sore.

If you are premenopausal or are taking hormones, your breast tissue will normally have some lumpiness or places where the tissue feels thicker. If the lumpiness is the same in both breasts, it is probably normal. If you find a lump that is different or much harder than the rest of your breast tissue, or if you find anything else that worries you, have it checked by your doctor.

If you are past menopause and are not taking hormones, any new lump you find should be checked by your doctor. Keep in mind that breast lumps can be caused by many things besides cancer.

Preparing for a Mammogram

- Do not wear deodorant, perfume, powder, or lotion, because they can affect the quality of the X-ray.

- Wear clothing that allows you to easily undress from the waist up.

- If you had a previous mammogram at a different facility, have it sent before your test or bring it with you on the day of your mammogram.

Clinical Breast Exam

During a clinical breast exam, a doctor or nurse looks at your breasts and gently feels them for lumps or other unusual changes. He or she may also examine your neck and armpits. During the exam, the doctor or nurse can teach you how to examine your breasts yourself or show you a video explaining breast self-exams.

A clinical breast exam is recommended every year starting at age 40 or whenever a woman has symptoms indicating that there may be a problem with her breasts.

Prevention and Early Detection of Breast Cancer

- Limit your alcohol intake to 1 drink per day. Moderate to heavy drinking increases your risk for breast cancer.

- Eat a low-fat diet. Fat in the diet is linked to an increased risk for breast cancer. Cut down on fried foods and high-fat meats and dairy products. Choose lean meats and low-fat dairy products instead.

- Eat foods that contain vitamins A and C, such as dark green and orange vegetables and fruits. Eat more cruciferous vegetables (broccoli, cabbage, kale). There is some evidence that a diet that includes these foods may reduce your risk for breast cancer.

- Have a mammogram every 1 to 2 years. Talk to your doctor about the best screening schedule for you. If you are over 70, talk with your doctor about whether to continue having mammograms.

- Have a clinical breast exam every year or according to a schedule that you and your doctor agree upon.

When to Call a Health Professional

- If you find a lump in your breast or armpit that concerns you, particularly if it is hard and unlike any other tissue in your breasts.

- If you find a breast lump and you are past menopause and not taking hormones.

- If you have a bloody or greenish discharge from a nipple, or a watery or milky discharge that leaks out when there is no pressure on your nipple or breast.

- If you notice that one of your nipples is inverted (does not point outward).

- If one of your breasts changes shape, or if it seems to pucker or "pull" when you raise your arms.

- If the skin of one breast becomes dimpled like an orange peel.

- If you notice a change in the color or feel of the skin of one breast or the darker area (areola) around the nipple.

- If you have a new pain in one breast that was not caused by an injury and that lasts longer than 1 or 2 weeks.

- If you have any signs of infection in a breast:
  - Pain, swelling, redness, heat, or tenderness in or around the breast.
  - Pus draining from the nipple or a sore or wound on the breast.
  - Fever of 100° or higher without another cause.
  - Swollen, tender lymph nodes under the arm.

Gynecological Health

Regular pelvic exams and Pap tests are vital components of women's health. These exams can detect signs of abnormalities in the reproductive organs. It is better to catch any disease in its early stages, when it may be easier to treat.

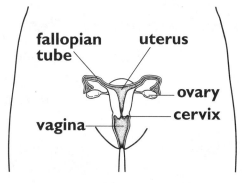

Female pelvic organs

Self-Exam

Self-exams will help you better understand your own body and what is normal for you. Periodically examine your entire genital area for any sores, warts, red swollen areas, or unusual discharge. A normal vaginal discharge may be white to yellowish white and smell slightly like vinegar. It can be either thick or thin and may vary in amount; every woman is different. Your vaginal discharge will change gradually as you age and at menopause. If your discharge seems unusual in amount, smell, or texture, see Vaginitis on page 264.

There should be no pain or straining when you urinate, and the urine should come out in a fairly steady stream. The urine should be pale yellow, and it should not have a strong ammonia smell. If you experience pain or burning when you urinate, see Urinary Tract Infections on page 94 or Vaginitis on page 264. If you have problems with bladder control, see Urinary Incontinence on page 92.

Pelvic Exam and Pap Test

A pelvic exam will generally include an external genital exam, a Pap test, and a manual examination of the uterus and ovaries.

The Pap test is used to screen women for cancer of the cervix (the opening of the uterus). The test is very reliable for detecting abnormal cell changes that could lead to cancer. To do the test, your health professional will insert an instrument called a speculum into your vagina to spread apart your vaginal walls. Then, using a cotton swab, small brush, or wooden or plastic spatula, your health professional will gather several samples of cells from your cervix. The cells are put on a slide or into a solution and sent to a lab for examination under a microscope. Your health professional should let you know the results of your Pap test when they return from the lab. Ask for an explanation of your results if you don't understand them.

 If your Pap test results are abnormal, you will be asked to return for more testing. Your doctor may do another Pap test or may try to find the area in your cervix that contains abnormal cells by using a special magnifying device (colposcopy).

To do a manual exam, your health professional will insert two gloved and lubricated fingers into your vagina and press on your lower abdomen with his or her other hand to feel for any abnormalities in the shape or size of your ovaries and uterus. A digital rectal exam may be done for the same reason as the manual pelvic exam. To do this exam, your health professional will insert one gloved, lubricated finger into your rectum and another into your vagina while pressing on your lower abdomen with his or her other hand.

Scheduling a Pelvic Exam

Pap tests are recommended every 1 to 3 years, depending on whether you have risk factors for cervical cancer. Factors that may increase your risk for cervical cancer include:

- Being infected with the human papillomavirus (HPV), which may cause genital warts or abnormal cervical cells.

- Being infected with the human immunodeficiency virus (HIV).

- Having sexual intercourse with a person who has had many sex partners.

- Having sexual intercourse before age 18.

- Smoking cigarettes.

- Having three or more sex partners in your lifetime.

- Using birth control pills.

If you have risk factors for cervical cancer or a history of abnormal Pap tests, it is recommended that you have a Pap test each year.

You and your doctor may decide that it is appropriate for you to have Pap tests less often if:

- You have had several normal Pap tests in a row (done annually).

- You have only one sex partner.

- You do not have a history of abnormal Pap tests, cervical cancer, or a sexually transmitted disease such as genital warts.

- You have had a hysterectomy with removal of your cervix for a reason other than cancer.

- You are older than 65 years of age.

Do not douche, have sexual intercourse, or use feminine hygiene products for at least 24 hours before a Pap test, because doing any of these things can alter the test results.

Screening for Endometrial Cancer

Endometrial (uterine) cancer affects the lining of the uterus. It can be successfully treated if it is detected early.

Irregular vaginal bleeding or vaginal bleeding that occurs after you have completed menopause may be a warning sign of endometrial cancer.

The pelvic exam (see page 258) is an important part of the exam for endometrial cancer. If a pelvic exam reveals changes in the shape or size of your uterus or if you are having abnormal vaginal bleeding, further testing, such as an ultrasound exam or an endometrial biopsy, will probably be necessary. Ultrasound is a procedure that uses sound waves to create pictures of an organ in your body. An ultrasound exam of the uterus can detect uterine tumors and thickening of the uterine lining. An endometrial biopsy is an outpatient procedure in which small samples of tissue are removed from the uterine lining. The tissue samples are examined under a microscope to see if any cancerous changes have occurred.

Taking estrogen-only replacement therapy (ERT) to treat menopause symptoms and prevent osteoporosis increases your risk for endometrial cancer. If you take estrogen and you still have your uterus, you also need to take the female hormone progesterone for protection against endometrial cancer. If you do not take progesterone, your doctor may recommend annual ultrasound exams to screen for endometrial cancer.

Screening for Ovarian Cancer

Ovarian cancer is the second most common cancer of the female reproductive organs. When detected early, ovarian cancer may be successfully treated. Unfortunately, ovarian cancer is difficult to detect until it has grown and spread. Regular pelvic exams may detect ovarian cancer before it causes symptoms.

Menopause

Menopause is a normal part of life, marking the end of a woman's menstrual periods and her ability to become pregnant. It occurs as a result of the body's producing smaller amounts of the female hormones estrogen and progesterone. Menopause is a process that usually begins 2 to 5 years before a woman's last menstrual period and is complete when she has gone 1 full year without having a menstrual period. Most women go through menopause between the ages of 45 and 55.

Hysterectomy Guidelines

Hysterectomy is the surgical removal of the uterus. It is generally done to treat disease. However, there are times when other treatments may work as well with fewer risks.

Hysterectomy is often the best treatment for:

- Uterine, cervical, or ovarian cancer.
- Severe endometriosis.
- Severe uterine bleeding.
- Large, noncancerous tumors (fibroids) that cause severe bleeding and pain or press on the bladder.
- Severe uterine prolapse (uterus falls into the opening of the vagina).

Conditions that may respond to nonsurgical treatments include:

- Precancerous changes on the cervix.
- Abnormal uterine bleeding.
- Fibroids that cause mild symptoms.
- Mild to moderate uterine prolapse.
- Pelvic inflammatory disease.

 Getting all the facts and thinking about your own needs and values will help you make the best decision about hysterectomy.

MORE INFO For more information, see the back cover.

Decreasing levels of estrogen are responsible for many of the symptoms associated with menopause and for long-term health problems that can develop after menopause, such as osteoporosis. Hormone therapy can ease some menopause symptoms and reduce your risk for osteoporosis. See Hormone Therapy on page 263. At the onset of menopause, you and your health professional can develop a plan to help you deal with menopause symptoms and protect yourself against long-term health problems. The plan you and your health professional develop may address one or more of the following menopause-related issues.

Irregular periods. The hormonal changes that occur during menopause may cause you to have irregular periods before your periods stop altogether. This may mean that your menstrual flow will be lighter or heavier than usual; that the intervals between your periods will be shorter or longer; or that you will have spotting between periods. Some women have regular periods until their periods stop suddenly, and others have irregular periods for a long time until menopause.

Birth control. Although you may be less fertile during the years just before the onset of menopause, you may continue to release eggs (ovulate) and could become pregnant. If you do not wish to become pregnant, continue to use birth control until your doctor confirms that you have reached menopause or until you have not had a menstrual period for 12 months.

Hot flashes. Hot flashes are sudden periods of intense heat, sweating, and flushing. A hot flash usually begins in the chest and spreads out to the neck, face, and arms. Seventy-five to 80 percent of women going through menopause will have hot flashes. Hot flashes may occur as frequently as once an hour and last from a few minutes to an hour. If they occur at night, they may disrupt your sleep patterns. Disrupted sleep can lead to insomnia, fatigue, irritability, or inability to concentrate.

Hot flashes usually stop within 1 or 2 years but may persist for several years. They are rarely noticed by others.

Vaginal changes. Vaginal changes that occur during menopause include vaginal dryness caused by the loss of lubrication and moisture in the vagina; thinning of the vaginal walls and loss of elasticity in them; and shrinkage of the outer lips (labia) of the vagina. Pain, irritation, and discharge resulting from these changes is known as atrophic vaginitis. These vaginal changes can lead to soreness during and after sexual intercourse and may also increase your risk for vaginal infections and urinary incontinence. See Vaginitis on page 264 and Urinary Incontinence on page 92.

Mood changes. The hormonal and physical changes of menopause can cause mood changes. Symptoms such as nervousness, lack of energy, insomnia, moodiness, or depression are common.

Many women think that menopause means emotional upset and the loss of sexuality. Other women feel positive about the changes that occur with menopause, such as freedom from menstruation and the risk of pregnancy. Understanding what is happening to you and having a plan for dealing with symptoms will help you through menopause. You may want to include some of the home care tips that follow in your own menopause plan.

Home Treatment

Irregular Periods

Keep a written record of your periods in case you need to discuss them with a health professional.

Hot Flashes

Hot flashes usually improve after 1 to 2 years. In the meantime:

- Keep your home and workplace cool, or use a fan.

- Wear layers of loose clothing that can be easily removed. Wear natural fibers such as silk and cotton.

- Drink cold beverages rather than hot ones, and limit your intake of caffeine and alcohol.

- Eat smaller, more frequent meals to avoid heat generated by digesting large amounts of food.

- Exercise regularly and try some of the relaxation techniques discussed on page 344.

Vaginal Dryness

- Use a water-soluble vaginal lubricant, such as Astroglide or Replens, to ease discomfort during sexual intercourse. Vegetable oil will also work. Do not use petroleum-based products such as Vaseline.

- Frequent sexual intercourse will help maintain muscle tone in your vagina. Firm muscle tone in the vagina may also help problems such as urinary incontinence.

Mood Changes

The best thing you can do for yourself is to realize that you are not alone. Discuss your symptoms with other women. Give yourself, and ask others for, abundant amounts of love, caring, and understanding. Try to develop a relaxed attitude about menopause. Tension and anxiety may make your symptoms worse.

Hormone therapy may improve hot flashes, vaginal dryness, and mood changes in addition to protecting you from osteoporosis, but it also has potential side effects and risks. See Hormone Therapy on page 263. Some women find that progesterone cream eases menopause symptoms such as irregular bleeding, hot flashes, and memory problems. Progesterone cream is available with or without a prescription.

Hormone Therapy

During and after menopause, a woman's body produces much less of the hormones estrogen and progesterone. Hormone therapy may be prescribed to treat symptoms of menopause. There are two types of hormone therapy:

- Estrogen replacement therapy (ERT). ERT is estrogen alone. Because ERT may increase the risk of endometrial (uterine) cancer, it is usually prescribed only for women who have had a hysterectomy.

- Hormone replacement therapy (HRT). HRT combines estrogen with progestin, another female hormone. Progestin reduces the effect of estrogen on the uterine lining and protects against endometrial cancer.

Hormone pills are taken every day. Some forms of hormone therapy are available as skin patches, vaginal creams, or vaginal rings.

 <u>Hormone therapy</u> reduces the discomfort of menopausal symptoms such as hot flashes and vaginal dryness and helps maintain bone density. It can also have unpleasant side effects such as bloating, breast tenderness, and irregular vaginal bleeding. Hormone therapy appears to have significant risks, including an increased risk of breast cancer, stroke, and heart conditions. (It is not clear to what extent estrogen alone carries these risks.) For some women, however, the short-term benefit of reducing menopausal symptoms may outweigh the risks. Talk with your doctor about whether starting or continuing hormone therapy is a good idea for you.

Hormone therapy usually is not recommended for women who have had breast cancer, endometrial cancer, problems with blood clots, heart attack, stroke, liver disease, or undiagnosed uterine bleeding.

There are other approaches to relieving menopause symptoms that you may want to learn more about and discuss with your doctor. These include exercise, diet therapy, and herbal therapy. Ongoing studies are evaluating the effectiveness of foods that contain chemicals called phytoestrogens for relieving menopause symptoms. Phytoestrogens are found in soy-based foods (tofu, soy milk), legumes, fennel, and parsley. Soy-based foods contain other substances that may protect against heart disease, osteoporosis, and cancer. Herbs such as black cohosh (for relief of hot flashes) and ginkgo biloba (for improving memory) are widely used, but they have not been approved by the Food and Drug Administration (FDA) for the treatment of menopause symptoms.

When to Call a Health Professional

- If your menstrual periods are unusually heavy, irregular, or prolonged (1½ to 2 times longer than usual).

- If bleeding occurs between periods when your periods have been regular.

- If bleeding recurs after periods have stopped for 6 months.

- If vaginal dryness is not relieved with a vaginal lubricant. Your doctor may prescribe a vaginal cream or suppositories that contain estrogen.

- If your symptoms are interfering with your life and home treatment does not help.

- If you are considering hormone therapy or other medical treatment.

- If you have unexplained vaginal bleeding that is different from what your health professional told you to expect while you are taking hormones.

Vaginitis

Vaginitis is any vaginal infection, inflammation, or irritation that causes a change in normal vaginal discharge. Vaginitis is a common problem, and some women are more prone to it than others. Postmenopausal women are more likely to get vaginitis because of the decreased estrogen level in their bodies. An aggravating fact about vaginitis is that it can recur.

Vaginal yeast (candidiasis) infections are the most common cause of vaginitis in older women. A yeast infection is caused by an excess growth of yeast organisms in the vagina.

Yeast infections can cause severe discomfort, but they rarely cause serious problems. Typical symptoms of a vaginal yeast infection include vaginal itching that may be severe; a white, curdy, usually odorless vaginal discharge; and pain or burning when urinating and during sexual intercourse.

Yeast infections are often associated with taking antibiotics or corticosteroids, having diabetes, or having an illness that weakens the immune system.

Other causes of vaginitis include bacterial vaginosis and trichomoniasis, which is caused by a parasite spread through sexual contact. Some other sexually transmitted diseases can cause unusual vaginal discharge or vaginal irritation. See Sexually Transmitted Diseases on page 279.

Irritation caused by douching frequently, wearing tight clothing, or using strong soaps or perfumed feminine hygiene products may also contribute to vaginitis.

If you have burning and pain when you urinate and feel the need to urinate often, see Urinary Tract Infections on page 94.

Prevention

- Wash your vaginal area once a day with plain water or a mild, nonperfumed soap. Rinse well and dry thoroughly. Don't douche unless your health professional advises you to do so.

- Avoid the use of feminine deodorant sprays and other perfumed products. They dry and irritate tender skin.

- Wipe from front to back after using the toilet, to avoid spreading bacteria from your anus to your vagina.

- Limit the number of your sex partners, and use condoms during sexual intercourse. Having multiple sex partners may increase your risk for vaginitis by changing the normal environment of your vagina. It also increases your risk of becoming infected with a sexually transmitted disease.

- Wear cotton or cotton-lined underpants. Avoid tight-fitting pants and undergarments, including panty hose. They increase heat and moisture in the vaginal area, and these conditions may allow yeast to grow more easily in your vagina.

- Drink acidophilus milk or eat yogurt that contains live *Lactobacillus* organisms. Yogurt may prevent vaginal infections. This is especially helpful if you are taking antibiotics, which can kill the healthy bacteria that grow in your vagina.

- If you have diabetes, controlling your blood sugar levels will help prevent yeast infections.

Home Treatment

A vaginal infection may clear up without treatment in 3 or 4 days. If your symptoms do not improve, call your doctor.

- Follow the prevention guidelines.

- Avoid sexual intercourse in order to give irritated vaginal tissues time to heal.

- Don't scratch. Relieve itching by applying cold water compresses or taking cool baths.

- If you are very sure that you have a yeast infection (you have had one before and the symptoms are exactly the same), use a nonprescription antifungal medication that contains clotrimazole or miconazole (such as Gyne-Lotrimin or Monistat 7) as directed.

When to Call a Health Professional

- If you have pelvic or lower abdominal pain, fever, and unusual vaginal discharge.

- If you have pain or bleeding after sexual intercourse (and the pain is not eased by a vaginal lubricant, such as Astroglide).

- If you have an unusual or foul-smelling vaginal discharge.

- If you have vaginal itching that does not go away after you use a nonprescription medication for yeast infections.

- If you think you've been exposed to a sexually transmitted disease (see page 279). Your sex partner may need to be treated too.

If you plan to see a health professional, do not douche, use vaginal creams, or have sexual intercourse for 48 hours or longer before your appointment. Doing any of these things may make it difficult to diagnose the problem.

*My doctor says I'm on the verge of becoming an
old man. I place no stock in that. I've been
on the verge of becoming an angel all my life.*
Mark Twain

17

Men's Health

This chapter focuses on health problems
that are unique to men. If you are looking
for general guidelines for making
healthy lifestyle choices to prevent illness
and injury, see Aging With Vitality starting on page 15. Use the index to find
other information you may need.

Genital Health

Daily cleansing of the penis, particularly
under the foreskin covering an uncir-
cumcised penis, can prevent bacterial
infections.

Daily washing also reduces the already
low risk of penile cancer. Because the risk
of testicular cancer is very low in older
men, testicular self-exams are usually not
recommended after age 50.

Call a health professional:

• If you have unexplained groin pain.

• If you notice any penile discharge. Also
see Sexually Transmitted Diseases on
page 279.

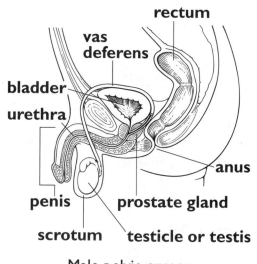

Male pelvic organs

Erection Problems

As a man ages, the speed of his sexual
response slows, his drive to reach orgasm
is delayed, and the force of his ejacula-
tions gradually decreases. These physical
changes need not be seen as problems. In
many cases, they can prolong sensual
enjoyment prior to orgasm.

Although occasional erection problems are common, healthy men of all ages are able to have erections.

A man has erectile dysfunction when he has persistent difficulty achieving or maintaining an erection that is sufficient to have satisfactory sexual intercourse.

Most erection problems are caused by a combination of physical and psychological factors. Physical causes of erection problems include illnesses, injuries, or complications of surgery (such as prostate surgery) that interfere with nerve impulses or blood flow to the penis. The use of certain medications, tobacco, alcohol, or illegal drugs may also lead to erection problems.

Psychological causes of erection problems include depression, anxiety, stress, grief, or problems with relationships. These problems interfere with the erection process by distracting a man from things that would normally arouse him.

Prevention

Most erection problems can be prevented or resolved by taking a more relaxed approach to lovemaking and by watching for possible side effects from medications or illnesses. Follow the tips outlined in Home Treatment.

Home Treatment

• First rule out medications as a cause of erection problems. Many drugs, especially blood pressure medicines, water pills (diuretics), and mood-altering drugs, can cause erection problems.

Ask your doctor or pharmacist to check your prescription medications for possible side effects on sexual function. You may be able to take different drugs that do not have this side effect. Do not stop taking any medication without talking to your doctor first.

• Avoid alcohol and tobacco products, which can make erection problems worse.

• Cope with stress. Tension in your life can distract you and make getting erections difficult. Regular exercise and other stress-relieving activities may help ease tension.

• Talk to your partner about your problems and concerns. Sexual intimacy is a form of communication. If you and your partner aren't talking outside the bedroom, it's unlikely that you will have good sexual intimacy.

• Take time for more foreplay. Let your partner know that you would enjoy more stroking. Slow down; then slow down some more.

• Make sure you're ready. If you are grieving over a loss, you may not be ready for erections and sexual intercourse. Give yourself some time. Worrying about sexual performance may only worsen erection problems.

• Find out if you can have erections at other times. If you can have an erection on awakening or during masturbation, the problem may be related to stress or an emotional factor.

- Avoid unproven remedies. Many products available in health food stores or through magazine advertisements promise relief of erection problems. They have never been medically proven to work and can also be expensive.

 If you have tried home treatment for a few months but your symptoms have not improved, you may wish to talk with your doctor about erection-producing medications or injections, a vacuum device, or a penile implant.

Getting all the facts and thinking about your own and your partner's needs and values will help you make a wise decision about treatment for <u>erection problems</u>.

When to Call a Health Professional

Seek care immediately:

- If an erection lasts longer than 4 hours after you use an erection-producing medication.

- If you have taken an erection-producing medication (such as Viagra, Levitra, or Cialis) in the past 24 hours and you are having chest pain. Do not take nitroglycerin tablets if you have taken Viagra, Levitra, or Cialis in the past 24 hours.

Call a health professional:

- If an erection problem develops after you start taking a new medication or change the dose of a medication.

- If your symptoms develop after a recent injury.

- If erection problems occur with signs of a hormonal imbalance, such as loss of pubic or armpit hair or breast enlargement.

- If you have other symptoms such as urinary problems, pain in the lower abdomen or lower back, or fever.

- If an erection problem is affecting your self-image or sense of well-being.

- If the problem has not improved despite home treatment.

Prostate Infection (Prostatitis)

The prostate is a small gland that lies under the bladder, about halfway between the rectum and the base of the penis. It encircles the urethra, the tube that carries urine from the bladder out through the penis. The prostate produces some of the fluid that transports sperm during ejaculation.

Prostatitis is a painful condition of the prostate gland. Types of prostatitis include acute and chronic bacterial prostatitis, inflammatory chronic pelvic pain, and noninflammatory pelvic pain. With the exception of acute bacterial prostatitis (in which the symptoms are severe, come on suddenly, and include fever and chills), it is difficult to determine the type of prostatitis a man has based on symptoms alone.

Symptoms associated with prostatitis include:

• Having a frequent urge to urinate, especially at night, but passing only small amounts of urine.

• Feeling a burning sensation when you urinate.

• Having difficulty starting a urine stream; having an interrupted or weaker-than-usual urine stream; being unable to empty your bladder completely; and dribbling after you urinate.

• Feeling pain or discomfort in your lower back, scrotum, the area between your scrotum and anus, your lower abdomen, upper thighs, or above your pubic area (this pain may get worse when you pass stools).

• Having prostate pain or vague discomfort during or after ejaculation.

Bacterial prostate infections usually respond well to self-care and antibiotics. If the infection recurs, long-term antibiotic treatment may be needed. Pelvic pain and prostate inflammation that are not caused by bacterial infection usually respond to home treatment.

Prevention

• Wash your penis daily.

• Drink enough water and other fluids so that you urinate regularly.

• If you develop symptoms of a urinary tract infection, seek treatment promptly. See Urinary Tract Infections on page 94.

• If your doctor prescribes an antibiotic for bacterial prostatitis, take the full amount prescribed. This can reduce your risk of having another infection in the future.

Home Treatment

• Avoid alcohol, caffeine, and spicy foods, especially if they make your symptoms worse.

• Take hot baths to help soothe pain and relieve stress.

• Eat plenty of high-fiber foods, and drink enough water to avoid becoming constipated. Straining to pass stools can be very painful when your prostate is inflamed.

• Take aspirin, ibuprofen, or acetaminophen to help relieve pain.

When to Call a Health Professional

• If symptoms of prostatitis are severe, come on suddenly, and occur with fever and chills.

• If your urine is bloody, red, or pink and there is no dietary reason why your urine might look this way (for example, if you had eaten beets). Always call your doctor if you have blood in your urine.

• If urinary symptoms (frequent urge to urinate, a burning sensation when urinating) occur with:

  - Persistent low back pain.

  - Lower abdominal pain.

- Pain in the area between your scrotum and anus.

- Pain in your upper thighs or above your pubic area (may get worse when you pass stools).

- Pain when you ejaculate.

• If you have recurrent urinary tract infections.

• If there is an unusual discharge from your penis. Also see Sexually Transmitted Diseases on page 279.

• If you have symptoms such as difficulty getting a urine stream started, inability to empty your bladder completely, or a frequent urge to urinate (especially at night).

• If symptoms continue for 5 days despite home treatment.

Prostate Enlargement

As a man ages, his prostate may grow larger. This condition is called benign prostatic hyperplasia, or BPH. This seems to a be natural process and is not really a disease. As the prostate gets bigger, however, it may squeeze the urethra and cause urinary problems, such as:

• Difficulty getting a urine stream started and completely stopped.

• A frequent urge to urinate, or being awakened by the urge to urinate.

• Decreased force of the urine stream, or splitting of the stream.

• Dribbling after urinating. (A small amount of dribbling after urinating is common and is not necessarily a sign of prostate problems.)

• A sensation that the bladder is not completely empty after urinating.

An enlarged prostate is not a serious problem unless it makes urination extremely difficult or causes urine to get backed up in the urinary tract, which can lead to bladder infections or kidney damage. BPH does not cause prostate cancer, and it has no effect on a man's ability to have erections or father children.

 Surgery is usually not necessary for an enlarged prostate. Many men find that their symptoms are stable, and symptoms sometimes clear up on their own. In these cases, the best treatment may be no treatment at all. Medications are available that may help minimize your symptoms. Your doctor can advise you about the various treatment options.

Home Treatment

• Avoid antihistamines, decongestants, and nasal sprays, which can make urinary problems worse. Check with your doctor or pharmacist to find out if urinary retention is a side effect of any prescription medications you are taking. You may be able to take different drugs that do not have this side effect. Do not stop taking any prescription medication without talking to your doctor first.

- The berries of the saw palmetto plant contain substances that can relieve urinary symptoms related to prostate enlargement. Saw palmetto extract is available in capsule, tablet, and liquid forms and as a tea. Saw palmetto has not been approved by the Food and Drug Administration (FDA) for the treatment of symptoms of prostate enlargement. Herbal remedies are not subject to the same testing or purity standards that prescription and non-prescription medications are. The amount of drug in herbal preparations varies widely, and herbs may be contaminated with metals and other harmful substances. If you choose to use saw palmetto, let your health professional know. For more information about the risks and benefits of using herbs to treat your health problems, see Complementary Medicine starting on page 347.

- Drink plenty of fluids throughout the day to help prevent urinary tract infections. If you are bothered by a frequent need to urinate at night, cut down on beverages before bedtime, especially those containing alcohol or caffeine.

- Don't postpone urinating, and take plenty of time. Try sitting on the toilet instead of standing to urinate.

- Also see Urinary Incontinence on page 92.

When to Call a Health Professional

- If you are unable to urinate, or if you feel as if you cannot empty your bladder completely.

- If you develop a fever, lower back or lower abdominal pain, or chills.

- If there is blood or pus in your urine.

- If you take water pills (diuretics), tranquilizers, antihistamines, decongestants, or antidepressants. Some of these medications can aggravate urinary problems. Ask your doctor if there are different medications you could take that will not cause urinary side effects.

- If the symptoms of an enlarged prostate come on quickly, are bothersome enough that you want help, or last longer than 2 months.

Prostate Cancer

Prostate cancer is the second leading cause of cancer deaths in men. When detected early, before it has spread to other organs, prostate cancer may be curable. A man's risk for prostate cancer increases with age, and most cases develop in men over age 65. Prostate cancer sometimes runs in families, is more common in African-American men, and tends to be more common in men who eat a high-fat diet.

Since prostate cancer tends to develop late in life and usually grows slowly, most older men who have prostate cancer don't die from the disease. Men younger than 65 who have prostate cancer (but no other serious health problems) are more likely to die of the cancer than older men are.

There are no specific symptoms of prostate cancer. Most men have no symptoms at all. In a few cases, prostate cancer may cause urinary symptoms similar to those associated with prostate enlargement (see page 271). In advanced cases, symptoms such as pain may develop if the cancer spreads to other organs or to the bones.

Prostate cancer treatment is tailored to each individual. Learn all you can about the available treatment options—which may include watchful waiting—so that you and your doctor can select one that will give you the greatest long-term benefit. Your age, overall health, other medical conditions, and the characteristics of your cancer are all important factors to consider when you make treatment decisions.

Prevention

There is no known way to prevent prostate cancer. However, you may reduce your risk of developing prostate cancer by:

- Eating a low-fat diet that includes plenty of fruits and vegetables.

- Including foods that contain tomatoes or tomato sauce in your diet.

- Increasing your intake of soy products.

- Taking certain dietary supplements. Researchers are studying the possibility that vitamin E, selenium, and green tea may help prevent prostate cancer. Talk to your doctor before taking any type of supplement.

 There is controversy about the value of using digital rectal exams and the prostate-specific antigen (PSA) blood test to screen all men for <u>prostate cancer</u>. Detecting early prostate cancer may not improve quality of life or prolong life, especially in men who are older or have other serious health problems. Therefore, many experts are uncertain whether routine screening is appropriate for all men. Talk with your doctor about your risks for prostate cancer and whether screening tests are appropriate for you.

When to Call a Health Professional

- If you have blood or pus in your urine.

- If any urinary symptoms (see Prostate Enlargement on page 271) come on quickly, are bothersome enough that you want help, or last longer than 2 months.

- If you want to discuss screening for prostate cancer, especially if you have a relative who developed prostate cancer.

Age may well offer the opportunity to understand sex as intimate communication in its finest sense.
Norman M. Lobsenz

18

Sexual Health

Sex and sexuality communicate a great deal: affection, love, esteem, warmth, sharing, and bonding. These gifts are as much the birthright of those in their 80s and 90s as of those who are much younger.

Three aspects of sexuality are covered in this chapter: the changes that come with aging, suggestions on how to adjust to these changes, and information about sexually transmitted diseases.

Sexuality and Physical Changes With Aging

In most healthy adults, pleasure and interest in sex do not diminish with age. Age alone is no reason to change the sexual practices that you have enjoyed throughout your life. However, you may have to make a few minor adjustments to accommodate any physical limitations you may have or the effects of certain illnesses or medications.

Common Physical Changes in Men

- A man's sexual response begins to slow down after age 50. However, a man's sexual drive is more likely to be affected by his health and his attitude about sex and intimacy than by his age.

- It may take longer for a man to get an erection, and more time needs to pass between erections.

- Erections will be less firm. However, a man who has good blood flow to his penis will be able to have erections that are firm enough for sexual intercourse throughout his entire life. For information about erection problems, see page 267.

- Older men are able to delay ejaculation for a longer time.

Common Physical Changes in Women

Most physical changes take place after menopause and are the result of decreased estrogen levels. These changes can be altered if a woman is taking hormone therapy.

- It may take longer for a woman to become sexually excited.

- A woman's skin may feel more sensitive and irritable, making caressing and skin-to-skin contact less pleasurable.

- The walls of the vagina become thinner and drier and are more easily irritated during sexual intercourse. Use a water-based vaginal lubricant, such as Astro-glide, K-Y Jelly, or Replens, to reduce the irritation. Do not use petroleum jelly. A doctor can also prescribe a vaginal cream containing estrogen, which will help reverse the changes in the vaginal tissues.

- Orgasms may be somewhat shorter than they used to be, and the contractions experienced during orgasm can be uncomfortable.

Not all women experience these problems. Those who do can experiment to find ways to enjoy sex despite these physical changes.

Sexuality and Cultural and Psychological Changes

In addition to physical changes, there are cultural and psychological factors that affect sexuality in later years. For example, in our culture, sexuality is equated with youthful looks and youthful vigor. Too many people seem to think that as a person ages, he or she becomes less desirable and less of a sexual being. Older adults may accept this stereotype and buy into the notion that they are not permitted or expected to be sexual.

Joy in sex and loving knows no age barriers. Almost everyone has the capacity to find lifelong pleasure in sex. To believe in the myth that older people have no interest in sex is to miss out on wonderful possibilities.

Being single through choice, divorce, or widowhood can present a problem as well. By the time a person reaches age 60, there are 5 single women for every single man, and that ratio goes up with increasing years. Women and men who are single may not know how to deal with their sexual feelings. Generally speaking, it is better to express your desires than to suppress them until you are no longer aware that they exist.

Physical and emotional needs change with time and circumstance. Intimacy and sexuality may or may not be important to you. The issue here is one of choice. If you freely decide that sex is no longer right for you, then that is the correct decision. It is possible to live a fulfilling life without sex. However, if you choose to continue enjoying your sexuality, you deserve support and encouragement. You may still find uncharted sensual territories to explore.

Use It or Lose It: Staying Sexual

Just as exercise is the key to maintaining fitness and health, having sex on a regular basis is the best way to maintain sexual capacity.

And just as it's never too late to start an exercise program, it's never too late to start having sex. Many older people who have been celibate for years develop satisfying sexual practices within new loving relationships. For others, self-stimulation is common and poses no health risks or side effects.

Here are some additional considerations:

• To enhance sexual response, use more foreplay and direct contact with sex organs.

• The mind is an erogenous zone. Fantasy and imagination help arouse some people. Try setting the mood with candlelight and soft music, or whatever else "turns you on."

• Many medications, especially high blood pressure medications, tranquilizers, and some heart medications, inhibit sexual response. Ask your doctor about these side effects. Your doctor may be able to reduce your dosage or prescribe different medications. Do not stop taking prescription medications without consulting your doctor first.

• Colostomies, mastectomies, and other procedures that involve changes in physical appearance need not put an end to sexual pleasure. Communicating openly about your fears and expectations can bring you and your partner closer together and help you overcome barriers. If necessary, a little counseling for both of you can help you adjust.

• People who have heart conditions can enjoy full, satisfying sex lives. Most doctors recommend that you abstain from sex for only a brief time following a heart attack. If you have angina, ask your doctor about taking nitroglycerin before you have sex. Do not take Viagra if you are using nitroglycerin.

• If arthritis keeps you from enjoying sex, experiment with different positions. Try placing cushions under your hips. Also try home treatment for arthritis pain. See page 113.

• Use lubricants such as K-Y Jelly or Replens if vaginal dryness or irritation is a problem.

• Drink alcohol only in moderation. Small amounts of alcohol may heighten your sexual responsiveness by squelching your inhibitions. Larger amounts of alcohol may increase your sexual desire, but they decrease sexual performance.

- Prescription medications that can enhance the sexual response—such as sildenafil citrate (Viagra) for men and testosterone for women—are available. Some people find that herbs such as ginkgo biloba and ginseng enhance their sexual function. Both prescription drugs and herbal remedies carry the risk of side effects. Your health professional can help you decide whether these options are right for you.

Other Aspects of Sexuality

Sexuality goes far beyond the physical act itself. It is part of who we are. It involves our needs for touch, affection, and intimacy.

Touch

Touch is a wonderful and needed sensation. Babies who are not touched do not thrive. Children who are not touched develop emotional problems. Touch is important to older adults as well. Touch helps us feel connected with others and enhances our sexuality.

- Get a massage. Professional massages are wonderful, but simple shoulder and neck rubs feel great too. Find a friend who will trade shoulder rubs with you. See page 354 for instructions on massage.

- Look for hugs. Everybody needs them. Some people are a little shy about hugs, but it's okay to ask, "Would you like a hug?"

- Consider getting a pet. Caring for a pet can help meet your needs for touch. Some studies have shown that older people who have pets to care for live longer.

Affection

To give and receive affection is a wonderful feeling. If you like someone, be sure to let them know. If someone seems to like you, appreciate it. It is never too late to make new friends and strengthen bonds with longtime companions.

Intimacy

Intimacy is the capacity for a close physical or emotional connection with another person. Intimacy is a great protector against depression.

Talking with a confidant can help ease life's problems. When you lose a loved one, intimacy may be what you miss most. You may not find someone to fully replace a loved one who died, but you can begin to rebuild intimacy in your life in the following ways:

- Turn to your children, siblings, or old and new friends.

- Look for another person who is in the same situation as you are. One of the richest benefits of support groups is that members often find intimacy with one another.

- Be available to others. Just as you need people, there are people who need you too.

Sexually Transmitted Diseases

Sexually transmitted diseases—also known as STDs or venereal diseases—are infections passed from person to person through sexual intercourse, genital contact, or contact with semen, vaginal fluids, or blood. Many of these diseases can also be spread by sharing needles and other items that may be contaminated with infected blood or body fluids. STDs can affect anyone, no matter what his or her age. Talk openly with your partner about STDs and take whatever precautions are necessary to protect yourself before you engage in any form of sexual contact (see Prevention on page 282).

Chlamydia

Chlamydia is a bacterial infection that affects millions of men and women. It may be difficult to detect chlamydia; up to 80 percent of women and 50 percent of men with the disease have no symptoms, but they can still infect their sex partners. If symptoms do show up, they occur 1 to 3 weeks after exposure to the bacteria. In women, symptoms may include vaginal discharge or irregular menstrual bleeding, pain or burning when urinating, or lower abdominal pain. In men, there may be a discharge from the penis and pain or burning when urinating.

Chlamydia is easily treated with antibiotics. If undetected and untreated, chlamydia can cause pelvic inflammatory disease in women and inflammation of the epididymis (a coiled tube at the top of the testicle) in men. Both partners need to be treated.

Genital herpes

Genital herpes is caused by the herpes simplex virus, which also causes cold sores. Genital herpes is easily spread through sexual contact and any other direct contact with genital herpes sores. Symptoms of the first genital herpes outbreak occur 2 to 7 days after contact with an infected person. It is also possible to be infected with genital herpes and have no symptoms.

The first outbreak of genital herpes may be quite severe, with many painful sores or blisters. Fever, swollen glands, headache, and muscle aches may also occur. If herpes sores develop inside the urethra or anus, you may have pain when you urinate or pass stools. Sores in the vagina can cause vaginal discharge. The sores crust over and disappear in 2 to 3 weeks.

 There is no known cure for genital herpes, although medication can reduce pain and speed healing of sores during an outbreak. Most people with genital herpes have recurrent outbreaks. Having four outbreaks per year is typical. Outbreaks tend to become less frequent and less severe over time. Itching, burning, or tingling may occur at the place where the sores will later appear. If you have very frequent or severe outbreaks, taking medication every day can reduce how often outbreaks occur and how long they last.

Genital warts

Genital warts are caused by the human papillomavirus (HPV), which is spread through sexual contact. The warts generally look like small, fleshy bumps or flat, white patches and appear on the lips (labia) around the vagina, inside the vagina, on the penis or scrotum, or around the anus. A person infected with HPV may never develop genital warts, or the warts may be too small to be seen. Certain types of HPV increase a woman's risk for cervical cancer. A Pap test may detect HPV if it is infecting the cervix.

 If genital warts are bothersome or develop on the cervix, they can be treated by a health professional. However, treatment does not cure HPV infection, and the warts may persist or recur. There does not appear to be an effective cure for HPV infection at this time. However, in many people the infection goes away by itself and does not cause further problems.

Gonorrhea

Gonorrhea is a bacterial infection that is spread through sexual contact. Symptoms appear 2 days to 2 weeks after infection and may include pain or burning with urination, vaginal discharge, irregular menstrual bleeding, or a thick discharge from the penis. Many people who are infected with gonorrhea have no symptoms.

Untreated gonorrhea can lead to pelvic inflammatory disease in women and prostate infection in men. It sometimes spreads to a person's joints, causing arthritis. Antibiotic treatment cures the infection. Both sex partners need to be treated to keep from passing the infection back and forth.

Hepatitis B

Hepatitis B is a viral infection that is spread through contact with infected blood, semen, or vaginal fluid. The hepatitis B virus is very contagious and may be spread to household contacts other than sex partners by sharing such things as razors and toothbrushes. Most people with hepatitis B recover completely after 4 to 8 weeks, but a small percentage of adults remain infected for months or years. Chronic infection can lead to life-threatening liver damage or cancer. For more information, see Hepatitis on page 85.

Medication for chronic hepatitis B infection is not very effective. People at risk for hepatitis B infection should receive the hepatitis B vaccine. Those at risk include people with more than one sex partner; men who have sex with men; people who use intravenous drugs; and health care workers.

Human immunodeficiency virus (HIV)

Human immunodeficiency virus (HIV) is spread when blood, semen, or vaginal fluids from an infected person enter someone else's body. Once a person becomes infected, the virus attacks and gradually weakens his or her immune system. Acquired immunodeficiency syndrome, or AIDS, is the last phase in HIV disease, when the body is no longer able to fight infection or disease. Without treatment, AIDS develops in most people 12 to 13 years after they first become infected with HIV. With treatment, AIDS may be delayed for many more years.

A person is said to be HIV-positive if antibodies to the virus are detected in his or her blood. Antibodies may not appear for up to 6 months after a person is exposed to the virus. However, the virus can be spread to others before antibodies or symptoms are apparent.

The specific behaviors that spread HIV include:

• Having more than one sex partner.

• Having sex without using condoms properly. Unprotected sex between men (other than in a relationship in which both sex partners have sex only with each other and neither is infected) is especially risky.

• Sharing needles, syringes, or other "drug works" with someone who is HIV-positive.

• Having a sex partner with a history of any of the above risk factors.

Because all donated blood has been tested for HIV since 1985, the risk of getting the virus from transfused blood or blood products is extremely low.

HIV is not spread by mosquitoes, toilet seats, being coughed on by an infected person, having casual contact with someone who is HIV-positive or who has AIDS, or donating blood. Being touched, hugged, or lightly kissed by someone who is HIV-positive will not transfer the virus to you.

A simple, confidential blood test can determine if you are HIV-positive. You can have the test done in your doctor's office or at the local health department. A saliva test is available for home use as well. If you engage in activities that put you at risk for HIV infection, have an HIV test every 6 months. Early diagnosis and treatment of HIV are important even before symptoms develop. If you think you have been exposed to HIV but you test negative, you should be tested again 6 months after your last known exposure to HIV.

People who educate themselves about <u>HIV</u> infection learn how to make wise health decisions about preventing the spread of the virus and seek treatments that may improve their chances for staying healthy longer.

Syphilis

Syphilis is a bacterial infection spread by sexual contact and through sharing needles that are contaminated with an infected person's blood. When syphilis is spread through sexual contact, symptoms appear about 3 weeks after infection occurs. The first symptom is a red, painless sore that appears on the genitals, rectal area, or mouth. The sore may go unnoticed and go away on its own. Swollen lymph nodes near the sore are another possible symptom.

If syphilis is not treated early, it can proceed to a second phase after about 2 months. Symptoms of the second phase include skin rash, patchy hair loss, fever, swollen lymph nodes, and flulike symptoms that are easily confused with other illnesses.

Syphilis can be cured with antibiotics; both partners need to be treated. If left untreated, syphilis may cause serious health problems and death.

Trichomoniasis

Trichomoniasis is a bacterial infection that is spread by sexual contact. In women, the bacteria usually infect the vagina or urethra. In men, infections can develop in the urethra or under the foreskin of the penis. Up to 50 percent of women who have trichomoniasis have no symptoms, and symptoms in infected men are rare. If symptoms do appear, they do so 4 to 28 days after infection occurs. Symptoms in women may include vaginal discharge, itching, and irritation and pain during sexual intercourse and when urinating. In men there may be a discharge from the penis and pain or burning when urinating.

Trichomoniasis usually does not lead to serious illness. However, the infected person and his or her sex partner need to be treated with antibiotics to keep from passing the infection back and forth. Condoms should be used or intercourse avoided until treatment is completed.

Prevention

Preventing a sexually transmitted disease is easier than treating an infection once it occurs. Only monogamy between uninfected partners or sexual abstinence completely eliminates the risk. The following **safer sex guidelines** will help you reduce your risk of becoming infected with an STD or spreading an infection to someone else.

- If you are beginning a new sexual relationship:

  - Take time before having sex to talk about HIV and other STDs. Find out if your partner has ever been exposed to or infected with an STD or if your partner's behavior puts him or her at risk for HIV infection. Tell your partner if you've ever engaged in high-risk behavior. Remember that it is possible to be infected with an STD without knowing it.

  - Use latex condoms every time you have sex (vaginal, anal, or oral) until you are certain that neither you nor your partner has any STDs and that neither of you will have unprotected sexual contact with anyone else while your relationship lasts. Spermicide does not prevent STDs. If it irritates the skin or tissues in your genital area, it may increase your risk of becoming infected.

  - If you plan to use HIV testing to decide whether it is safe to have unprotected sex, have the test done 6 months after the last time you engaged in high-risk behavior. In the meantime, use condoms every time you have sexual contact.

- Avoid unprotected sexual contact with anyone who has symptoms of or has been exposed to an STD or with anyone whose behavior puts him or her at risk for HIV infection. Keep in mind that a person may still be able to transmit STDs, including HIV, even if no symptoms are present.

- Avoid unprotected vaginal, anal, or oral sex with anyone whose sexual history may not be risk-free or who has sores on the genitals or mouth. Use latex condoms from the beginning to the end of sexual contact. "Natural" or lambskin condoms do not protect against HIV infection or other STDs.

- Do not rely on spermicides or a diaphragm to protect against STDs. Except for abstinence, latex condoms provide the best protection against STDs, including HIV.

- Avoid sexual contact while you or your partner is being treated for an STD.

- If you or your partner has genital herpes, avoid sexual contact when a blister or open sore is present. Use condoms unless you are in a stable, monogamous relationship and you have considered the risks associated with having unprotected sex with a person who has genital herpes. Remember that herpes can be spread even when sores are not present.

- Avoid activities that may spread HIV. Safer activities include closed-mouth kissing, hugging, massage, and other pleasurable touching.

- Never share needles, syringes, razors, or other personal items that could be contaminated with blood.

If your job or behavior puts you at risk for HIV infection, or if you come in contact with HIV-infected blood (for example, an accidental needle stick), contact a health professional immediately.

In some cases, medications may prevent HIV infection if they are started within a few hours after you are exposed to the virus. Have a blood test 6 months after any activity or accident that puts you at risk for HIV infection.

For more information, call the National AIDS Hotline at 1-800-342-AIDS.

When to Call a Health Professional

All STDs need to be diagnosed and treated by a health professional. Your sex partner may also need to be treated, even if he or she has no symptoms. Otherwise, your partner may reinfect you or develop serious complications.

Call a health professional:

- If you notice any unusual discharge from the vagina or penis; if you notice sores, redness, or growths on the genitals; or if you suspect that you have been exposed to an STD.

- If your behavior puts you at risk for exposure to HIV, or if your sex partner has high-risk behavior or is HIV-positive.

- If you have symptoms, including fatigue, weight loss, fever, diarrhea, cough, or swollen lymph nodes, that do not go away after a short period of time and do not seem to be related to another illness. Early symptoms of HIV infection may mimic the flu.

- If you are HIV-positive and you develop any of the following:

  - Fever higher than 103°.

  - Fever higher than 101° that lasts 3 days or longer.

  - Increased outbreaks of cold sores or any unusual skin or mouth sores.

  - Severe numbness or pain in the hands and feet.

  - Rapid, unexplained weight loss.

  - Unexplained fever and night sweats.

  - Severe fatigue.

  - Diarrhea or other bowel changes.

  - Shortness of breath and a persistent dry cough.

  - Swollen lymph nodes in the neck, armpits, or groin.

  - Personality changes, difficulty concentrating, confusion, or severe headache.

Even if you are on the right track, you will get
run over if you just sit there.
Will Rogers

19

Fitness

What would you say if someone told you there is a simple thing you can do that would:

- Make you stronger and more flexible and improve your balance?

- Reduce your risk of heart disease?

- Help you maintain a healthy body weight?

- Improve your mood and give you more energy?

Would you do it? Of course you would! A famous doctor who studies older adults once said that if this thing could be put into a pill, it would be the most widely prescribed drug in the world. What is it? It's exercise!

But what if it's been years since you've exercised? Can you still benefit? Definitely! Even if you have health problems that limit your mobility or your endurance, you can still find enjoyable activities to help you get results that will make a difference. It's absolutely guaranteed.

Your Personal Fitness Plan

No one can prescribe the perfect fitness plan for you. You have to figure it out based on what you enjoy doing and what you will continue to do. The next few pages can be a big help.

Consistency is the most important, most basic, and most often neglected part of people's fitness efforts. No matter which activities you choose to do, you need to do them regularly in order to get the most benefit.

A good fitness plan has three parts: aerobic fitness, muscle strengthening, and flexibility. Many physical activities stress two or all three of these aspects of fitness. Read the sections that follow to learn about each aspect of fitness; then see Setting Your Fitness Goals on page 290.

Don't forget the important role that nutrition plays in your healthy lifestyle. A balanced diet and regular physical activity go hand in hand to help you maintain a healthy body weight. Good nutrition also plays an important role in keeping your bones healthy so you can stay active. Review Nutrition starting on page 301 to learn how to plan a healthy diet.

Benefits of Exercise

Exercise is one of your best defenses against many problems that are associated with aging.

Problem	How Exercise Helps
Arthritis	Improves flexibility and range of motion; improves muscle strength; helps protect joints.
Chronic obstructive pulmonary disease (COPD)	Improves endurance and feeling of well-being.
Constipation	Regular activity keeps waste moving through your bowels.
Depression	Improves self-image; increases energy level; often improves mood.
Diabetes (type 2)	Helps the body use blood sugar more efficiently; helps control weight; increases longevity.
Heart disease	Helps lower cholesterol; improves the heart's ability to pump blood; increases longevity.
High blood pressure	Lowers blood pressure; improves heart and lung health.
Insomnia	Reduces stress and promotes relaxation. Exercising early in the day often improves sleep.
Obesity	Reduces weight by burning calories; helps maintain a healthy body weight.
Osteoporosis	Weight-bearing exercise (walking, lifting weights) helps maintain bone strength.

Aerobic Fitness

Aerobic exercise improves the function of your heart and lungs. The purpose of aerobic conditioning is to increase the amount of oxygen that is delivered to your muscles, which allows them to do more work. It also helps you avoid weight gain.

Generally speaking, any activity that raises your heart rate can be considered aerobic exercise. Some of the more common and easy-to-do aerobic exercises are discussed in the pages that follow.

You don't have to go out of your way to improve your aerobic fitness. Many activities that you do each day raise your heart rate. If you do them regularly and long enough, they will help you become more fit. Current recommendations are to be physically active for at least 30 minutes a day. If 30 minutes seems like a lot, you can accumulate it in several 5- to 10-minute sessions. The following ordinary activities all count as aerobic activity:

- Sweeping or mopping floors (perhaps to fast-paced music)

- Raking leaves, shoveling snow, or pushing a lawn mower

- Taking the stairs instead of the elevator

- Walking across the parking lot at the shopping center instead of parking close to the entrance

When to Slow Down or Stop Exercising

Exercising to stay fit may cause minor muscle and joint soreness at first. That's not a problem. However, it's a good idea to stop exercising if any of the following symptoms develop:

- Chest or upper abdominal pain or pressure that may spread to the neck, jaw, upper back, shoulders, or arms. Many people mistake these symptoms of heart trouble for indigestion or heartburn. See Chest Pain on page 140.

- Panting or extreme shortness of breath.

- Nausea.

- Persistent pain, joint discomfort, or muscle cramps.

The effects of exercise last long after your workout is over. If you find you are having trouble sleeping, you may be exercising too late in the day.

Mild muscle aches and minor strains are to be expected when you first start an exercise program. However, if persistent muscle soreness does not go away after 1 to 2 weeks, you may need to modify your exercise routine.

Walking

Walking is a terrific form of aerobic exercise. It improves endurance and overall health. It causes few injuries. It is inexpensive, and it's enjoyable whether you are alone or in a group. You can do it almost anywhere.

If you want to start walking for health right now, great! Put this book down and go! It's as easy as that.

The following tips may increase the benefits and your enjoyment of walking:

• Walk at a steady pace, brisk enough to make your pulse and breathing increase, but not so fast that you can't talk comfortably. See How Hard Should I Exercise? on page 288.

• Don't worry about your duration at the beginning. Consistency is what's important. As time goes by and your fitness improves, you'll likely find yourself walking longer (and picking up your pace).

• If there is a shopping mall in your area, find out if there is a walking program there. Mall walking is a popular and safe way to exercise (and meet new friends) when the weather is bad.

• Find out about other organized walking groups in your community if you're looking for companionship. Ask at the local senior center, YMCA, or YWCA. Or simply ask a family member, friend, or neighbor to join you.

Dancing

Dancing is one of the most fun ways to exercise and meet people. Fast-paced dancing keeps your heart and lungs in shape, strengthens your leg muscles, and can help improve your balance. Check the Yellow Pages for businesses that offer dance lessons, or watch for dance classes being offered at the local senior center.

Swimming

Swimming, water aerobics, and water jogging are forms of aerobic exercise that are easy on your joints and muscles.

Check into what's available in your community. Organized classes are often available, as are open pool times when you can exercise by yourself.

Bicycling

Bicycling is another aerobic activity that is kind to joints and muscles. If you are not inclined to head out onto the open road (helmet firmly on your head), try a stationary bike (no helmet required). The health benefits are the same even if the scenery doesn't change.

How Hard Should I Exercise?

In order to benefit from aerobic exercise, you need to work hard enough to increase your heart rate. Work hard enough to feel the effort, but not so hard that you become out of breath. Above all, listen to your body. If the exercise feels too hard, slow down. You will reduce your risk of injury and enjoy the exercise much more.

Try the "talk-sing test" to determine your ideal exercise pace:

• If you can't talk and exercise at the same time, you are going too fast.

• If you can talk while you exercise, you are doing fine.

• If you can sing while you exercise, it would be reasonable to increase your pace a little.

Muscle Strengthening

When it comes to your muscles, the most important advice you can follow is this: Use it or lose it. Muscles become soft, flabby, and weak if they are not being used. Muscles that get regular use stay strong, no matter what your age.

If you're not likely to join a gym or an organized fitness class to pump iron, try doing resistance exercises at home using inexpensive rubber tubing (see page 295), books, or soup cans. Ordinary housework and yard work, such as scrubbing the bathtub, washing walls, tilling the garden, or pulling weeds, can become muscle-strengthening activities if you do them regularly. Walking up and down stairs is a great way to strengthen your legs (and build endurance).

Other simple, safe, and effective strengthening exercises can be found on pages 292 to 299. Most of the aerobic exercises discussed earlier will also help strengthen large muscle groups.

Flexibility

Many people notice a significant loss of flexibility as they grow older. Their legs, back, neck, and shoulders all seem so much stiffer than before. That stiff feeling can affect the way you walk and your sense of balance. Is this part of growing older? Maybe not.

Arthritis pain reduces joint mobility. However, if you want to be more flexible so that you can avoid injuries, garden more comfortably, walk more smoothly, or get out of bed more easily, you can. Only minutes per day of slow, pleasant, relaxing stretching will give you results you can feel immediately. Stretching after exercise, when your muscles are warmed up, is particularly helpful.

There are many classes that teach stretching. Yoga and tai chi classes are popular and effective. Swimming will help improve flexibility, and so will the exercises on pages 292 to 299.

• Stretch slowly and gradually. Don't bounce. Maintain a continuous tension on the muscle.

• Relax and hold each stretch for a count of 10.

• Exhale as you stretch to further relax your muscles. If stretching hurts, you are doing something wrong.

• Try to stretch a little every day, even if you don't have a regular exercise session planned.

Getting Started: Tips for Beginners

If you are just starting a new exercise program, congratulations! You've already accomplished the most difficult task—deciding to do something to improve your fitness. Here are a few things to keep in mind as you begin your adventure.

- Start your new routine gradually. See the section called How Often and How Long Should I Exercise? on page 291.

- Remember that you can accumulate 30 minutes or more of physical activity each day with multiple short activity sessions.

- If you're going to exercise for more than just a few minutes, spend the first 5 or 10 minutes of your exercise routine warming up your muscles by walking and then doing some of the stretches on pages 292 to 299. Slowing your pace and adding some gentle stretches at the end of your routine will lower your heart rate gradually, improve your flexibility, and reduce the chance of stiffness and injury.

- Expect some minor muscle and joint soreness and stiffness at first. Muscles that are not used to strenuous exercise will be sore for a day or two after you exercise. Adding new exercises and increasing the duration of your exercise routine also can cause soreness. This is normal and is not a cause for concern as long as the discomfort is not severe and does not last. Stretching before and after you exercise will help prevent soreness and stiffness. See When to Slow Down or Stop Exercising on page 287.

- Drink water before, during, and after exercise to avoid dehydration.

- Let your doctor know that you plan to start a new fitness routine, especially if you have a chronic health problem. He or she may have special recommendations for you. See Exercise Cautions on page 291.

- If you join an organized exercise class, let your instructor know about any health conditions you have. He or she may ask you to modify or avoid certain exercises that could cause you problems.

Setting Your Fitness Goals

If you want to improve your physical fitness, here's one piece of advice: Try to improve a little bit at a time.

- Pick one aspect of fitness (aerobic, strength, flexibility) that you want to improve first.

- Pick an activity that you enjoy. You're more likely to keep doing something you like.

- Set a 1-week goal that you think you can reach. For example, plan to walk for 10 minutes a day, 3 days a week, or to stretch for 5 minutes each morning.

- Start today. Keep a record of what you do.

- When you reach your first goal, reward yourself! Then set a new goal. Once you get used to meeting weekly goals, try setting a monthly goal.

- If you haven't met your goal, think about why you haven't met it. What changes do you need to make to be successful?

Exercise Cautions

Moderate exercise is safe for most people. However, if you answer yes to any of the following questions, talk with your doctor before starting an exercise program.

- Do you have heart trouble?

- Do you often have pain or pressure in your heart or chest?

- Do you have high blood pressure?

- Do you often feel faint or have dizzy spells?

- Do you have arthritis or other bone or joint problems that might be made worse by exercise?

- Do you have diabetes? (Increased exercise affects your insulin needs.)

- Do you have 2 or more risk factors* for heart disease?

- Are you over 40 and planning to do hard exercise?

*Cholesterol over 200 mg/dl, blood pressure over 140/90, smoking, diabetes, obesity, inactive lifestyle, family history of heart disease before age 50

How Often and How Long Should I Exercise?

The three factors you need to consider when planning a fitness routine are:

- Frequency (how often you exercise).

- Duration (how long you exercise).

- Intensity (how hard you exercise).

Achieving a balance between these three factors will give you better results than if you take any one of them to an extreme. You may choose to do a vigorously paced physical activity, such as swimming, fast dancing, or cycling, 3 times a week for 30 minutes per session. Or you may choose moderate exercise, such as walking or yard work, and do it 5 to 6 times a week for 30 minutes per session. The first routine stresses intensity while the second stresses frequency. Both routines are probably equally effective for improving your overall fitness.

If 30 minutes of exercise a day is an unrealistic goal for you, aim for 15 to 20 minutes or several short sessions. You don't have to do the exercise all at once. Three 10-minute walks are probably as good for you as one 30-minute walk.

If you are doing a repetitive activity, such as the strength and flexibility exercises described later in this chapter, start by doing 3 to 5 repetitions. Increase the number of repetitions when you can do 5 repetitions with ease. Always take time to rest between exercises.

It's all right to exercise every day (after you've built up your endurance) as long as you don't start feeling extremely fatigued and don't have persistent muscle or joint pain. These problems are your body's way of telling you that it needs more rest.

Fit Fitness Into Your Life

Whether you're just starting a new fitness routine or you've been physically active for years, there will be days when exercising just doesn't feel good. Oncoming illness, a poor night's sleep, worry, or a busy schedule can all keep you from getting the most out of your exercise routine. Listen to what your body and mind are trying to tell you. Try to keep going, but if you feel like you are struggling, stop and forget about it for that day. Don't feel guilty about taking a day off.

Unless you are ill, start your routine again the very next day. Chances are, you'll enjoy the activity even more because you've given your body the rest it was asking for. If you do end up taking a short break from your fitness routine, start again at a lower level of exertion. Even a short layoff can result in a loss of conditioning, but you'll soon regain what was lost. Coming back gradually will reduce your risk of injury.

One of the simplest ways to stay on track is to record your progress in a notebook or on a calendar. Each day write down:

• What you did.

• How long you did it.

• How hard you felt your effort was.

• Your attitude or motivation for that day.

Exercises for Muscle Strength and Flexibility

The exercises on the following pages will help improve your strength and flexibility. Try to do some of these exercises every day. Try them first thing in the morning for an invigorating wake-up!

• Do these exercises slowly.

• Breathe deeply and don't hold your breath.

For exercises that help strengthen your back and abdominal muscles, see pages 101 to 104.

Neck

Slow Neck Stretches

• Gently lower your right ear toward your right shoulder. Hold for 5 counts.

• Bring your head back to center.

• Gently lower your chin to your chest. Hold for 5 counts.

• Return to center.

• Gently lower your left ear toward your left shoulder. Hold for 5 counts.

• Return to center.

• Do this exercise 5 times.

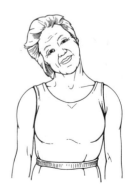

Slow neck stretches

Half-Circles

- Keep your chin level.

- Gently turn your head to the right. (Try to look over your shoulder.) Hold for 2 counts.

- Gently turn your head to the left. Hold for 2 counts.

- Do this exercise 5 times.

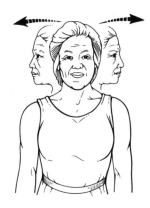

Half-circles

Shoulders and Upper Back

Shoulder Rolls

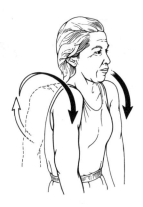

Shoulder rolls

- Keep your arms relaxed and at your sides.

- Trace large circles in the air with your shoulders.

- Roll forward 5 times, backward 5 times.

Arm Circles

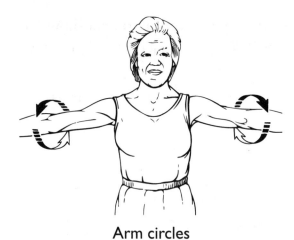

Arm circles

- Raise your arms out from your sides to shoulder level. Keep your elbows straight.

- Rotate your arms from the shoulders in small circles.

- Do 10 circles forward, 10 backward.

Hands and Wrists

Finger Squeezes

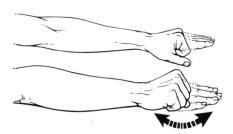

Finger squeezes

- Extend your arms in front at shoulder level, palms down.

293

Healthwise for Life

- Slowly squeeze your fingers to form a fist; then release. Do this 5 times.

- Turn your palms up. Squeeze and release. Do this 5 times.

Hand Circles

- Extend your arms in front at shoulder level. Keep your elbows straight, but not locked.

- Rotate your wrists in small circles.

- Do 10 circles to the right, 10 to the left.

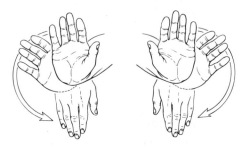

Hand circles

Torso

Spine Twists

- Sit or stand with your back straight, head high.

- Raise your arms out from your sides to shoulder level. Bend your elbows so your forearms are upright, with palms facing forward.

- Keep your hips and knees facing forward.

- Slowly twist your upper body to the right. Hold for 5 counts.

- Return to center; then twist to the left. Hold for 5 counts.

- Do this exercise 5 times.

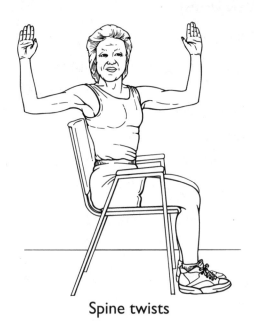

Spine twists

Knee Flexors and Lower Abdomen

Knee Lifts

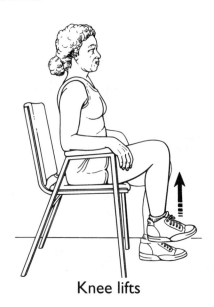

Knee lifts

- Sit in a chair with both feet on the floor.

- Raise your right knee to your chest or as far up as possible. Do not pull up or push down on the chair with your hands.

- Return to the starting position.

- Bring your left knee to your chest or as far up as possible.

- Do this exercise 5 times.

Ankles

Ankle and Foot Circles

- Sit in a chair and cross your right leg over your left knee.

- Slowly rotate your right foot, making large circles.

- Repeat with your left foot by crossing your left leg over your right knee.

- For each ankle, do 10 rotations to the right, 10 to the left.

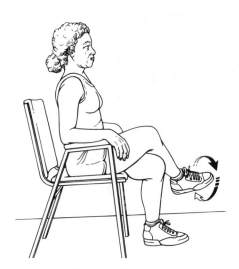

Ankle and foot circles

Rubber Tubing Exercises

These exercises will improve strength and flexibility in the arms and shoulders. They will also build strength in the chest and back. To do these exercises, you will need a 24-inch length of surgical latex tubing with knots tied at each end. Some exercise "stretchies" (such as Thera-Band or REP Band) are sold at fitness and home medical supply stores. Go slowly and be careful not to overstretch the tubing. Keep a firm grip on the tubing; you don't want it snapping back at you!

Start by holding each stretch for a count of 5. You may increase the time as you get stronger.

Stretch and Reach

- Shorten the tubing by holding one end with one hand and gripping the middle of the tubing with the other hand.

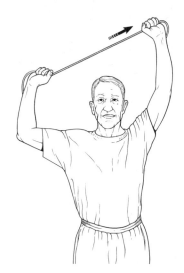

Stretch and reach

- Raise both arms overhead, hands facing forward.
- Reach for the ceiling with alternate hands.
- Do this 5 times with each hand.

Overhead Pull

- Raise both arms overhead, hands facing forward.
- Tighten the tubing by slowly pulling both arms away from center. Do not overstretch.
- Do this 5 times.

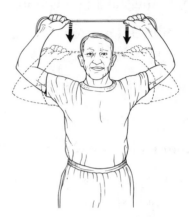

Up-down pull

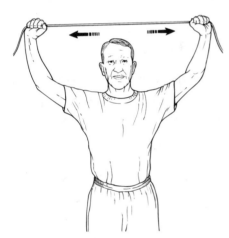

Overhead pull

Chest-Level/Lap-Level Pull

- Raise your arms in front of you to shoulder level.
- Pull your hands apart, stretching the tubing.
- Do this 5 times.
- Drop your arms to the level of your lap.
- Pull your hands and arms apart, away from your body.
- Do this 5 times.

Up-Down Pull

- Raise both arms overhead.
- Stretch the tubing slightly.
- Bend your elbows and forearms to bring the tubing to rest on your shoulders behind your head.
- Do this exercise 5 times.

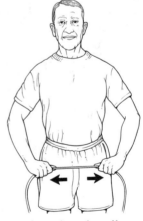

Lap-level pull

Additional Stretching and Strengthening Exercises

For safety, you may want to hold on to the back of a chair or a door frame to do some of these exercises. You may need to hold on to a piece of furniture that will support your weight as you lower yourself to the floor to do some of the exercises (and again as you get up).

Some people become mildly dizzy when rising from the floor after exercising. To keep yourself from falling, sit up for a moment and let any dizziness pass before you try to stand up.

Side Stretch

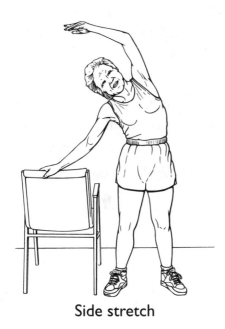

Side stretch

- Hold on to the back of a chair with your right hand.
- Stand with your feet shoulder-width apart.

- Bring your left arm up and over your head. Slowly bend over to the right. Feel the stretch in your left side. Hold for a count of 10.

- Slowly return to an upright position.

- Do this exercise 5 times on each side.

Calf Stretch

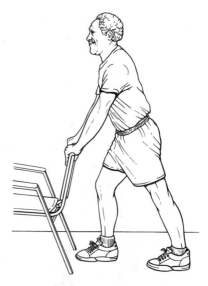

Calf stretch

- Face the back of a chair, with your hands on the backrest, and point your toes straight ahead.

- Stretch your left leg behind you. Keep your right leg slightly bent.

- Press your left heel to the floor. (You should feel the stretch in your left calf muscle.)

- If you cannot get your heel down to the floor, move your left leg forward a little. Hold for a count of 5.

- Do this exercise 5 times with each leg.

Heel Raises

- Hold on to the back of a chair for support.

- Rise up on your toes. Hold for a count of 5; then lower your heels to the ground.

- Do this 10 times.

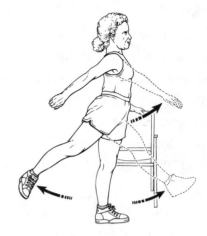

Leg swings

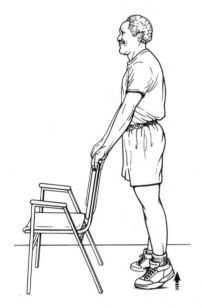

Heel raises

Hamstring Stretch

This exercise stretches the muscles in the back of your thigh, which will allow you to bend your legs without putting stress on your back.

- Lie on your back in a doorway with one leg through the doorway on the floor. Put the leg you want to stretch straight up, with the heel resting on the wall next to the doorway.

Leg Swings

- Stand up straight with your left leg next to the back of a chair. Hold on to the chair with your left hand.

- Gently swing your right leg forward and backward. Use controlled movements. Don't let your body move to the back or front when you swing your leg.

- Do this exercise 10 times with each leg.

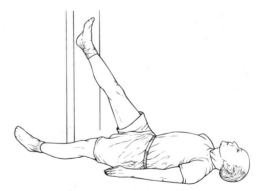

Hamstring stretch

- Keep the leg straight and slowly move your heel up the wall until you feel a gentle pull in the back of your thigh. Do not overstretch.

- Relax in this position for 30 seconds; then bend the knee to relieve the stretch. Repeat with the other leg.

Head and Shoulder Curl

This exercise will strengthen your neck and stomach muscles.

- Lie on your back with your knees slightly bent.

- Keep your arms at your sides.

- Curl your head and shoulders off the floor. Hold for 5 counts.

- Return to the starting position.

- Do this exercise 10 times.

Side-Lying Leg Lifts

- Lie on your side, legs extended.

- Raise your upper leg as high as is comfortable.

- Lower the leg to the starting position.

- Do this exercise 10 times on each side.

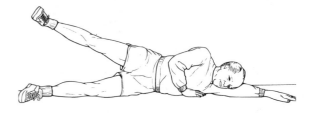

Side-lying leg lift

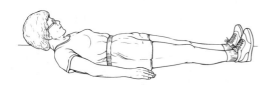

Head and shoulder curl

Eat less sugar.
Eat less fat.
Beans and grains
Are where it's at.
Unknown

20

Nutrition

As you age, certain things can happen that may change both what you need and what you choose to eat.

- Your metabolism slows down and you are likely to be less physically active, so you don't need to take in as many calories as you did when you were younger.

- Physical changes may make different foods more attractive to you. For example, soft foods may be more appealing if you have dental problems. Sweet or salty foods may appeal to you if your senses of taste and smell have changed.

- If you are less physically active than you were before, you are more likely to become constipated. You may find it helpful to increase the amount of fiber in your diet.

- Your lifestyle may change. You may eat alone more often, which may make you less inclined to prepare complete meals. Arthritis and other health problems may make shopping and meal preparation difficult.

Although your body needs fewer calories, it still needs plenty of vitamins, minerals, protein, and fiber to stay healthy. That's why planning a nutritious diet becomes even more important as you get older. Use the checklist on page 308 to determine how healthy your diet is.

Build a Base for Good Health

The Dietary Guidelines for Americans, developed by the U.S. Department of Agriculture (USDA) and the Department of Health and Human Services (DHHS), aim to improve your health and reduce your risk for disease, especially high blood pressure, heart disease, stroke, type 2 diabetes, osteoporosis, and certain types of cancer. The guidelines recommend the following ways to build a base for good health:

1. Aim for a healthy weight. Healthy bodies come in a variety of shapes and sizes. Work toward achieving and maintaining the weight that is best for you by choosing a variety of healthy foods and exercising regularly. If you would like to lose weight, work with your doctor or a registered dietitian to develop a plan that is tailored to your unique needs. For more information, see Maintain a Healthy Body Weight on page 16 and the Fitness chapter starting on page 285.

2. Be physically active every day. Regular physical activity that is vigorous enough to raise your heart rate has many benefits. The combination of a balanced diet and regular exercise is the best way to stay healthy.

3. Let the Food Guide Pyramid (see page 304) guide your food choices. The Pyramid is a simple, flexible tool designed to help you follow a balanced diet. It encourages you to eat a variety of foods in balance with one another so your body gets the nutrients it needs each day.

4. Choose a variety of grains daily, especially whole grains. Foods made from grains, such as wheat, rice, and oats, are the foundation of good nutrition. They provide vitamins, minerals, and fiber and are often low in fat. The fiber in whole grains helps prevent constipation. Whole grains may also help protect against heart disease and high blood pressure.

5. Choose a variety of fruits and vegetables daily. Fruits and vegetables are key parts of your daily diet, but most people eat fewer than the 5 servings a day that are recommended for good health. Fruits and vegetables taste great, are easy to prepare, and may help protect you from some types of cancer and heart disease.

6. Keep food safe to eat. Prevent food poisoning by keeping hot foods hot and cold foods cold. Bacteria can grow rapidly when food is not stored or handled properly. For tips on food safety, see Stomach Flu and Food Poisoning on page 88.

7. Choose a diet low in saturated fat and cholesterol and moderate in total fat. Limiting your fat intake can reduce your risk for heart disease, cancer, and high blood pressure. Eating more grains, fruits, and vegetables can help you reduce the amount of total fat in your diet.

8. Choose beverages and foods with little or no added sugar. Added sugars contain few other useful nutrients, and when consumed in excess, they crowd healthier foods out of your diet.

9. Choose and prepare foods with less salt. You can reduce your risk of high blood pressure by eating less salt. Reducing your salt intake can also help you lower your blood pressure if it is already high.

10. Drink alcoholic beverages only in moderation. Alcohol supplies calories but few nutrients. Drinking alcohol is the cause of many health problems and accidents and can lead to addiction. Moderate alcohol consumption is defined as no more than 2 drinks per day if you are a man and 1 drink per day if you are a woman.

Eating Well: A Basic Plan

Eat a variety of foods from the Food Guide Pyramid each day. Most people who follow the diet outlined by the Pyramid (see page 304) will get all the vitamins, minerals, and other nutrients their bodies need. When combined with a regular exercise program, the diet outlined by the Pyramid is helpful in maintaining a healthy body weight. If you avoid all foods from one or more of the food groups in the Pyramid, work with your health professional or a registered dietitian to plan a diet that meets all your nutritional needs.

Grain Products

Grains are the foundation of the Food Guide Pyramid. The Food Guide Pyramid recommends that you eat 6 to 11 servings from the bread, cereal, rice, and pasta group each day. As often as possible, choose foods made from whole grains. Whole grains like whole wheat, oats, and brown rice contain large amounts of vitamins, minerals, fiber, and complex carbohydrates for energy. Refined grains, such as products made with white flour, white rice, and pasta, also contain complex carbohydrates and some vitamins and minerals, but most of the fiber has been removed from them.

Whole-grain foods are filling because of their high fiber content and by themselves are low in fat. Be careful not to add too much fat to the whole-grain foods you eat. Use butter, mayonnaise, and other spreads in moderation, and top pasta with a tomato-based sauce instead of a cream-based sauce.

Fruits and Vegetables

Fruits and vegetables make up the second tier of the Food Guide Pyramid. Notice that the plant-based foods in this group and the grain group represent about two-thirds of what you should eat each day. Aim to eat at least 5 daily servings of fruits and vegetables.

Fruits and vegetables provide vitamins, minerals, fiber, and carbohydrates and are naturally low in fat. They also contain compounds that appear to protect against heart disease, high blood pressure, and some types of cancer. These compounds include antioxidants, such as vitamin C, vitamin A (beta-carotene), and other carotenoids, as well as nonnutrient compounds called phytochemicals.

Guide to Eating Well

Grains (breads, cereals, rice, pasta) form the foundation of a healthy diet. Serving sizes: 1 slice of bread, 1 oz. of cereal, ½ bagel, ½ cup of pasta or rice.

Eat plenty of fruits and vegetables. Serving sizes: ¾ cup fruit or vegetable juice; ½ cup raw, canned, or cooked fruits or vegetables; 1 medium apple or banana; 1 cup raw leafy vegetables.

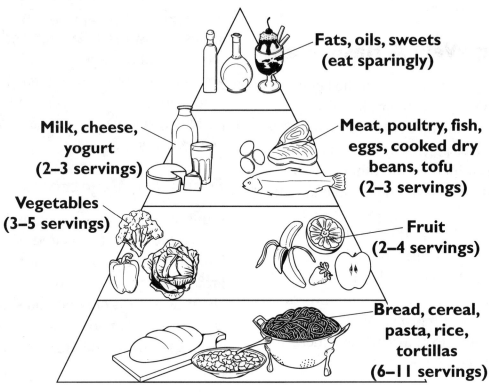

Fats, oils, sweets (eat sparingly)

Milk, cheese, yogurt (2–3 servings)

Meat, poultry, fish, eggs, cooked dry beans, tofu (2–3 servings)

Vegetables (3–5 servings)

Fruit (2–4 servings)

Bread, cereal, pasta, rice, tortillas (6–11 servings)

The Food Guide Pyramid (USDA)

Choose lean meats, fish, or poultry and cooked dry beans to reduce fat. Serving sizes: 2–3 oz. cooked lean meat, poultry, or fish; ½ cup cooked dry beans; 1 egg; 2 tbsp. peanut butter.

Choose nonfat or low-fat dairy products. Serving sizes: 1 cup milk or yogurt, 1½–2 oz. low-fat cheese, ½ cup cottage cheese.

Eat foods from the top of the Pyramid only in moderation. Examples: cooking oil, butter or margarine, high-fat salty snacks, alcohol, candy.

To make the most of the nutrients and healthy compounds in fruits and vegetables:

- Avoid damaged and wilted produce when shopping for fruits and vegetables. Choose produce that is in season and locally grown, if possible. Frozen or canned fruits and vegetables are also good choices.

- Store most fruits and vegetables in the crisper drawer of your refrigerator, or store them in a cool, dry, dark place. If they are not ripe yet, you can leave them at room temperature until they are ripened.

- Before eating fruits and vegetables, rinse them well but don't soak them. Chop vegetables into large pieces just before cooking. Microwave, steam, stir-fry, or sauté vegetables in a small amount of water or oil until they are just tender.

Meat, Fish, Poultry, and Milk Products

The Food Guide Pyramid recommends that you eat 2 to 3 servings from the meat, poultry, and fish group (this group also includes eggs, cooked dry beans, tofu, nuts, and seeds) and 2 to 3 servings from the milk and milk products group each day. These foods are important sources of protein and minerals such as iron and zinc. Protein is important for maintaining healthy muscles, tendons, bones, skin, hair, blood, and internal organs.

> ## Tips for People Who Are Underweight
>
> If you have trouble gaining weight or maintaining your minimum healthy weight, try the following:
>
> - Eat 3 meals plus 3 snacks a day. Don't skip meals.
> - Use liquid supplements, such as Ensure, between meals to add calories.
> - Choose the higher-calorie items from each food group (for example, whole milk instead of skim milk).
> - Eat the highest-calorie items first in a meal.
> - Add extra fat to the foods you prepare.

The need for protein does not decrease with age. Fortunately, most older adults get all the protein they need in their diets. If you eat animal products, such as milk, cheese, eggs, fish, and meat, your diet will contain plenty of protein. However, if you eat little meat, poultry, or fish and use no milk products, you need to plan your diet carefully to ensure that you get all the protein and other nutrients you need.

Milk products also supply your body with the calcium it needs to maintain bone strength. For more information about calcium, see page 310.

Fiber

Fiber is the indigestible part of plants. It is not absorbed into the bloodstream like other nutrients are, but it plays an important role in keeping your digestive tract healthy.

Insoluble fiber, found in whole-grain products, such as whole-wheat flour, provides bulk for your diet. Together with fluids, insoluble fiber stimulates your colon to keep waste moving out of your bowels. Without fiber, waste moves too slowly, increasing your risk for constipation, diverticulosis, and possibly colon cancer. If your stools are hard and difficult to pass, more fiber and water may help. See Constipation on page 72.

Soluble fiber, found in fruit, legumes, and oats, helps lower blood cholesterol, reducing your risk for heart disease. Soluble fiber, especially the fiber in legumes, can also help regulate your blood glucose level.

To increase fiber in your diet:

• Eat at least 5 servings of fruits or vegetables each day. Eat fruits with edible skins and seeds: kiwi fruit, figs, blueberries, apples, and raspberries. Eat more raw or lightly cooked vegetables.

• Switch to whole-grain and whole-wheat breads, pasta, tortillas, and cereals. The first ingredient listed should be whole-wheat flour.

• Eat more cooked dry beans, dry peas, and lentils. These high-fiber, high-protein foods can replace some of the high-fat, no-fiber meats in your diet.

Foods that come from animal sources, such as meat and milk products, tend to be high in fat. However, that doesn't mean you have to exclude these foods from your diet. You can get the protein and calcium your body needs without going overboard on fat if you follow some simple guidelines.

When eating meat:

• Keep serving sizes at 2 or 3 ounces (about the size of a deck of cards), and don't eat second helpings. If you eat red meat, choose the leanest cuts, such as tenderloin, flank steak, chuck, or top and bottom round.

• Regularly eat poultry (without the skin) and fish instead of beef and pork. These foods contain less saturated fat than red meat does.

• Remove all visible fat from meat, poultry, and fish before cooking. Remove poultry skin either before or after cooking.

• Bake, broil, or sauté meats, poultry, and fish instead of frying in butter or fat.

• A couple of times a week, serve a combination of legumes (dry beans, peas, lentils) and grains in place of a meat entree.

When using milk products:

• Use skim, ½, or 1% milk.

• Choose cheeses made with skim or part-skim milk, or look for cheeses that contain no more than 5 grams of fat per ounce.

- Try low-fat cottage cheese or yogurt in place of cream and sour cream; or use fat-free sour cream and fat-free cream cheese.

Lactose Intolerance

People whose bodies produce too little of the enzyme lactase have trouble digesting the lactose (sugar) in milk. Symptoms of lactose intolerance include gas, bloating, cramps, and diarrhea after drinking milk or eating milk products.

If you have mild to moderate lactose intolerance:

- Eat small amounts of milk products at any one time.

- Try eating cheese. Most of the lactose in cheese is removed during processing.

- Eat yogurts made with active cultures, which provide their own enzymes that digest the lactose in milk.

- Drink pretreated milk (such as Lactaid), or try enzyme tablets (such as Lactaid or Dairy Ease), which will help you digest lactose.

- You may be able to tolerate milk if you drink it with snacks or meals.

If you have severe lactose intolerance, be sure to include non-dairy sources of calcium in your diet. See page 310. Ask your doctor or a dietitian whether you need to take a calcium supplement.

Fats, Oils, and Sweets

Despite all the bad things you hear about fat, it is still essential to your body. Fats help maintain healthy skin and provide your body with certain (fat-soluble) vitamins.

Fats found in food are a mixture of three types: saturated, monounsaturated, and polyunsaturated. Saturated fats are found in meats (especially red meat), eggs, and milk fats (butter, cheese, cream). Many processed foods contain saturated fats. Coconut oil, palm oil, and cocoa butter are vegetable fats that are naturally saturated and are often found in processed foods. "Hydrogenated" fats are also saturated fats. A diet that includes a lot of saturated fat will cause increased levels of LDL ("bad") cholesterol in the blood (see High Cholesterol on page 312).

Unsaturated fats, especially mono-unsaturated fats, help lower cholesterol. Monounsaturated fats are found in canola, olive, and peanut oil; avocados; most nuts; and fish. Polyunsaturated fats are found in corn, sunflower, safflower, walnut, and cottonseed oil.

The Dietary Guidelines for Americans recommend that 20 to 35 percent of your total calorie intake come from fat. Reducing your dietary fat intake to 30 percent will slow the development of heart disease, reduce your cancer risk, and improve your overall diet. No more than 10 percent of total calories should come from saturated fats.

Determine Your Nutritional Health

The warning signs of poor nutritional health are often overlooked. Use this checklist to find out if you or someone you know is at risk for poor nutrition. Read the statements below. Circle the number in the "yes" column for those statements that apply to you or someone you know. Add up the numbers you circled for your total nutritional score.

	Yes
I have an illness or condition that made me change the kind or amount of food I eat.	2
I eat fewer than 2 meals per day.	3
I eat few fruits, vegetables, or milk products.	2
I have 3 or more drinks of beer, liquor, or wine almost every day.	2
I have tooth or mouth problems that make it hard for me to eat.	2
I don't always have enough money to buy the food I need.	4
I eat alone most of the time.	1
I take 3 or more different prescription or nonprescription drugs a day.	1
Without wanting to, I have lost or gained 10 pounds in the last 6 months.	2
I am not always physically able to shop, cook, or feed myself.	2
Total	____

Score	
0–2	**Good!** Recheck your nutritional score in 6 months.
3–5	**You are at moderate nutritional risk.** See what you can do to improve your eating habits and lifestyle. Your office on aging, senior nutrition program, senior citizen center, or health department can help. Recheck your nutritional score in 3 months.
6+	**You are at high nutritional risk.** Bring this checklist the next time you see your doctor, dietitian, or other qualified health or social service professional. Talk with him or her about any problems you have. Ask for help in improving your nutritional health.

Developed and distributed by the Nutrition Screening Initiative, a project of the American Academy of Family Physicians, the American Dietetic Association, and the National Council on the Aging, Inc., 1994.

The Food Guide Pyramid is designed to help you eat a low-fat diet. If you need additional help reducing fat in your diet, a registered dietitian can create a menu plan that will help you meet your goal. You can also make use of the following tips for preparing foods:

- Steam vegetables. If you choose to sauté them, use 1 tablespoon of oil (or less), or try using other liquids such as wine, defatted broth, or cooking sherry.

- Use nonstick pans, or add a small amount of oil to a preheated pan (less oil goes farther this way).

- Season vegetables with herbs and spices instead of butter and sauces; or try a butter substitute such as Butter Buds or Molly McButter. Dress salads with lemon juice, fat-free mayonnaise, or fat-free dressing.

- Use a cooking oil that is liquid at room temperature, such as canola, olive, or peanut oil. Use cooking oil sparingly (1 teaspoon at a time).

- Experiment with using less oil than is called for in recipes. You may need to increase other liquids. Use applesauce, prune puree, or mashed bananas to replace some or all of the fat in baked goods.

Sugar

In moderation, sugar does little harm. However, if too many of your calories come from sugar, your body may not get enough of the nutrients you need from other foods, and you may gain weight. Sugar also contributes to dental cavities.

To reduce sugar in your diet:

- Be aware that all sugars are basically alike. Honey and brown or raw sugar are no better for you than other sugars. Corn syrup is another form of sugar that is commonly found in processed foods.

- Processed foods and drinks can be full of sugar. Flavored yogurt, breakfast cereals, and canned fruits often have sugar added. Shop for breakfast cereals that have 6 grams or less of added sugar per serving. Limit the number of foods you buy that list sugar among the first few ingredients.

- You lose taste buds as you age. Foods may need more sugar or other seasonings to taste like they used to. Try using less sugar and more sweet spices, like cinnamon, vanilla, and nutmeg, in your favorite recipes.

- Make it a habit to eat a sweet piece of fruit instead of a sugary dessert most of the time.

- Drink water, sparkling water, or milk instead of soft drinks or sweetened fruit drinks.

Artificial Sweeteners

Although artificial sweeteners help you avoid sugar, they don't necessarily help with weight management. Avoid using artificial sweeteners to justify eating more high-fat food.

Aspartame (found in products that contain NutraSweet) and saccharin (found in products such as Sweet 'n Low) are considered safe when used in moderation. People who have PKU (phenylketonuria—an inherited disorder caused by the absence or a very low level of the enzyme needed to process phenylalanine) should not use aspartame.

Vitamins and Minerals

Vitamins are tiny elements of food that have no calories, yet are essential to good health. Vitamins A, D, E, and K are fat-soluble and can be stored in the liver or in fat tissue for a relatively long time. Other vitamins, including all the B vitamins and vitamin C, are water-soluble, and your body can only retain them for a short time. It is important that you consume these water-soluble vitamins often.

Most people who eat a variety of foods from the Food Guide Pyramid (page 304) get all the necessary vitamins. However, if you typically eat fewer than 1,500 calories per day, you may want to consider taking a vitamin-mineral supplement. Choose a balanced, multivitamin-mineral supplement rather than a specific vitamin or mineral, unless your doctor prescribes a specific supplement. Avoid taking much more than 100 percent of the Daily Value (DV) of any vitamin or mineral unless it is prescribed by a doctor.

Certain vitamins found in foods have been shown to prevent some diseases. However, researchers are still trying to determine whether those vitamins have the same preventive effects when taken as supplements. If possible, add more variety and balance to your diet rather than trying to make up for a poor diet by taking supplements.

Minerals have many important roles in the structure and function of your body. You need minerals to maintain healthy teeth and bones, carry nerve signals to and from your brain, carry oxygen to your cells, regulate your blood sugar level, and maintain a healthy immune system.

Sixty minerals have been discovered in the body, and 22 are essential to health. Two minerals—calcium and sodium (as salt)—are particularly important to older adults. Eating a variety of foods is the best way to get all the minerals you need.

Calcium

Calcium is the primary mineral needed to maintain strong bones. Women rapidly lose calcium from their bones after menopause. Eating a diet rich in calcium and vitamin D and exercising regularly may help you prevent or postpone osteoporosis (see page 126) and the bone fractures that it can cause.

Adults age 51 and older need 1,200 mg of calcium per day. Fat-free or low-fat milk products are the best source of dietary calcium. Each serving provides about 300 mg of calcium. Milk products provide other nutrients in addition to calcium, such as protein and vitamin D. The Food Guide Pyramid (see page 304) recommends 2 to 3 servings a day from the milk group to meet your calcium needs. Other foods, such as tofu, fortified soy milk, broccoli, certain greens, and calcium-fortified orange juice, provide calcium in varying amounts and can also help meet your body's calcium needs.

While dietary calcium is preferred, low-dose calcium supplements can also help keep bones strong. One 500-mg Tums (calcium carbonate) tablet provides about 200 mg of calcium. Calcium citrate (another form of calcium supplement) contains acids that help your body absorb calcium, and it is less likely than other calcium supplements to cause constipation. Avoid calcium supplements that are made from bonemeal or dolomite calcium, which may contain lead, arsenic, or other heavy metals.

Salt

Most people get far more salt than they need. The Dietary Guidelines for Americans recommend no more than 6 grams (about 1 teaspoon) of salt each day. For some people, including those of African-American descent, those over age 50, and those who have a family history of high blood pressure, excess salt causes high blood pressure. See High Blood Pressure on page 165. Eating less salt can help you avoid or control high blood pressure and may also help your bones retain calcium.

In general, processed foods contain the most salt, while unprocessed foods, such as fresh fruits and vegetables, have the least. If you want to cut back on the salt in your diet:

- Read the Nutrition Facts labels on foods for sodium content. Choose foods that contain less sodium.

- Limit ready-mixed sauces and seasonings, frozen dinners, and canned or dehydrated soups. These foods are usually packed with salt. Also watch out for salty chips, pretzels, and popcorn. Products labeled "low sodium" contain less than 140 mg of sodium per serving.

- Eat lots of fresh or frozen fruits and vegetables. These foods contain very little salt.

- Don't put the saltshaker on the table, or get a saltshaker that allows very little salt to come out. Use salt substitute or "lite salt" sparingly.

- Always measure the salt in recipes, and use half of what is called for.

- Avoid fast foods, which are usually very high in salt. In a restaurant, ask the chef not to salt food during cooking.

Water

As you age, your kidneys' ability to help your body retain water diminishes and your ability to sense thirst decreases. So, as you get older you need to drink plenty of water to avoid dehydration. Along with fiber, water is important in preventing constipation.

One easy way to make sure you're getting enough water is to drink a big glassful when you first get up in the morning; then drink 6 to 8 more glasses (8 ounces each) throughout the day. If you drink other liquids, you can get by with less water, but plain water is best. (Milk is another good choice, with the added bonus of a boost of calcium.)

If you are concerned about overloading your bladder, follow these tips:

- Gradually increase your water intake by 1 glass per week to give your body a chance to adjust.

- Drink most of your water in the morning and early afternoon.

High Cholesterol

Cholesterol is a type of fat that is produced by your body and is also found in foods that come from animal sources (meat, milk products, eggs, poultry, and fish). Your body's cells need cholesterol to function properly. However, excess cholesterol in the blood can build up inside your arteries (atherosclerosis), causing them to narrow. Atherosclerosis is the starting point for most heart and circulation problems (see page 157).

Good and Bad Cholesterol

Cholesterol travels through your bloodstream attached to protein, in a combination called a lipoprotein. Two lipoproteins are the main carriers of cholesterol: low-density lipoprotein (LDL) and high-density lipoprotein (HDL). High-density lipoproteins contain more protein than they do fat.

- LDL ("bad cholesterol") carries cholesterol from the liver to other parts of the body. When LDL levels are high, cholesterol can build up on the walls of the arteries. Having a high LDL cholesterol level increases your risk for coronary artery disease (CAD), heart attack, and stroke.

- HDL ("good cholesterol") helps clear cholesterol from the body by picking up cholesterol from the bloodstream and taking it back to the liver for disposal. Increasing your HDL cholesterol level may reduce your risk for heart disease, stroke, and peripheral vascular disease.

Triglycerides are another type of fat that can be found in the bloodstream. A high triglyceride level may also increase your risk of coronary artery disease and stroke.

What Do the Numbers Mean?

There are guidelines doctors rely on to evaluate your cholesterol numbers and assess your risk for heart disease. The importance of the numbers varies from person to person, depending on whether a person has additional risk factors for heart disease or actually has heart disease. The following ranges apply to people who are at average risk for heart disease.*

Total cholesterol

Desirable: less than 200

Borderline high: 200 to 239

High: 240 and above

HDL cholesterol

High (desirable): Above 60

Acceptable: 40 to 60

Low (not desirable): Less than 40

LDL cholesterol

Optimal: Less than 100

Near optimal: 100 to 129

Borderline high: 130 to 159

High: 160 to 189

Very high: 190 and above

Triglycerides

Normal: less than 150

Borderline high: 150 to 199

High: 200 to 500

Very high: Above 500

Figures provided by the National Cholesterol Education Program (NCEP) of the National Institutes of Health (NIH)

Cholesterol Screening

Basic cholesterol screening tests are easy, quick, and inexpensive. Call your local health department to find out when free or low-cost cholesterol tests may be available.

You and your doctor can determine the schedule that is best for you based on your risk factors for coronary artery disease. A test every 5 years is appropriate for most people between the ages of 50 and 75 who are not at high risk.

You may want to have your cholesterol checked more often if your total cholesterol is greater than 200 mg/dl (milligrams per deciliter), or if you have any of the following risk factors for coronary artery disease:

• You have a family history of early heart attack (before age 55 in father or brother; before age 65 in mother or sister).

• You are a smoker.

- You have high blood pressure (above 140/90) or take high blood pressure medication.

- You have diabetes.

- You had an HDL level below 40 or a triglyceride level over 150 in your previous cholesterol test.

If your total cholesterol is over 200 mg/dl and you don't know what your HDL and LDL levels are, more extensive testing can help you better estimate your actual risk.

How to Reduce Your Blood Cholesterol

A diet low in saturated fat and regular exercise are all that most people need to lower cholesterol. People with very high cholesterol, diabetes, or coronary artery disease (or who are at very high risk for it) may need medication as well as exercise and a low-fat diet to lower their cholesterol.

To reduce your cholesterol:

- Get less than 30 percent of your daily calories from fat. Follow the guidelines that start on page 307.

- Attend a low-fat diet workshop or consult a registered dietitian to learn ways to lower your saturated fat intake to 7 percent or less of total calories and your dietary cholesterol intake to less than 200 mg per day.

- Eat at least 5 servings of fruits and vegetables each day.

- Eat 2 to 3 servings (3 to 4 ounces) of baked or broiled fish per week. The safety and value of fish oil supplements is not yet known.

- Eat more soluble fiber (fruit, dry beans and peas, oats). See page 306.

- Exercise more. Exercise increases your HDL cholesterol level and may decrease your LDL level.

- Quit smoking. Smoking increases the risk of heart attack and stroke, even in people with low cholesterol.

- Lose weight if you are overweight. Losing even 5 to 10 pounds can lower triglyceride levels and raise HDL levels. In some people, LDL levels may fall as well.

The DASH Diet for High Blood Pressure

If you have mild to moderate high blood pressure (hypertension), you may benefit from the Dietary Approaches to Stop Hypertension—or DASH—diet. The diet includes:

- Eating 8 to 10 servings of fruits and vegetables.

- Eating 7 to 8 servings of grains.

- Eating 3 or more servings of low-fat milk products.

- Limiting your total fat intake to less than 30 percent of your caloric intake and limiting your saturated fat intake to less than 10 percent of your caloric intake.

Medication for High Cholesterol

 Several medications are effective in lowering cholesterol. However, they may have side effects, they are expensive, and they require lifelong use. Unless your LDL level is very high, your doctor will probably recommend changes to your diet to try to lower cholesterol before prescribing medications.

Medications may be prescribed sooner if you have diabetes, high blood pressure, or other conditions that increase your risk for heart attack or stroke. Even if you are taking medication to lower your cholesterol, you must still follow a low-fat diet.

Eating Alone?

Many older adults live and eat alone. This can affect your nutritional status, since you may not eat as well alone as you would when dining with others. You may not take the time to make balanced meals, or you may skip meals. If you often eat alone, consider the following:

• Plan your meals for the week, and shop from a list. You are more likely to eat meals for which you have planned and have all the ingredients.

• Take turns with friends preparing meals and eating together.

• Make a big pot of hearty stew or soup that you can enjoy for several meals. Freeze leftover portions.

• Contact your local or state health department to find out about community meal programs in your area. They provide low-cost, nutritious meals and opportunities to be with other people.

• Find out if your community has a Meals on Wheels program. If you are temporarily or permanently homebound, this service will deliver a hot, nutritious, and inexpensive meal once a day.

• If you sometimes don't have enough money to buy the food you need, you may be eligible for food stamps or Supplemental Security Income (SSI).

To be 70 years young is sometimes far more cheerful
and hopeful than to be 40 years old.
Oliver Wendell Holmes on the 70th birthday of
Julia Ward Howe

21

Mental Health

Mental health problems are common among older adults, but they are not a "normal" part of aging. Like other illnesses, many mental health problems can be prevented, and those that do occur can often be successfully treated. Unfortunately, far too many older adults never have their mental health problems diagnosed by a health professional, so they don't get the treatment they need to feel better.

Without treatment, conditions like depression, anxiety, and drug and alcohol abuse can make other health problems worse and take a toll on a person's independence. Many older adults pay the ultimate price for not getting treatment for mental health problems— they commit suicide. In fact, suicide is more prevalent among older adults than among any other age group in the United States.

Having symptoms of a mental health problem is nothing to keep hidden or be ashamed of. Today it is known that mental health problems often have underlying physical causes that can be treated. For example, illnesses such as thyroid disease and chronic anemia can cause depression. Arthritis and other problems that cause chronic pain commonly lead to depression and, for some people, may increase the likelihood of drug or alcohol abuse.

Mental health problems can also begin when physical stress (such as an illness or injury) or emotional stress (such as the loss of a loved one) triggers chemical changes in the brain. While some people can withstand more stress than others, no one is immune to mental health problems.

In order to take care of your mental health, you need to be aware of the symptoms of mental health problems. If you can recognize symptoms early and are willing to address their underlying causes, you can often prevent major mental health problems. If a problem has already developed, recognition of symptoms may allow you to seek help before the problem causes serious disruptions in your life.

In general, it is a good idea to seek professional help for a mental health problem when:

- A symptom becomes severe or disruptive.

- A symptom becomes a continuous or permanent pattern of behavior and does not respond to self-care.

- Symptoms become numerous, affect all areas of your life, and do not respond to self-care or communication efforts.

- You are thinking about hurting yourself or someone else.

There is a wide range of professional and lay resources to choose from for help with mental health problems. You may need to talk to more than one counselor before you find one with whom you feel comfortable and who you think can help you.

Family doctors or internists: Mental health problems often have physical causes. Your doctor can review your medical history and medications for clues, provide some counseling, prescribe medications when necessary, or refer you to other resources.

Psychiatrists: Psychiatrists are medical doctors who specialize in mental disorders. They counsel people, prescribe medications, and order medical treatments.

Psychologists, social workers, and counselors: These professionals receive special training in helping people deal with mental health problems. They help people identify, understand, and work through disturbing thoughts and emotions.

Nurse specialists: Some nurses have advanced training to treat mental disorders. Nurse specialists can provide both medication and counseling.

Clergy: People often turn to their clergy for counseling and advice in times of emotional distress. Some clergy have formal training in counseling.

Are You a Problem User?

Answer the following questions honestly. They refer to your use of alcohol and drugs, including prescribed and illegal drugs.

- Have you ever felt that you ought to cut down on your drinking or drug use?

- Do you get annoyed at criticism of your drinking or drug use?

- Do you ever feel guilty about your drinking or drug use?

- Do you ever take an early morning drink or use drugs first thing in the morning to get the day started or to eliminate the "shakes"?

A person who answers yes to any of these questions may have a problem with alcohol or drugs. Call a health professional to arrange for other tests to diagnose alcohol or drug dependence.

Alcohol and Drug Problems

The overuse or abuse of alcohol or other drugs is called substance abuse. It is common, costly, and associated with many medical problems.

Alcohol Problems

A person has an alcohol use problem if he or she continues to drink even though alcohol is interfering with his or her health or daily living. Alcoholism is defined as a physical or psychological dependence on alcohol.

Alcohol abuse patterns vary. Some people get drunk every day. Some drink large amounts of alcohol at specific times, such as weekends. Others may be sober for long periods and then go on drinking binges that last for weeks or months.

 Long-term heavy drinking causes liver, nerve, heart, and brain damage; high blood pressure; stomach problems; sexual problems; and cancer. Alcohol abuse can also lead to violence, accidents, social isolation, and difficulties at work, at home, or with the law.

For older adults, it is especially important to remember that:

• Alcohol slows brain activity.

• Alcohol impairs mental alertness, memory, judgment, physical coordination, and reaction time.

• Heavy alcohol use can lead to loss of employment, friends, and loved ones.

• As a person gets older, it takes the body longer to break down alcohol, and the body's tolerance for alcohol decreases. Drinking the same amount that you drank 20 years ago can cause a lot more damage.

• Alcohol can make existing medical problems worse.

• Tranquilizers, barbiturates, certain painkillers, and antihistamines all increase the intoxicating effect of alcohol.

• Alcohol interferes with the medical benefits of many drugs, including anticonvulsants, anticoagulants, and diabetes medications.

Signs that a person is dependent on alcohol include blackouts, drinking more and more for the same "high," and being uncomfortable in situations where alcohol isn't served. A person with alcoholism may gulp or sneak drinks, drink alone or early in the morning, and suffer from the shakes.

A person whose body is dependent on alcohol may suffer serious withdrawal symptoms (such as trembling, hallucinations, sweating, and seizures) if he or she suddenly quits drinking alcohol or tries to reduce his or her alcohol intake. Once alcohol dependency develops, it is very difficult for a person to stop drinking without outside help. Medical detoxification may be needed.

Drug Problems

Most people think of drug abuse as the use of marijuana, cocaine, heroin, or other "street drugs." Drug problems among older adults are more likely to result from drug misuse—the intentional or unintentional overuse of legal prescription drugs. Tranquilizers, sedatives, painkillers, and amphetamines are misused most often. A person with a drug addiction will continue to abuse drugs even though drug use is damaging his or her health or daily living.

Drug dependence (addiction) occurs when a person develops a physical or psychological need for a drug. A person may not be aware that he or she has become dependent on a drug until he or she tries to suddenly stop taking it. Withdrawing from the drug can cause uncomfortable symptoms such as muscle aches, diarrhea, or depression. The usual treatment for drug dependence is to reduce the dose of the drug gradually until it can be stopped completely.

The symptoms of drug misuse vary widely, depending upon the kind of drug being used. Often, symptoms develop slowly over a long period of time, and they can be confused with symptoms of other health problems.

Prevention

- Stay active and maintain your daily responsibilities.

- Look for signs of mental stress. Try to understand and resolve sources of depression, anxiety, or loneliness. Don't use alcohol or drugs to deal with these problems. Ask for support from friends or family after you have suffered any major loss or life change.

- Seek friendships with people who do not rely on alcohol or drugs to enjoy themselves.

- If you drink, do so in moderation: not more than 2 drinks a day if you are a man and not more than 1 drink a day if you are a woman. One drink is 12 ounces of beer, 5 ounces of wine, or 1 ounce of hard liquor.

- Do not regularly use medications to help you sleep, lose weight, or relax. Look for nondrug solutions.

- Be especially cautious about taking any of the following types of medications:

  - Painkillers, such as codeine, Darvocet, Demerol, Norco, Percodan, Vicodin, and others.

  - Tranquilizers, such as Ativan, Librium, Valium, Xanax, and other benzodiazepines.

  - Sedatives or sleeping pills, such as Seconal, phenobarbital, Nembutal, and other barbiturates; Dalmane, Doriden, Halcion, and other non-barbiturates; and nonprescription sleep aids.

- Talk to your doctor about all the prescription and nonprescription medications you take. If you and your doctor decide some of the medications are not necessary, gradually reduce the dosages. Do not suddenly stop taking any medication unless your doctor advises you to do so.

• Avoid alcohol when you are taking medications. Alcohol can react with many drugs and cause serious complications.

• See pages 378 to 380 for tips on how to take your medications correctly and avoid adverse reactions. Also see Medication Problems on page 390 for more prevention guidelines.

Home Treatment

• Recognize early signs that alcohol or drug use is becoming a problem. See Are You a Problem User? on page 318.

• Attend an Alcoholics Anonymous or Narcotics Anonymous meeting. These are self-help groups devoted to helping members get and stay sober.

• If you are concerned about another person's alcohol or drug use:

- Never ignore the problem. Discuss it as a medical problem.

- Build up the person's self-esteem and reaffirm his or her value as a person. Help the person see that he or she can be successful without alcohol or drugs. Let the person know you will support his or her efforts to change.

- Ask if the person will accept help. Don't give up if you get a negative response; keep asking periodically. If the person eventually agrees, act that very day to arrange for help. Call a health professional, Alcoholics Anonymous, or Narcotics Anonymous for an immediate appointment.

- Attend a few meetings of Al-Anon, a support group for family members and friends of alcoholics. Read some 12-step program information.

When to Call a Health Professional

• If a person loses consciousness after drinking alcohol or taking drugs. See Fainting and Unconsciousness on page 46.

• If a person who has been drinking alcohol or using drugs threatens to harm him- or herself or others.

• If a person who suddenly stops using alcohol has withdrawal symptoms (trembling, hallucinations, seizures).

• If you answer yes to any of the questions under Are You a Problem User? on page 318.

• If you recognize an alcohol or drug problem in yourself and are ready to accept help. Both outpatient and inpatient programs are available.

Anger and Hostility

Anger is a normal response to upsetting events and an appropriate response to any situation that poses a threat. It signals your body to prepare for a fight. When you get angry, adrenaline and other hormones are released into your bloodstream. Your blood pressure, pulse, and respiration rate all go up. Anger can be directed to become a positive, driving force behind your actions.

Hostility is being ready for a fight all the time. Continual hostility keeps your blood pressure high and may increase your risk for heart attack and other illnesses. Being hostile also isolates you from other people.

Home Treatment

• Try to understand the real reason why you are angry. Is it the current situation that is making you angry or something that happened earlier in the day?

• Notice when you start to become angry, and take steps to deal with your anger in a positive way. Don't ignore your anger until you "blow up." Express your anger in healthy ways:

  - Count to 10, go for a short walk or jog, or practice some other form of mental relaxation (see page 344). When you have calmed down, you will be better able to discuss the conflict rationally.

  - Talk with a friend about your anger.

  - Draw or paint to release the anger, or write about it in a journal.

• Use "I" statements, not "you" statements, to discuss your anger. Say "I feel angry when my needs are not being met," instead of "You make me mad when you are so inconsiderate."

• If you are angry with someone, listen to what the other person has to say. Try to understand his or her point of view.

• Forgive and forget. Forgiving helps lower blood pressure and ease muscle tension so you can feel more relaxed.

When to Call a Health Professional

• If anger has led or could lead to violence or harm to you or someone else.

• If anger or hostility interferes with your work, family life, or friendships.

Anxiety and Panic Disorder

Feeling worried, anxious, and nervous is a normal part of everyday life. Everyone frets or feels anxious from time to time.

Anxiety can cause both physical and emotional symptoms. A specific situation or fear can cause some or all of these symptoms for a short time. When the situation passes, the symptoms go away.

Physical Symptoms

• Trembling, twitching, or shaking

• Lightheadedness or dizziness

• A feeling of fullness in the throat or chest

• Muscle tension, aches, or soreness

• Restlessness

• Fatigue

• Insomnia

• Breathlessness or rapid heartbeat

• Sweating or cold, clammy hands

Emotional Symptoms

- Feeling keyed up and on edge

- Excessive worrying

- Fearing that something bad is going to happen

- Poor concentration

- Irritability or agitation

- Constant sadness

Many people develop anxiety disorders in which these symptoms occur for no identifiable or rational reason. This type of anxiety can become overwhelming and is not normal. People with an anxiety disorder may develop irrational and involuntary fears (phobias) of common places, objects, or situations.

Panic disorder is a common anxiety-related disorder. People with panic disorder go through periods of sudden, intense fear and anxiety when there is no clear cause or danger. These panic attacks can cause frightening (but not life-threatening) symptoms, including feelings of choking or suffocation, nausea, shaking, sweating, a pounding heart, and dizziness or faintness. People who have had panic attacks may try to avoid any situations or behaviors that might trigger another attack. This often results in a higher level of anxiety.

Some medical conditions, such as hyperthyroidism (see Thyroid Problems on page 181), can also cause the physical and emotional symptoms of anxiety.

Self-care, often combined with professional treatment, can be effective in managing anxiety and panic disorder.

Home Treatment

The following home treatment tips can relieve simple anxiety and can also help if you are receiving medical treatment for anxiety.

- Recognize and accept your anxiety about specific fears or situations. Then say to yourself, "This is not an emergency. I feel uncomfortable, but I am not in danger. I can keep going even if I feel anxious."

- Be kind to your body:

  - Relieve tension by exercising or getting a massage.

  - Practice relaxation techniques. See page 344.

  - Get enough rest. If you have trouble sleeping, see Sleep Problems on page 333.

  - Avoid alcohol, caffeine, and nicotine. They may increase your anxiety level or trigger a panic attack.

- Engage your mind:

  - Get out and do something you enjoy, such as going to a funny movie or taking a walk or a hike.

  - Plan your day. Having too much or too little to do can make you more anxious.

- Keep a record of your symptoms. Discuss your fears with a good friend or join a support group. Confiding with others sometimes relieves stress.

- Get involved in social groups or volunteer to help others. Being alone sometimes makes things seem worse than they are.

- Talk to your doctor or pharmacist if you think a medication may be causing your anxiety symptoms. Don't stop taking any medication unless your doctor tells you it is safe to do so.

When to Call a Health Professional

- If you are seriously considering harming yourself or someone else.

- If anxiety or irrational fear interferes with your daily activities.

- If sudden, severe attacks of fear or anxiety with intense physical symptoms (shaking, sweating) seem to occur for no reason.

- If symptoms of anxiety are still severe after 1 week of home treatment.

- If you suffer from nightmares or flashbacks to traumatic events.

- If you are unable to feel certain about things (for example, whether you unplugged the iron) no matter how many times you check.

- If you cannot resist your urge to perform repetitive actions and they interfere with your daily activities.

Sadness or Depression?

If you have experienced 4 or more of the following symptoms nearly every day for more than 2 weeks, you may be suffering from depression:

- Feeling sad or hopeless

- Feeling nervous or "empty"

- Not enjoying things the way you used to

- Eating more or less than usual

- Having persistent backaches, headaches, stomach problems, or other aches that don't respond to treatment

- Sleeping more or less than usual

- Feeling very tired or run-down

- Feeling restless or irritable

- Feeling worthless or guilty

- Being unable to concentrate, remember, or make decisions

- Feeling like nobody loves you

- Thinking often about death or suicide

Home treatment may be all that is needed for mild depression. However, if you are feeling suicidal or if home treatment doesn't help lift your mood within 2 weeks, contact a health professional. With counseling, medication, and continued home treatment, you can overcome most cases of depression.

Depression

Depression is a common yet under-treated health problem in older adults. Depression often goes undiagnosed in older adults because they either don't recognize their feelings as signs of depression or they don't want to admit that they are feeling depressed. Many people are convinced that feeling sad all the time, having persistent aches and pains, and becoming forgetful are just part of growing older—that nothing can be done about it. Others may fear that a diagnosis of depression is a sign of weakness, or that it means they no longer have a "sound mind" and are a step closer to losing their independence.

Doctors sometimes have a hard time diagnosing depression in older adults. Symptoms of depression in older adults may differ from those that are typically seen in younger people. To further complicate matters, other health conditions that affect older adults have symptoms similar to those caused by depression, and depression can occur along with other health problems. It may take a while for a doctor to sort through all the symptoms and recognize depression as part of the picture.

You don't have to live with depression. It is not a character flaw. Depression is almost always treatable, either with self-care or a combination of self-care and professional treatment. If you have a better understanding of what causes depression and are able to recognize its symptoms, you can get the help you need and keep yourself from suffering.

While the exact cause of depression is not known, it is believed to involve a combination of factors, including problems with the balance of chemical messengers (neurotransmitters) in the brain and increased production of certain hormones that put the body "on alert." Depression tends to run in families and is more common in people who have low self-esteem. The amount of stress in a person's life and the way a person copes with stress also contribute to depression.

Many things can trigger depression, including:

- Having a major illness, injury, or surgery.

- Grieving the death of a loved one.

- Going through major life changes (loss of a job, divorce, children leaving home, retirement).

- Being under long-term stress, such as having a family member with a chronic illness.

- Taking certain medications or having certain health conditions, such as cancer, diabetes, or stroke.

- Drinking alcohol, using illegal drugs, or misusing prescription drugs.

Reduced daylight during the winter seems to cause a form of depression called seasonal affective disorder in some people. See Seasonal Affective Disorder on page 328.

What About St. John's Wort?

The herbal supplement St. John's wort has become a popular alternative to anti-depressant medications. Hypericum, the active ingredient in St. John's wort, is extracted from the flower of a plant (*Hypericum perforatum*). St. John's wort is not classified as a drug by the U.S. Food and Drug Administration. Therefore, it has not gone through the same tests for safety and effectiveness that prescription and nonprescription drugs have.

A standard effective dosage for St. John's wort has not been determined. This means that the products you find in health food stores and pharmacies may contain varying amounts of hypericum, and that some products may be more pure and more potent than others.

Although St. John's wort seems to be a promising new treatment for depression, the verdict is still out. Studies to determine the safety and effectiveness of St. John's wort are under way.

If you are thinking about trying St. John's wort, let your health professional know, especially if you have a chronic illness or are taking other medications. Be aware that some people experience side effects, such as mild stomach upset, rash, and increased sensitivity to sunlight, when using St. John's wort. Do not use St. John's wort in combination with other antidepressant medications. Doing so can result in serious side effects.

When purchasing St. John's wort, look for the words "standardized extract" on the product label. This means the product is more likely to have an exact, effective amount of hypericum in each dose.

Everyone gets sad. Gauging how deep and pervasive your sad feelings are can help you decide what to do. See Sadness or Depression? on page 324 to learn the symptoms of depression.

 Because many factors can contribute to depression, the best approach to treatment often involves a combination of self-care, counseling (psychotherapy), and medication. If a person is severely depressed and at risk of harming him- or herself or someone else, treatment in a hospital may be necessary.

Home Treatment

For some people, self-care alone can improve symptoms of mild depression. For more serious depression, self-care can add to the benefits of professional treatment.

- Consider what might be causing or adding to your depression:

  - Are medications causing it? Review your prescription and nonprescription medications with a pharmacist or doctor. Don't stop taking any medication unless your doctor tells you to do so.

  For more information, see the back cover.

- If it's wintertime or you haven't been out in the sun for a while, read about seasonal affective disorder on page 328.

• Pace yourself according to your energy level. Choose what is most important to get done, and do those things first.

• Don't make major life decisions when you are depressed. If you must make a major decision, ask someone you trust to help you.

• Don't drink alcohol, use medications that have not been prescribed by your doctor, or take more medication than has been prescribed.

• Spend time with other people. Do things you usually enjoy, even if you don't feel like doing them.

• Get enough sleep. If you are having difficulty sleeping, see Sleep Problems on page 333.

• Eat a healthy diet (see the Nutrition chapter starting on page 301). If you don't feel like eating, try small snacks rather than large meals.

• Exercise regularly. Getting 20 to 30 minutes of exercise each day is good for your body and your mind. Go for a walk. Take the stairs instead of the elevator. Dance.

• Believe that this mood will pass. Then look for signs that it is ending.

• Give yourself time to heal. Do not expect too much from yourself too soon.

• Read books about self-care for depression. Look in the self-help section of your library or bookstore.

Caregiver Tips for Depression

• Help the person rebuild his or her self-esteem. Help the person remember the positive things he or she has done and good times he or she has had.

• Help the person identify the situations over which he or she has control.

• Encourage activity with others.

• Depressed people can lose objectivity about themselves. If signs of major depression are present, insist that the person talk with a health professional.

• Caregivers get depressed too. If you develop symptoms of depression, see Home Treatment on page 326 for tips to help you get back on track.

• Remember that symptoms of dementia often resemble those of depression. You may be able to rule out depression if the person seems confused or withdrawn or has other symptoms of dementia (see page 196).

When to Call a Health Professional

- If you are planning to hurt yourself or someone else.

- If you hear voices.

- If you have a sudden change in your behavior or start to do things that you wouldn't usually do (especially impulsive, irresponsible behavior).

- If symptoms of depression (see Sadness or Depression? on page 324) last longer than 2 weeks despite home treatment.

- If grieving continues without improvement for more than 4 weeks. See Grief on page 328.

Grief

Grief is a natural healing process that enables you to adjust to significant change or loss. Although painful, grief is also of great benefit. It provides a period of adjustment and an opportunity to build a foundation for a meaningful future.

Grief can be expressed physically as well as emotionally. Physical symptoms include crying, sighing, exhaustion, insomnia, restlessness, headaches, loss of appetite, and nausea. Emotional responses to loss can include sadness and yearning, denial, anger, guilt, depression, and many other strong feelings.

Seasonal Affective Disorder

Seasonal affective disorder (SAD), sometimes called the winter blues, is a mental health problem that usually occurs in the months when there is less sunlight. There is no known cure for the disorder, but it can be controlled. It improves in the spring when there are more hours of daylight. The main symptoms include depressed mood, decreased energy, and food cravings. If you notice such a pattern developing during the winter, consider trying the following:

- Go out into the sun as often as possible. Protect your skin—it's your eyes' exposure to the sun that will help.

- Take a vacation to a sunny place.

- Get regular exercise, either outdoors or indoors near a window that lets in sunlight.

 Light therapy (phototherapy) is sometimes successful in treating SAD. It involves sitting, working, or reading in front of special high-intensity lights for up to several hours a day.

Medication and counseling can also be helpful. Some people benefit from an approach that involves medication, counseling, and light therapy.

For more information, see the back cover.

It is not uncommon to be preoccupied with the image of a loved one who has died. Survivors often report seeing, having conversations with, or even being touched by the deceased person. This is normal.

No person or book can tell you what your grief should be like. How long and in what ways you grieve will be unique to you. Remember, losses are seldom "gotten over"; they're "gotten through." Your life may not ever be the same as it was before the loss. A time will come, however, when you regain your balance and start to reconnect with the world.

The Stages of Grief

Grief is different for everyone. Your grief may not progress directly from one stage to the next. However, there are stages of grief that are more or less common to many who suffer a loss. Understanding what others have experienced can help you deal with your own emotions.

Shock and Denial: The "Not Me" Stage

If your loss is sudden, your first reaction may be shock. Shock is a natural anesthetic that protects you from overwhelming pain.

You may even act as if nothing happened. You may feel numb. Later, you may not remember how you felt or acted during this period.

Denial is normal. You understand what has happened, but on a deeper level you don't really believe it.

Caregiver Tips for Grief

At every stage of the grieving process, caregivers and friends can provide valuable support.

Shock and Denial Stage

- Give hugs; hold hands. Send cards, notes, flowers.
- Provide food, transportation.
- Do chores, but expect the person to help too.
- Talk to the person about his or her loss to help the person acknowledge that it really happened.

Guilt and Anger Stage

- Listen, listen, listen. Show no judgment unless asked.
- Call or visit often. Be together in silence.
- Accept abrupt mood shifts.
- Provide assurance that the person was not to blame.
- Recommend and help arrange for support groups.

Adjustment and Acceptance Stage

- Invite the person to go places with you.
- Encourage exercise.
- Offer to listen.
- Reinforce your friendship.
- Encourage rebuilding friendships.
- Offer opportunities for recreation.

Denial may pass quickly, or it may last for months or even years. Denial is all right for a while. It provides a brief respite before you have to gear up to deal with the loss. However, if denial lasts too long, it may separate you from reality.

Guilt and Anger: The "Why Me?" Stage

Few people experience the loss of someone or something important to them without some feeling of guilt. You tell yourself that you should have done things differently. "If only . . ." is a common thought. You may feel there was more you could have done. Eventually, feelings of guilt will be put in proper perspective.

Anger is also a normal response. Many people feel rage or at least mild anger. This anger needs to be expressed. However, lashing out at others can cause misunderstandings. Some therapists recommend screaming or yelling in a private place to vent angry feelings without hurting those around you. See Anger and Hostility on page 321 for other ways to deal with anger.

Adjustment and Acceptance: The "Let's Get On With It" Stage

Life goes on. At some point in the grieving process, you will be better able to come to terms with your loss. Grief will loosen its hold on you, and in struggling to get on with life, you may discover new opportunities.

Loss teaches us new lessons. You may gain wisdom from your experience and be better able to help others.

Home Treatment

These home treatment guidelines are meant to help when you have lost a loved one. The same basic principles apply for other losses as well.

- Take as much time as you need to grieve. Review mementos, play nostalgic music, or read old letters.

- Let yourself cry.

- Try to cut back on some of your usual responsibilities and activities until your grieving period is past. Postpone any major decisions.

- Discuss your feelings with friends who will listen to and support you while encouraging you to reconnect with the world. Joining a support group or talking to a clergyperson may also help.

- Exercise. Take a walk. Exercise can help release pent-up emotions.

- Get enough rest and sleep. Try activities to help you relax.

- Write down your thoughts in a journal, or paint or draw your grief. Find any way possible to express your feelings.

- Friends may feel awkward about mentioning your loss. Let them know it's all right to talk about it.

- As you begin to move beyond your grief, renew old interests and pursue new ones. Do things that give you a sense of control and hope.

When to Call a Health Professional

In some cases, normal grieving can last for years. Call a health professional if you have any of the following problems after a reasonable amount of time has passed since the loss occurred. (This will vary from person to person.)

- You feel hopeless or cannot stop yourself from thinking about death or suicide.

- You are starting to behave in physically or financially self-destructive ways.

- You are feeling excessive anger toward specific people whom you blame for the loss.

- You have undiminished and overwhelming feelings of guilt.

- You are feeling more and more isolated from other people.

- You have been grieving longer than you think is good for you.

Memory Loss

Contrary to what many people believe, normal aging does not contribute to memory loss. When you think about all the information your brain collects and stores over a lifetime, doesn't it seem logical that it should take more time to retrieve some memories? With a little training ("use it or lose it" definitely applies here), you can improve your ability to concentrate and keep your memory sharp.

Sometimes memory lapses indicate a medical problem. The following symptoms could be cause for concern:

- Increasing forgetfulness accompanied by behavior changes

- Ignorance about familiar things like the alphabet, numbers, or the names of common objects

- Inability to remember a short name or phone number long enough to write it down. (This could also be caused by a hearing problem or failure to pay attention.)

Prevention

The best way to prevent memory loss is to stay healthy and actively use your mind. The following guidelines can be helpful:

- Eat well and drink plenty of fluids. A balanced, low-fat diet with ample sources of vitamins B_{12} and folate will help protect memory. Drinking plenty of water prevents dehydration and the confusion and memory problems that dehydration can cause.

- Exercise regularly. Keeping your body healthy will help protect your memory.

- Get plenty of rest. Many memory problems are the result of being overtired. If you have difficulty sleeping, see page 333.

- Minimize your use of medications. Overuse of medications may be the single biggest cause of memory loss among older adults.

- Get help if you are depressed. Long-term depression has a powerful impact on memory and can cause other symptoms that mimic dementia (see page 325).

- Limit your alcohol intake. Alcohol can affect memory long after you sober up.

- Be a social butterfly. Spend time with others discussing current events (bonus points if you take a walk while talking) or playing cards or word games. If you don't think you get out enough, get a part-time job or check out the social activities at your church or local senior center.

- Develop a positive attitude about your memory. Reject the notion that memory declines with age. If you expect to keep a strong memory, it will be there when you need it.

Home Treatment

- Follow the prevention guidelines. If you are concerned that memory loss may be caused by Alzheimer's disease or dementia, see pages 193 and 196.

- Deal with reversible causes of memory loss:

  - Acute illnesses will affect your memory. If you have a fever or any other signs of infection, see page 146.

  - Chronic problems with any major organ system, such as heart or kidney disease, can cause memory loss. If

these problems are corrected through medical treatment, your memory problems may improve.

  - Consider having your hearing or vision tested. If you do not hear or see well, your brain will have a more difficult time recording information that is heard or seen.

- Learn new techniques to improve your memory:

  - Take a memory improvement course.

  - Strive to increase your attention span and ability to concentrate. Older people have more difficulty than younger people in dividing their attention between two or more activities, so don't try to focus on too many things at once.

  - Keep written notes. Write all your plans on a calendar that you can refer to often.

  - To keep track of your eyeglasses, keep them on a cord around your neck.

  - To avoid misplacing your keys, keep them in a special place by the door.

  - Use a timer with a loud bell whenever you have something on the stove or in the oven.

  - To remember medications, use a pill organizer with compartments for each day.

When to Call a Health Professional

- If you are concerned that memory loss is caused by prescription drugs or specific medical problems.

- If there are obvious behavior changes, or memory problems related to immediate recall; or if a person has difficulty remembering familiar things like the alphabet or how to read a clock.

- If memory loss starts to interfere with your work, hobbies, or friendships, or if it is becoming a safety hazard (for example, if you forget to turn off the stove).

- If you are concerned about memory loss, or if memory loss has not responded to home treatment, discuss it with your doctor during your next appointment.

Sleep Problems

The term **insomnia** can mean:

- Trouble getting to sleep (taking more than 45 minutes to fall asleep).

- Frequent awakenings with inability to fall back asleep.

- Early morning awakening.

None of these are problems unless they make you feel chronically tired. If you are less sleepy at night or wake up early in the morning, but still feel rested and alert, there is little need to worry.

Short-term insomnia, lasting from a few nights to a few weeks, is usually caused by worry over a stressful situation. Long-term insomnia, which can last months or even years, is often caused by general anxiety, medications, chronic pain, depression, or other physical disorders.

Sleep apnea is a sleep disorder that is usually caused by a blockage in the upper airways. When airflow through the nose and mouth is blocked, breathing repeatedly stops for 10 to 15 seconds or longer. People who have sleep apnea usually snore loudly. They may toss and turn during the night, have a headache when they wake up, and complain of being tired during the day. Sleep apnea is common in older men who are overweight.

 Mild sleep apnea may be cured by changing some of your pre-bedtime habits. More severe sleep apnea may require medical treatment.

Prevention

- Get regular exercise, but avoid strenuous exercise within 2 hours before bedtime.

- Avoid alcohol and smoking before bedtime. Drink caffeine in moderation and not after noon.

- Drink a glass of warm milk at bedtime. (But don't drink more than 1 glass of fluid before going to bed.)

Home Treatment

- Don't take sleeping pills. They can cause daytime confusion, memory loss, and dizziness. Continued use of sleeping pills actually increases sleeplessness in many people.

- Try the following 7-step formula for 2 weeks:

  1. Engage in relaxing activities in the evening. For example, take a warm bath, read, or do some slow, easy stretches.

  2. Use your bed for sleeping and sex only. Don't eat, watch TV, or read in bed.

  3. Sleep only at bedtime. Don't take naps.

  4. Go to bed only when you feel sleepy.

  5. If you lie awake for more than 15 minutes, get up and leave the bedroom.

  6. Repeat steps 4 and 5 until it is time to get up.

  7. Get up at the same time each day, no matter how sleepy you are.

- Review the sleeping tips for snorers on page 155.

- Review all of your prescription and nonprescription medications with a pharmacist or doctor to rule out drug-related sleep problems.

- Read about anxiety and depression on pages 322 and 325. Either condition can cause sleep problems.

When to Call a Health Professional

- If you regularly take sleeping pills and are unable to stop taking them.

- If you suspect medication or a health problem is causing sleep problems.

- If you or your partner snores loudly and heavily and feels excessively sleepy during the day.

- If you or your partner has many episodes of sleep apnea (stops breathing, gasps, and chokes during sleep).

- If you wake up frequently because your legs move or get cramps.

- If a full month of self-care doesn't solve the problem.

Suicide

The suicide rate among older adults is higher than that of any other age group in the United States. Many older adults who commit suicide have mental health problems, such as depression, alcohol abuse, or drug abuse. However, most people who have mental health problems don't kill themselves. Life-changing events such as the diagnosis of a serious illness, the loss or illness of a loved one, and physical disabilities also increase an older person's risk for suicide.

Many people have fleeting thoughts about death. Having such thoughts is much different from actively planning to commit suicide and having the means to carry out the plan. Most people who seriously consider suicide do so because they can't think of any way to solve their problems or end their pain. With the right kind of help, such as counseling and drug treatment for mental health problems, there is a good chance that a suicidal person will find answers to his or her problems and choose to live.

Prevention

If you are thinking about committing suicide:

- Talk about your thoughts with someone you trust—a friend or family member, a clergyperson, or your doctor. If you don't think anyone you know would be willing to listen to you, contact your community mental health agency or suicide prevention or crisis center. Don't keep your thoughts and plans to yourself.

- Stay away from alcohol and drugs. Alcohol and drugs can impair your judgment and lead you to do things that you might not have done if you weren't using them.

If you are a friend of or caregiver for a person who is at risk for suicide:

- Watch for warning signs of suicide. For older adults, such warning signs include:

  - Social isolation.

  - Frequently talking about death and dying.

- Take all warning signs of suicide seriously. Anytime a person talks about suicide or wanting to die or disappear, even in a joking manner, take the person seriously.

- Encourage the person to see a mental health professional immediately. Since a suicidal person may feel that he or she cannot be helped, you may have to contact a mental health professional and take the person to the appointment.

- Make sure someone stays with the person at all times until he or she is seen by a mental health professional.

- Follow up to find out how the person's treatment is going. A suicidal person may be reluctant to seek help and may not continue with treatment after the first visit with a mental health professional. With your support and encouragement, the person may decide to continue with his or her treatment.

When to Call a Health Professional

Call 911 or other emergency services immediately:

- If you or someone you know has set a time and place to commit suicide.

- If you think suicide is the only way to solve a problem or end your pain.

- If you are having these thoughts and possess the means, such as weapons or medications, to harm yourself or another person.

Call your doctor, your local suicide hot line, or the national suicide hot line at 1-800-784-2433:

• If you are considering suicide but you do not have a suicide plan.

• If you have frequent thoughts about suicide.

• If you suspect that someone you know has made suicide plans.

You've got to accentuate the positive.
Eliminate the negative.
Latch on to the affirmative.
Don't mess with Mr. In-Between!
From a song by Johnny Mercer

22

Mind-Body Wellness

The first part of this chapter will help you understand how your mind and body work together and how you can maximize your health—even if you have a chronic illness—by keeping a positive frame of mind. The second section discusses how devastating stress can be to your mental and physical health; it also provides tips you can use to recognize and manage stress before it takes its toll on your well-being.

The Mind-Body Connection

Medical science is making remarkable discoveries about the relationship between your state of mind and your mental and physical health. Researchers have found that one function of the brain is to produce substances that can improve your health. Your brain can create endorphins, which are natural painkillers; gamma globulin, which fortifies your immune system; and interferon, which combats infections, viruses, and even cancer. Your brain can combine these and other substances into a vast number of tailor-made prescriptions for whatever ails you.

The substances that your brain produces depend in part on your thoughts, feelings, and expectations. If your attitude about an illness (or life in general) is negative and you don't have expectations that your condition will get better, your brain may not produce enough of the substances your body needs to heal. On the other hand, if your attitude and expectations are more positive, your brain is likely to produce sufficient amounts of the substances that will boost your body's healing power.

Your physical health also has an impact on your brain's ability to produce substances that affect your mental well-being. An illness or injury that causes long-term physical stress can lead to chemical imbalances in the brain. These imbalances may lead to depression and other mental health problems.

Visualization

Visualization adds mental pictures to your affirmations. Focus on your affirmation and start thinking of mental images that support it.

- Select one specific affirmation, for example, "My hands are flexible and pain-free."

- Develop a mental image of your affirmation. For example, for pain-free hands, picture cool, soothing water pouring over your hands, making them more and more flexible. Be as creative as you like, but keep it simple.

- Repeat the mental picture over and over. Combine several longer sessions with short replays of the visual picture throughout the day.

- This time is for positive thoughts only. If any doubts arise, dismiss them until after you have finished the exercise.

- Practice makes perfect. Create visualizations daily to help you meet your goals.

Positive Thinking

People with positive attitudes generally enjoy life more, but are they any healthier? The answer is often yes. Optimism is a resource for healing. Optimists are more likely to overcome pain and adversity in their efforts to improve their medical treatment outcomes. For example, optimistic coronary bypass patients generally recover more quickly and have fewer complications after surgery than do patients who are less hopeful.

Your body responds to your thoughts, emotions, and actions. In addition to staying fit, eating right, and managing stress, you can use the following three strategies to help maintain your health:

1. Create positive expectations for health and healing.

Mental and emotional expectations can influence medical outcomes. The effectiveness of any medical treatment depends in part on how useful you expect it to be. The "placebo effect" proves this. A placebo is a drug or treatment that provides no medical benefit except for the patient's belief that it will help. Many patients who receive placebos report satisfactory relief from their medical problem, even though they received no actual medication.

Changing your expectations from negative to positive may enhance your physical health. Here's how to make the change:

- Stop all negative self-talk. Make positive statements that promote your recovery.

- Send yourself a steady stream of affirmations. An affirmation is a phrase or sentence that sends strong, positive statements to you about yourself, such as, "I am a capable person" or "My joints are strong and flexible." See Affirmations on page 339.

- Visualize health and healing. Add mental pictures that support your affirmations. See Visualization on page 338.

- Don't feel guilty about health problems. While there is a lot you can do to reduce your risk for health problems and improve your chances of recovery, some illnesses may develop and persist no matter what you do. Some things just are. Do the best you can.

Affirmations

An affirmation is a phrase or statement that sends strong, positive messages to you about yourself. Affirmations can raise both conscious and subconscious expectations about your future. They allow you to improve the reality you create for yourself.

An affirmation can be any positive statement. It can be very general: "I am a capable person." Affirmations can also help you with a specific problem: "My memory serves me well."

To create an affirmation:

- Express your statement in positive terms. Instead of saying "My joints hurt less today," say "My joints are strong and flexible."

- Keep your statement simple, and put it in the present. Instead of saying "I am going to be more relaxed," say "I am completely and deeply relaxed."

- Phrase affirmations with "I" or "my." Say "I am a supportive husband," rather than "Mary appreciates the help I provide."

To practice your affirmation:

- Write it down 10 to 20 times. Then read and reread what you wrote.

- Repeat your affirmation silently or aloud at any time during the day (after waking, during housework, while walking, or just before bed). Repeat it slowly, and say it like you mean it.

- If you start using negative self-talk, develop affirmations to counteract these contrary thoughts.

Affirmations help build a more optimistic attitude. However, they are not meant to contradict your true feelings. For problems with depression, anger, anxiety, and emotions, see Mental Health starting on page 317.

2. Open yourself to humor, friendship, and love.

Positive emotions boost your health. Fortunately, almost anything that makes you feel good about yourself helps you stay healthy.

- Laugh. A little humor makes life richer and healthier. Laughter increases creativity, reduces pain, and speeds healing. Keep an emergency laughter kit that contains funny videotapes, jokes, cartoons, and photographs. Put it with your first aid supplies and keep it well stocked.

- Seek out friends. Friendships are vital to good health. Close social ties help you recover more quickly from illness and reduce your risk of developing diseases ranging from arthritis to depression.

- Volunteer. People who volunteer live longer and enjoy life more than those who do not volunteer. By helping others, we help ourselves.

- Plant a plant and pet a pet. Plants and pets can be highly therapeutic. When you stroke an animal, your blood pressure goes down and your heart rate slows. Animals and plants help us feel needed.

3. Appeal to a higher power.

If you believe in a higher power, ask for support in your pursuit of healing and health. Faith, prayer, and spiritual beliefs can play an important role in helping you recover from an illness. See Healing Touch on page 351.

Your sense of spiritual wellness can help you overcome personal trials and things you cannot change. If it suits you, use spiritual images in visualizations, affirmations, and expectations about your health and your life.

Mentally Managing a Chronic Illness

Many of the health problems discussed in this book, such as headaches, flu, and colds, get better with good home care or medical treatment. These **acute** illnesses go away after a short time and usually don't do any long-term harm to your body.

As people get older, they tend to get **chronic** health problems, such as arthritis, high blood pressure, heart disease, or diabetes. Unlike acute illnesses, chronic conditions persist. Generally, they can be managed, but not cured completely.

Your frame of mind can make a big difference in how much your chronic illness affects your life and how well you respond to treatment. People who decide not to let their health problems dominate their lives tend to be less bothered by their problems than are people who are overcome by fear and worry about their health.

Living with a chronic condition is not easy. In addition to their symptoms, chronic illnesses often bring on tension, depression, and fatigue. It's hard to feel positive when it seems like so much is going wrong. However, what you think can determine how good and how "in control" you feel.

Negative feelings can limit your body's ability to heal itself and fight disease. On the other hand, positive thoughts and expectations can boost your immune system and your mental powers to help you cope with the disease. If you are depressed because of your illness, see page 325.

Coping With Chronic Pain

Chronic pain is a common problem in many long-term illnesses. Chronic pain often has a mental as well as a physical component. Pain is not "all in your head," but your thoughts and feelings about the pain often affect how much pain you feel. Feeling anxious, angry, frustrated, or out of control about your pain may make the pain worse. Your mind and body are important allies in your efforts to manage pain.

You can train yourself to think and feel differently about chronic pain. These ideas are not a substitute for treatments or advice from your doctor, but they may be a helpful addition to your regular medical care.

- Take control of the pain. This may mean accepting that the pain is not going away, but deciding to take active steps toward managing it and keeping it from affecting your life too much.

- Track how your moods, thoughts, and feelings affect your pain. Record your pain level, activities, moods, thoughts, and feelings several times a day for several days. You may find that your pain is worse during or after certain activities or when you are feeling a certain emotion.

- Recognize negative or self-defeating thoughts you have about your pain, such as "This pain will never get better" or "I'll never be able to play with the grandkids with this pain." Your thoughts can affect your perception of pain.

- Practice positive self-talk. When you catch yourself in a negative thought, actively replace it with a positive statement, such as "I can manage this pain" or "I will relax before the kids get here."

- Try a relaxation technique. Chronic pain causes stress and tension, which in turn may increase pain. See pages 344 to 346 for relaxation techniques. Gentle exercise, such as walking, also helps relieve tension.

- Change the way you do daily activities so you can do them with less pain.

If you can put your mind to work against the pain, you may find that you can manage pain better and that it interferes less with your life. Also see Dealing With Chronic Pain on page 119.

Winning Over Serious Illness

A feeling of hopelessness often goes hand in hand with a diagnosis of chronic or life-threatening illness. The best way to triumph over cancer, heart disease, diabetes, or any other serious illness is to shake that feeling of hopelessness and stay in control of your life.

- Remember who you really are. Who you are does not change because of your illness.

- Keep communicating with family and friends. Talking openly about your illness will help them as well as you.

- Gather your support network around you. Forget any notion about being a burden. Letting people help you helps them feel good about themselves.

- Join a support group of other people who are coping with the same problem. Finding even one person who has overcome a problem similar to yours can raise your spirits and add to your confidence.

Lots of people win their struggles over serious illness, either by being cured or by not letting illness control their lives. While there are no guarantees, taking charge of your life will give both your body and your mind the best opportunity to be victorious.

Stress

Stress comes with all of life's daily hassles as well as with crises and life-changing events. Stress can sometimes be motivating and energizing, and you feel a sense of relief after you have gotten through a stressful time. At certain times in your life, however, you may find yourself experiencing mounting levels of stress—brought on by changes in your health, your job or financial situation, your family, or events in the world—from which there seems to be little or

no relief. This is chronic stress, and it can greatly increase your risk for physical and mental illness.

What Stress Does to Your Body

The stress response is a natural reaction to a threat. At the first sign of alarm, chemicals released by your pituitary and adrenal glands and nerve endings automatically trigger these physical reactions:

- Your heart rate increases to move blood to your muscles and brain.

- Your blood pressure goes up.

- You start to breathe more rapidly.

- Your digestion slows down.

- You start to perspire more heavily.

- Your pupils dilate.

- You feel a rush of strength.

Your body is tense, alert, and ready for action and will stay that way until you feel that the danger has passed. Then your brain will signal an "all clear" to your body, and your body will stop producing the chemicals that cause the stress response and gradually return to normal. You feel this as a sense of relief.

In chronic stress, your body fails to give the "all clear" signal, and your body and mind don't return to a relaxed state for prolonged periods of time. This can be very harmful to your physical body, your immune system, and your emotional health. You may find it difficult to see the relationship between chronic stress and physical health problems, because the long-term effects of stress are subtle and slow to develop. However, experts in every area of medicine are discovering the links between stress and disease. By changing the way you respond to stressful situations and finding ways to regularly relieve the tension caused by stress, you can decrease your risk for stress-related health problems.

Becoming More Stress-Hardy

Some people seem to be more resistant to stress, and studies indicate that these people are less likely than others to get sick. Researchers have identified four personality factors that stand out in stress-hardy people:

• They have a strong commitment to self, work, family, and other values.

• They have a sense of control over their lives.

• They generally see change in their lives as a challenge rather than a threat.

• They have a strong network of support and close relationships.

It's never too late to develop a more stress-hardy personality. The first step is to believe that you can do it (remember, think positive!). Approach one challenging area of your life at a time. Be committed to making things better for yourself and those around you. Identify the things you can control and those you cannot. Accept that changes will occur, and know that you will be able to deal with them. Call upon your support

network to get the help you need, whether it's someone to watch your children for a few hours so you can run errands or someone who will just listen to your plans. As you begin to gain control over one challenging area of your life, you will find more time and energy for tackling additional areas.

Recognizing Stress

Classic signs of unrelieved stress include headache, stiff neck, or a nagging backache. You may start to breathe rapidly or get sweaty palms or an upset stomach. You may become irritable and intolerant of even minor disturbances. You may lose your temper more often and yell at your family for no good reason. Your pulse rate may increase, and you may feel jumpy or exhausted all the time. You may find it hard to concentrate.

When these symptoms appear, recognize them as signs of stress and find a way to deal with them. Just knowing why you're feeling the way you do may be the first step in coping with the problem. It is your attitude toward stress, not the stress itself, that affects your health the most.

Managing Symptoms of Stress

 Some people try to relieve the symptoms of <u>stress</u> by smoking, drinking, overeating, using drugs, or just "shutting down." Some people become violent or abusive in response to stress. These methods of coping have harmful side effects. By learning other ways to deal with symptoms of stress, you can avoid problems that may affect yourself or others and improve your overall quality of life.

- Express yourself. Stress and tension affect your emotions. By expressing your feelings to others, you may be better able to understand and cope with the feelings. Talking about a problem with a spouse or a good friend is a valuable way to reduce tension and stress. Expressing yourself through writing, doing crafts, singing, playing an instrument, drawing, or painting may also relieve tension.

- Cry. Crying can relieve tension. It's part of your emotional healing process.

- Get moving. Regular, moderate physical activity may be the single best approach to managing stress. Walking briskly will take advantage of your rapid pulse and tensed muscles and release your pent-up energy. After a long walk, your stress level is usually lower and more manageable. Stretching is also a good way to release muscle tension; or you might try yoga or tai chi to help relieve stress and relax your body.

- Be kind to your body and mind. Getting enough sleep, eating a nutritious diet, and taking time to do things you enjoy can all contribute to an overall feeling of balance in your life and help reduce stress.

Relaxation Skills

Whatever you do to manage stress, you can benefit from the regular use of relaxation skills.

The relaxation and meditation techniques that follow are among the simplest and most effective. Try doing them once or twice a day for about 20 minutes each time. Pick a time and place carefully, so you won't be disturbed or distracted. Once you've trained your body and mind to relax, you'll be able to achieve a relaxed state whenever you want.

Roll Breathing

The way you breathe affects your whole body. Full, deep breathing is a good way to reduce tension and feel relaxed. The object of roll breathing is to develop full use of your lungs and get in touch with the rhythm of your breathing. It can be practiced in any position, but it is best to learn it while lying on your back, with your knees bent.

1. Place your left hand on your abdomen and your right hand on your chest. Notice how your hands move as you breathe in and out.

2. Practice filling your lower lungs by breathing so that your left hand goes up when you inhale and your right hand remains still. Always inhale through your nose and exhale through your mouth.

3. When you have filled and emptied your lower lungs 8 to 10 times, add the next step to your breathing: inhale first into your lower lungs as before; then continue inhaling into your upper chest. As you do so, your right hand will rise and your left hand will fall a little as your abdomen falls.

4. When you exhale slowly through your mouth, make a quiet, whooshing sound, as first your left hand, and then your right hand falls. As you exhale, feel the tension leaving your body as you become more and more relaxed.

5. Practice breathing in and out in this manner for 3 to 5 minutes. Notice that the movement of your abdomen and chest is like rolling waves rising and falling in a rhythmic motion.

Practice roll breathing daily for several weeks until you can do it almost anywhere. Then you'll have an instant relaxation tool anytime you need one.

Caution: Some people get dizzy the first few times they try roll breathing. If you begin to hyperventilate or become light-headed, slow your breathing. Get up slowly.

Progressive Muscle Relaxation

Your body responds to stressful thoughts or situations with muscle tension, which can cause pain or discomfort. Deep muscle relaxation reduces muscle tension and general mental anxiety too. Progressive muscle relaxation is effective in combating stress-related health problems and often helps people get to sleep.

Muscle Groups and Procedure

You can use a prerecorded audiotape to help you go through all the muscle groups, or you can do it by just tensing and relaxing each muscle group. Choose a place where you can lie down on your back and stretch out comfortably, such as a carpeted floor. Tense each muscle group (hard, but not to the point of cramping) for 4 to 10 seconds; then give yourself 10 to 20 seconds to release it and relax. At various points, check the muscle groups you've already done and relax each one a little more each time.

Hands: Clench them.

Wrists and forearms: Extend them and bend the hands back at the wrist.

Biceps and upper arms: Clench your hands into fists, bend your arms at the elbows, and flex your biceps.

Shoulders: Shrug them. (Check your arms and shoulders for tension.)

Forehead: Wrinkle it into a deep frown.

Around the eyes and bridge of the nose: Close your eyes as tightly as possible. (Remove contact lenses before beginning the exercise.)

Cheeks and jaws: Grin from ear to ear.

Around the mouth: Press your lips together tightly. (Check your facial area for tension.)

Back of the neck: Press the back of your head against the floor.

Front of the neck: Touch your chin to your chest. (Check your neck and head for tension.)

Chest: Take a deep breath and hold it; then exhale.

Back: Arch your back up and away from the floor.

Stomach: Suck it into a tight knot. (Check your chest and stomach area for tension.)

Hips and buttocks: Squeeze your buttocks together tightly.

Thighs: Clench them.

Lower legs: Point your toes toward your face, as if trying to bring your toes up to touch your head. Then point your toes away and curl them downward at the same time. (Check the area from your waist down for tension.)

When you are finished, return to alertness by counting backwards from 5 to 1.

Relaxation Response

The relaxation response is the exact opposite of the stress response. It slows your heart rate and breathing, lowers your blood pressure, and helps relieve muscle tension.

Technique (adapted from Herbert Benson, MD)

1. Lie down in a place where you can stretch out comfortably. Close your eyes.

2. Begin progressive muscle relaxation. See page 345.

3. Become aware of your breathing. Each time you exhale, say the word "one" (or any other word or phrase) silently or aloud. Concentrate on breathing from your abdomen, not from your chest.

Instead of focusing on a repeated word, you can fix your gaze on a stationary object or just focus on your breathing. Any mental stimulus will help clear your mind.

Continue this for 10 to 20 minutes. As distracting thoughts enter your mind, don't dwell on them. Allow them to drift away.

4. Sit quietly for several minutes, until you are ready to open your eyes.

5. Notice the difference in your breathing and your pulse rate.

Don't worry about becoming deeply relaxed. The key to this exercise is to remain passive, to let distracting thoughts slip away like waves on the beach.

You may want to try combining **imagery** with the relaxation response:

1. Once you have begun the relaxation response and you feel relaxed and focused, create a vivid picture of a peaceful scene in your mind. The scene can be a sunny beach, a mountain meadow, or whatever works for you. Concentrate on the sights, sounds, and smells of your special place, letting the tranquility soothe your body and your mind. Stay as long as you like.

2. Continuing with your deep breathing, slowly come back to the present. Remember, the scene you create with your imagination is your special place to relax. Go there anytime you wish.

23

Complementary Medicine

The term "complementary medicine" broadly describes any health approach that is not part of the conventional medical approach of a particular society or culture. What is considered complementary or alternative varies from culture to culture. In the United States, many people use complementary therapies like acupuncture or herbal medicine along with mainstream medical treatments like medication or surgery to control pain, manage stress, and speed healing.

While complementary treatments are becoming more widely accepted, they are not right for everyone and every situation. As with any other treatment option, the decision to try complementary medicine should be made only after you gather as much reliable information as possible, understand the benefits and risks, and consider your personal needs and values. For more information, see Making Wise Health Decisions starting on page 3.

Here are some important things to consider when you're thinking about trying a complementary therapy:

• Think about what you want from complementary medicine. Are you looking for greater comfort and an improved quality of life? Or are you looking for a cure for illness? Seeking a cure through complementary medicine may be disappointing and, in some cases, harmful to your health. Discuss your expectations with the practitioner and make sure they are realistic.

• Do you think that complementary medicine has something special to offer you, or are you seeking an alternative treatment because you are fed up with conventional medicine? It is important to recognize the strengths and limitations of both conventional and complementary treatments.

• What is the practitioner's level of expertise? Check with state and local medical licensing agencies and departments of consumer affairs to see if the practitioner is licensed and in good standing. Talk to people who have had experience with the practitioner. Visit the practitioner and ask questions about his or her education, training, licenses, and certification.

• What does the evidence show? Have studies been done on this therapy? Are they good studies? Do they apply to your situation?

Your primary care doctor may be able to help you make informed decisions about complementary medicine. Some people think their doctors don't want them to try complementary medicine. But more and more doctors are realizing that complementary therapies can work with conventional medicine to improve health and help people feel better. Your doctor may be able to refer you to qualified complementary medicine practitioners.

If you do decide to try some form of complementary medicine, let your doctor know. Even if your doctor is not comfortable with your decision, it is important that he or she knows what you are doing about your health concerns. As much as possible, it is important that your conventional treatments work with your alternative treatments.

Health Fraud and Quackery

Millions of people are taken in each year by medical fraud and worthless health products.

Bogus cures are advertised for many chronic health problems, especially arthritis, cancer, baldness, obesity, and impotence. The ads target people who are ready to try anything. Unfortunately, many of these products cause harmful side effects. It is wise to be suspicious of products that:

• Are advertised by testimonials.

• Claim to have a secret ingredient.

• Have not been evaluated in prominent medical journals.

• Claim benefits that seem too good to be true.

• Are available only by mail.

Be suspicious of any practitioner who:

• Prescribes medicines or gives injections at every visit.

• Promises a no-risk cure.

• Suggests something that seems unethical or illegal.

The best way to protect yourself from medical fraud is to be observant and ask questions. If you don't like what you see or hear, find another practitioner or get a second opinion.

Risks and Benefits of Complementary Medicine

All treatments—whether conventional or complementary—have risks and benefits associated with them. In general, the risks and benefits of complementary therapies are as follows:

Risks

Overlooking effective conventional medicine: Perhaps greater than the concern for risks of a specific complementary therapy is the concern that a person will forgo effective medical treatment or neglect to get an accurate diagnosis. Some practitioners of complementary therapies do not refer people to conventional doctors even when it is possible that conventional medicine could help. And some people who choose complementary medicine refuse to consider conventional medicine for any problem. This can be dangerous. It is best to get as much information as possible and then make informed decisions, selecting from both conventional and complementary approaches for treatment of a specific health problem.

Potential dangers: Since many complementary therapies are not well studied, and the manufacture of complementary medicine products is not well regulated, you may be exposing yourself to unknown effects or possible dangerous interactions. The lack of regulation of products and practitioners may also expose you to additional health risks, especially if you have other medical conditions. In some cases it may be dangerous to combine complementary and conventional treatments. For example, taking St. John's wort while you are taking an antidepressant may overmedicate you and cause serious side effects.

Many options, and inadequate evidence: There are many different complementary treatments, and there is lots of evidence about them. Some of it is reliable. Very few complementary treatments have been studied for safety and effectiveness using traditional scientific methods. Unlike conventional medications, herbal medicines and nutritional supplements are not regulated by the Food and Drug Administration (FDA). Little reliable information is available, which makes it difficult to make an informed decision.

Cost: Many health insurance companies do not yet cover the costs of complementary therapies. As with conventional medical treatments, you must decide whether a complementary therapy is working for you and whether its benefits are worth the time and money you must invest.

Benefits

Holistic approach: When you see your conventional doctor, your visit usually lasts only 10 to 15 minutes. Practitioners of complementary medicine often take an hour or more to learn all about you—your beliefs, health expectations, family, friends, diet, activities, and work. Many health problems, especially chronic ones, may respond best to treatment that considers the whole person and his or her environment and lifestyle.

Active listening and touch: For many people, to be listened to and touched in a caring way can be very healing. People who provide complementary treatments are often taught to listen to and touch their patients.

Mind-body connection: Science has shown that people's emotional states can affect their health. See the Mind-Body Wellness chapter starting on page 337. People who describe themselves as happy tend to be healthier than those who describe themselves as unhappy. People who have a lot of stress in their lives are more likely to get sick. Conventional medicine does not have much to offer for these kinds of problems. Complementary practices like meditation and tai chi can help ease stress and improve a person's sense of well-being, which may improve the person's health.

Empowerment: Many people find that having the access and freedom to try complementary therapies is empowering. It gives them a stronger sense of control over their bodies and their health.

Choosing the Right Therapy for You

There are many types of complementary medicine. Choosing between different treatments can be confusing. This section describes several of the most widely available choices. Use this section to learn about different treatments and how they might work for you.

Acupuncture

Acupuncture is an ancient Chinese therapy based on the theory that there is energy called *qi* or *chi* (pronounced "chee") flowing through your body. Your *chi* flows along energy pathways called meridians. If the flow of *chi* is blocked or unbalanced at any point on a meridian, theoretically it may result in illness. Traditional practitioners believe acupuncture unblocks and balances the flow of *chi* to restore health. Western medicine practitioners who have studied acupuncture theorize that it reduces pain by acting on the biological mechanisms that control pain.

Traditional Chinese acupuncture is done by inserting very thin needles into the skin at specific points on the body to stimulate energy flow along the body's energy pathways. Other types of acupuncture may use heat, pressure, or a mild electrical current.

Acupuncture may be used to relieve pain and treat health conditions such as addiction, asthma, headache, menstrual cramps, and joint and muscle problems. Promising results have been found for the use of acupuncture in relieving pain after surgery and in treating nausea and vomiting related to chemotherapy.

Bodywork and Manual Therapy

Bodywork and manual therapy refer to a variety of body manipulation techniques used for relaxation and pain relief. Massage and chiropractic are well-known forms of bodywork. Other common forms include the Alexander Technique, the Feldenkrais Method, the Trager approach, Rolfing, and deep tissue massage.

The idea behind bodywork is that people learn (or are forced into by injury or stress) unnatural ways of moving or holding their bodies. Theoretically, these unnatural movements and postures change the natural alignment of bones. This in turn causes discomfort and may contribute to health problems.

The goal of bodywork is to realign and reposition the body to allow natural, graceful movement. Along with identifying possible causes of unnatural movement and posture, bodywork is thought to reduce stress and ease pain.

There has not been much scientific testing of bodywork. A few studies suggest good results for people with arthritis, stress-related problems, or low back pain, and for children with cerebral palsy.

Chiropractic Treatment

Chiropractic is a hands-on therapy based on the theory that many medical disorders may be caused by dislocations in the spine. The main goal of chiropractic therapy is to help the body heal itself by correcting misalignments or dislocations of the joints, particularly the bones of the spine.

Chiropractic treatments usually involve having a chiropractor twist, pull, or push your body to adjust your joints and the bones in your spine. Some chiropractors use heat, electrical stimulation, or ultrasound to relax your muscles before doing an adjustment.

Chiropractic treatment has been shown to be helpful in treating low back pain, neck pain, and headaches.

Healing Touch

Healing touch, spiritual or energy healing, therapeutic touch, prayer, and distant healing are terms used to describe the conscious focus on another person to promote healing and well-being without physical intervention. Spiritual healing is widely practiced and may or may not have anything to do with an established religion. Therapeutic touch is taught in many nursing schools, and nurses may use it in conventional medical settings to help comfort their patients.

Like many other complementary approaches, healing touch starts with the idea that people are naturally healthy. The way people live and think may disturb their natural health energy and make them ill. The aim of healing touch is to focus or channel healing energy to restore health and balance. Some forms of healing touch use physical touch as part of the healing, but many do not.

There has been almost no research on the effects of healing touch. It is a difficult form of therapy to study using traditional scientific methods. However, supporters of healing touch believe it is helpful in healing wounds, curing infection, and relieving pain. At the least, healing touch may help reduce anxiety and stress and provide comfort to a sick person.

The only known risk in using healing touch arises when people forgo effective medical treatment and rely only on healing touch. Healing touch is not appropriate for acute, life-threatening situations or as a replacement for other treatments that are known to improve a disease. Prayer, healing, and therapeutic touch can always be used along with more conventional treatments.

High-Dose Vitamin and Mineral Therapy

It has been suggested that high doses of vitamins and minerals—particularly antioxidant vitamins such as A, C, and E and minerals such as zinc—may be helpful in the prevention or treatment of health problems ranging from colds to cardiovascular disease to cancer.

Megavitamin and mineral therapies are the subject of a number of clinical studies. Until the safety and effectiveness of these therapies are better understood, it is important to use vitamins and minerals with caution. If you take vitamins or minerals in doses that exceed the Recommended Daily Value (RDV), you need to weigh the potential benefits against the risk of side effects and drug interactions. Find out as much as you can about the proper dosage of any vitamin or mineral you plan to take, and learn what forms are best used by your body.

Let your health professional know that you are considering using megavitamin or mineral therapy. This is especially important if you are taking medications or receiving other treatments for a health condition.

Herbal Medicine

Plants and other natural products have been used for thousands of years to maintain health and treat illness. They are the basis for many conventional medications. For example, willow bark tea was used for centuries to control fever. Drug companies learned to copy the chemical makeup of willow bark to produce aspirin.

Herbal medicines do many of the same things conventional drugs do. They may prevent illness. They may cure infection. They may soothe a fever or help wounds heal. They may keep your bowels regular or ease your pain. They may calm you down or perk you up.

Some herbal medicines have no effect at all. Others may even be harmful. Like conventional medicines, herbal medicines and natural supplements may cause side effects, trigger allergic reactions, or interact with other medications you are taking.

There have been thousands of studies on the effects of herbs. Most of the research has been done in Europe and China, where herbal medicine is widely practiced. In the United States, the analysis of this research began fairly recently, and many new studies are under way.

When shopping for herbal supplements, look for the USP (United States Pharmacopeia) or NF (National Formulary) symbols. These symbols indicate that the product has complied with the manufacturing and safety standards set by the USP. The USP symbol further indicates that the product has an FDA or USP endorsement for its intended use.

Be sure to tell your doctor about any herbs or natural supplements you are taking. If you have a serious health problem, do not use any herbal medicines or natural supplements without first consulting your doctor.

Homeopathy

Like other complementary treatments, homeopathy is based on the idea that the body has the ability to heal itself. Sometimes the body needs to be stimulated to start the healing process. In homeopathy, a treatment is chosen because it can cause a health problem just like the one that is troubling you. The treatment is given in such a small amount that, in theory, it does not cause the problem but does stimulate your body to heal the problem. Extremely dilute solutions containing only a trace of plant or mineral are given.

Homeopathy has been used to treat allergies, atopic dermatitis, rheumatoid arthritis, irritable bowel syndrome, and other chronic conditions. It is not considered appropriate for treatment of serious illnesses or emergencies.

Homeopathy is widely used in England and other European countries. It is not clearly understood how or to what extent homeopathy works.

Magnetic Field Therapy

The body naturally generates electric currents (which trigger heartbeats and nerve impulses) and emits a slight magnetic force.

Practitioners of magnetic field therapy believe that interactions between the body, the earth, and other electromagnetic fields can cause physical and emotional changes. They also believe the body's electromagnetic field must be in balance to maintain good health.

Magnetic field therapy uses magnets to stimulate areas of the body in an attempt to maintain health and treat illness. The magnets are applied to the outside of the body. They may be electrically charged to deliver an electrical pulse to the area being treated or used in combination with acupuncture needles. Static (not electrically charged) magnets may be inserted in pads and wraps of various sizes and shapes, belts, jewelry, shoe insoles, seat cushions, and mattresses. These magnets deliver continuous magnetic energy to the affected area as long as they are in contact with it.

Magnetic field therapy is being studied for use in treating a wide range of problems, including arthritis and other joint problems, migraine headaches, depression, and cancer. It may also be useful in treating postsurgical pain and chronic pain and in sports medicine to treat strains and sprains. Magnetic field therapy has not been proven effective in the treatment of any illness.

Magnetic field therapy is not thought to have any side effects when combined with conventional medical treatment. However, people who have implants with a magnetic field, such as pacemakers, should not use magnetic field therapy because it could interfere with the function of the implant.

Be sure to tell your doctor if you plan to use magnetic field therapy in addition to the treatment he or she prescribes.

Massage Therapy

Massage therapy is based on the idea that touch is healing. There are many different types of massage. Some are gentle, while others are active and intense. Some methods apply the same principles as acupuncture: the massage therapist will press on or stroke points on the body where energy is blocked.

Massage therapy has been and continues to be widely studied. Many studies have shown that massage therapy decreases stress and helps control pain. Health problems that are caused or made worse by stress, such as depression and inflammatory bowel disease, may also improve with massage treatment.

Current research is focusing on the effects of massage in treating conditions such as asthma, diabetes, skin disorders, fibromyalgia, high blood pressure, behavioral problems, and eating disorders.

Naturopathy

Naturopathy blends conventional medicine with complementary medicine. Schools of naturopathy teach anatomy, cell biology, pharmacology, and other sciences studied in conventional medical schools. They also teach herbal medicine, acupuncture, and bodywork. The goal of naturopathy is to help you become and stay well, which is believed to be your body's natural state.

Naturopathic medicine is used to promote health, prevent disease, and treat all kinds of health problems. Most naturopaths can treat earaches, allergies, and other common medical problems. A properly trained naturopath refers people to other practitioners for diagnosis or treatment when appropriate.

Two of the biggest concerns about naturopathic medicine are the use of fasting and its approach to immunization.

Fasting puts your body under stress and can be dangerous, especially if you have a disease like diabetes. Talk with your conventional doctor before you try fasting. If you start to feel sick while fasting, break your fast with small amounts of fruit or juice and then return to your normal diet.

Some naturopaths do not believe that immunization is necessary. This philosophy is very controversial. Talk with your conventional doctor or visit the Web site of the Centers for Disease Control and Prevention (www.cdc.gov) before deciding against immunization.

Tai Chi and Qi Gong

Tai chi (pronounced "tie chee") and qi gong ("chee goong") are traditional Chinese exercises. They are based on the idea that through gentle, graceful, repeated movements, deep concentration, and focused breathing, you can increase and improve the flow of energy (*chi* or *qi*) through your body and improve your health.

Tai chi and qi gong are also founded on the Chinese belief that nature consists of opposing forces called yin and yang. It suggests that good health results when yin and yang are balanced. Tai chi and qi gong movements are done in an attempt to help restore the body's balance of yin and yang.

Tai chi is a series of movements done in a rhythmic pattern, either very slowly or very quickly. Qi gong is a lot of different movements that can be done in any order. Qi gong is useful to know because you can do it anywhere, anytime, even if you are unable to sit up or stand. Some common qi gong movements include raising and lowering your arms, moving your head from side to side, and rubbing your ears, feet, and hands.

Both tai chi and qi gong can be done by people of all ages. Their primary benefits are improved muscle strength, balance, coordination, posture, and flexibility; they are excellent for older adults. They may increase stamina, lower blood pressure, and relieve stress. Possible muscle strains and sprains are their only harmful side effect. Gentle stretching before doing tai chi or qi gong can prevent most injuries.

Tai chi and qi gong usually can be used safely alongside conventional medicine, but they should not replace effective conventional treatment. Talk with your health professional so you can choose the tai chi or qi gong program that best suits your needs.

Yoga

Yoga is a meditation program that includes exercises to improve flexibility and breathing, decrease stress, and maintain health. It has been practiced in India for centuries and is based on the principle of mind-body unity.

Two basic components of yoga are proper posture and breathing. There are many different yoga exercises, called postures. These may be done while standing, lying down, or sitting in a chair; some are done in a headstand position. While practicing a posture, which stretches the body, you do breathing exercises to help relax muscles, maintain the posture, and focus your mind.

Most people who try yoga find that it helps them become more flexible and less stressed. Several studies have shown that yoga helps lower blood pressure and improves a person's sense of well-being. Research has also shown that yoga can help people who have asthma learn to breathe more easily. People with chronic medical conditions like migraine headaches, heart disease, arthritis, or cancer may benefit from combining yoga and their conventional medical treatment.

For more information about these and other alternative treatments, do some research at your local library, or contact the National Center for Complementary and Alternative Medicine (NCCAM) at the National Institutes of Health (NCCAM Clearinghouse, P.O. Box 8218, Silver Spring, MD 20907-8218, 1-888-644-6226). Visit the NCCAM Web site at nccam.nih.gov.

A great oak is only a little nut that held its ground.
Anonymous

24

Staying Independent

SCAN Health Plan® strives to help its members remain healthy, safe, independent, and in control of where and how they live. This chapter is all about living your life as you want and increasing the chances that your wishes are followed.

Your most basic right as an individual is to have control over your own life and make your own decisions. This means choosing where you live, how you spend your money, what health services you will accept, and what type of help you need (if any).

It is important to think about where you stand on issues regarding your health and independence and to communicate your feelings openly and clearly to your family and health professionals. Making plans now will help ensure that you receive the type of care you want later on, if you should become unable to express your wishes. If you would like your family or health professionals to help you make decisions about your future, listen carefully to the suggestions and options they offer, think them over, and then decide for yourself.

This chapter provides information about and tools for staying independent: tips on taking care of yourself and maintaining your health, information about services to help you in your home, and advice on planning for the future.

Plan to Age Well

When it comes to managing your health, you are in charge. For most of your medical care, you probably consult your doctor. But whether you are in tiptop health or have a chronic illness, you make decisions every day that affect your health and well-being.

Making good decisions requires belief in your ability to take care of yourself. To use a metaphor, we aren't simply cars maintained by mechanics; we are the car, the driver, and most often the mechanic too. Here are some routine "driving and maintenance" tips you can apply to your health.

Read the manual. Understand your own health needs. Learn to ask questions and use your doctor, nurse, and pharmacist as consultants. Don't be shy about it. If you find it hard to ask questions during an office visit, prepare a list of questions, or consider taking along a family member to help. If your doctor is short on time, ask the nurse or pharmacist. If you have a long list of questions, ask the doctor to help you prioritize which ones need to be answered now and which ones can wait.

Check the oil. See your doctor at least once a year for health screenings and immunizations.

Check the map and plan your trip. How do you plan to keep yourself in good health? What milestones are important for you to reach? Working towards achievement of your goals will help you feel good about yourself. If your health is changing, make plans for your needs. Will you need someone to help you after a surgery? Have you safely updated your home to suit your changing health and ability to get around?

Use premium fuel. Sustenance, both physical and emotional, is key. Maintaining relationships with friends and family can offer support. Spirituality can provide a sense of community and peace in both good and bad times. A variety of good foods will keep you running smoothly. (See the Nutrition chapter starting on page 301.) And don't forget to feed your brain. It thrives on a variety of ideas and challenges.

Engine light flashing? Don't ignore warning signs. It is far easier to add a little oil now than to replace a whole engine later. If you experience a new problem—a lump, bump, or other unexplained symptom—get it checked out. Instead of waiting to be told something is wrong, show and tell your doctor. If you turn out to be fine, you can stop worrying.

Participate in driver education. If you are diagnosed with a new condition, read reputable pamphlets, books, and articles to become knowledgeable. If the illness is complicated, consider taking a class to learn how to manage it, or join a support group. You will meet other people with similar problems to solve and solutions to share.

Use your turn signals. Keep your family and your doctor updated about changes in your health and your need for help. If you find it hard to do things you need to do, work with your health care consultants and family to find solutions you can live with. Medications, diets, therapies, and your living space can often be adapted.

Trade down. Take years off your physical age by exercising, eating healthy foods, not smoking, and limiting alcohol use. Participate in life by learning, volunteering, staying current on events in your community, and enjoying the arts. Keep a positive attitude and stay active.

Plan for the end of the journey. Have you told your family about your wishes for end-of-life care? When the time comes, it may be too late for your family to ask you what you want. Consider your spiritual and emotional needs, and those of your family, and make plans before a crisis occurs. Make out an Advance Health Care Directive, often called a "durable power of attorney for health care." Consider the situations in which you would want someone else to make decisions for you. It's okay to accept assistance from family or friends when you need it.

Enjoy the journey. Stop and smell the roses. Don't skip the scenic overlooks, the museums, the world's largest ball of string, and the orchards. Aging well means continuing to live each day, enjoying your world, learning, being amazed, and finding something to laugh about.

Services to Help You Stay Independent

Most people enjoy living in their own homes. They have family, friends, and neighbors with whom they share their lives. At some point, however, some individuals may need extra support to continue living at home safely and independently. Help with some daily activities, in the form of services or care from family members, can make it possible to remain in the familiar surroundings of their home.

The best way to remain independent is to know what your options are, when to ask for help, and where to find it. The following services may be available to you through SCAN or in your community.

Personal care coordination or care management: A program that provides staff, called care managers, to guide individuals and families in determining their needs and obtaining the services that address those needs.

Home health aides or personal care assistants: Staff who provide basic care such as assistance with bathing, dressing, and help in using the toilet. They can provide service in your home for short periods—after a hospitalization, for instance—or on an ongoing basis.

Homemaker services: Services that include light housekeeping, cooking, shopping, and laundry.

Chore services: Services that provide assistance with major house cleaning, yard work, and minor household repairs.

Personal Emergency Response System: A service that provides a device, usually worn around the neck or wrist, that you can activate if you have fallen or need urgent assistance. When activated, the device automatically calls a neighbor, a relative, or an emergency response center for help.

Adult day care: A setting that provides physical, social, or intellectual exercise and stimulation for impaired individuals, as well as relief for the regular caregiver.

Respite care: A service that provides temporary care for an impaired individual so that the regular caregiver can have some time to him- or herself to rest, do errands, or see friends. Respite services may range from a few hours to a week or two at a time, if the caregiver has to be away. (For more information, see the Caregiver Secrets chapter starting on page 367).

Home-delivered meals: Nutritionally balanced and affordable meals that are delivered to your home.

Congregate meals: Meals served at a central location, usually a senior center or meals site. These sites also offer social activities and discussion groups.

Senior centers: Community sites where older people gather for meals, social activities, trips, and educational programs.

Transportation: Taxi or van services provided by SCAN or your local government or community agency; they are often called Dial-A-Ride or ACCESS.

Friendly visitors or callers: Typically staffed by community volunteers, these services offer visits and companionship in your home or by phone.

Skilled home care: Professional nursing care that is carried out in your home rather than a hospital or nursing home. This level of care requires a physician's order/recommendation and is usually for a limited time. It is often supplemented with personal care provided by home health aides. In-home physical, respiratory, speech, and occupational therapy services are also available.

For help locating these services in your community, call SCAN Member Services at 1-800-559-3500. You can also ask senior center staff, social workers, clergy, physicians, nurses, and friends, or call the Elder Care Locator service provided by the U.S. Administration on Aging at 1-800-677-1116.

Independence and Control at the End of Life

One of the most difficult parts of aging is acknowledging that everyone passes through stages of life and all lives have an end point. The key is to plan ahead and empower yourself. That way your family and health care team will know your preferences and can carry them out in an informed manner. If you begin advance care planning early and make choices before a medical crisis occurs, you increase the chances that your wishes and directions will be honored.

Sometimes a medical crisis occurs suddenly and unexpectedly. Family and friends may be overwhelmed by the situation and feel uncomfortable making decisions on your behalf if they don't know your wishes and preferences. In this case, an advance directive can give them peace of mind about speaking for you or making decisions on your behalf. In other situations, changes in health can occur over time. Many people tend to put off or avoid thinking about "what if" or "someday." When that someday arrives, an advance directive guides your family in decision making.

Staying Safe When Using In-home Services

If you employ a caregiver or homemaker or have repairmen in your home, it's wise to be aware of a few safety tips. Unfortunately today, bad things occasionally happen, and the home environment offers temptations for some in-home workers. To keep your personal belongings, your identity, and yourself secure, take the precautions listed below. In doing so, you can make yourself less vulnerable to crime, further ensuring your independence and control of your home.

- Ask for identification before allowing any worker to enter your home.

- Only allow caregivers, homemakers, and home repair workers in your home at scheduled appointment times.

- Verify all unscheduled visits with the agency or repair service before allowing a worker into your home.

- Do not hide keys around the outside of your house for anyone to use while you are not home.

- Do not leave valuables in open view.

- Designate a closet or another area in your home where you can store valuables (purse, wallet, cash, credit cards, jewelry, checkbook) and important papers. Secure this area with a lock, and give a spare key to a loved one if possible. Make sure your valuables are locked away before allowing any workers into your home.

- NEVER give your Medicare/Medi-Cal or Social Security number to your caregiver.

- Do not leave house keys in the open.

- Do not leave strangers (caregivers, homemakers, repair persons, or sales people) unattended in your home.

- Do not allow the caregiver to use your car to do shopping for you.

- Do not discuss your financial affairs with your caregiver.

- If a caregiver asks inappropriate questions, report this to the caregiver's employer or agency.

- Keep money in a bank or financial institution, not at home.

- Do not rely on your caregiver to do your banking. If you are unable to do your own banking, entrust a relative or friend, not your caregiver. Make this person known to your bank manager, lawyer, and relatives.

- Arrange to have any incoming checks, such as your pension checks, deposited directly into your bank account.

- Do not loan your caregiver money. A request for a loan by a caregiver, no matter how friendly your relationship, is never appropriate. Report requests for a loan to the caregiver's employer.

- Be wary of anyone pressuring you to sell your house or sign any legal papers.

- Caregivers are professionals and should behave as such. Report any unprofessional behavior to the caregiver's employer. Your needs, not the caregiver's personal problems, should be the focus of the caregiver's visit.

Advance Care Planning

The process of talking with your doctor and your loved ones about your wishes for medical care at the end of your life is called advance care planning. When you write down your wishes, the document is called an advance directive.

An advance directive lets you specifically state what kind of treatments you do and don't want. It also enables you to name someone, such as your spouse, another close family member, or a group of family members, to make decisions for you if you lose your ability to communicate.

Probably the most commonly used form of advance directive is the "durable power of attorney for health care." A more limited type of advance directive is the living will; however, this is not considered legally binding in California. Both have recently been combined in California into a new form entitled Advance Health Care Directive.

How to Begin Thinking About Your Preferences, Beliefs and Hopes for End-of-Life Care

Start simply, by trying to list your fears and understand them. Do your concerns relate to leaving love ones or unfinished projects behind? To being in pain? Losing your dignity while undergoing treatment? Not being clearly understood by those around you? Being alone? Being overly sedated or in a lingering state of unconsciousness? Leaving your loved ones without adequate financial resources? Dying in a strange place?

Once you know that you want to explore these topics and make some plans, most experts suggest that you begin by talking. Talk openly to family and friends about your values and beliefs, your hopes and fears about the end stage of your life. Meet with your religious advisor or clergy about spiritual concerns. If a family member is uncomfortable with the subject, you can try starting the conversation with a related topic. Use "openings" in conversations, such as recalling a family event and talking about a future event where you might not be present. Talk about whom you wish to leave a possession to and whom you would like to have nearby if you were seriously ill.

Ask your doctor for a time when you can go over your ideas and questions about end-of-life treatment and medical decisions. Tell him or her you want guidance in preparing advance directives. If you are already ill, ask your doctor what you might expect to happen as the disease progresses. Let him or her know how much information you wish to receive about your illness, prognosis, care options, and hospice programs.

While initiating these conversations is uncomfortable for some, the risk of leaving these issues unresolved is greater. If you become unable to express your wishes and there is no clear indication about your preferences for treatment, these important decisions may be made by a court-appointed individual, who is unlikely to know you or your situation.

Financial Decisions

For some people, it is easier to start the process by focusing on your estate and financial planning. Make sure you have a valid, up-to-date will, or trust documents. Discuss with your lawyer or financial advisor whether your legal and financial affairs are in order. A "durable power of attorney for financial affairs" is a legally binding document that designates a trusted person to make financial decisions for you if you become unable to act for yourself. A lawyer should help you understand and complete these documents.

Medical Decisions

Advances in medical technology make it possible to keep alive a person who, in former times, would have died more quickly from the serious nature of his or her illness or injury. However, you have the right to make your own decisions about the extent of your care. You can request that medical treatment you do not want be withdrawn or withheld. For example, if you have a fatal illness and are near death, you may not want to have cardiopulmonary resuscitation (CPR) if your heart stops. You also have the right to insist on receiving treatments to relieve symptoms, such as medicine for pain.

California's Health Care Decisions Law, which became effective July 1, 2000, combines the "durable power of attorney for health care" and the instructions for health care decisions into one form called the Advance Health Care Directive. However, older forms executed before July 1, 2000, are still valid.

Things to Think About When Writing an Advance Directive

There are no right or wrong answers to these questions. Talk them over, then answer them according to your own beliefs and share your wishes with your health care agent, family, and doctor. Give copies of your advance directive to your attorney, your doctor, your family, and your health care agent.

- How important is independence and being in control in your life?

- How do you feel about the use of life-supporting medical treatments such as CPR, respirators or ventilators, kidney dialysis, artificial nutrition or hydration, and antibiotics to treat a life-threatening infection?

- Who do you feel should make the final decision about any medical treatments you might undergo?

- What will be important to you when you are dying (for example, physical comfort, no pain, family members present, etc.)?

- Where would you prefer to die?

- Do you want to donate parts of your body to someone else when you die?

- How do your spiritual beliefs affect your feelings about serious or terminal illness?

Remember that you can revisit these issues and change your advance directive at any time.

Advance Health Care Directive forms are available from several agencies and Web sites:

1. SCAN Health Plan Member Services, 1-800-559-3500

2. Your doctor's office or local hospital

3. California Medical Association, CMA Publications, P.O. Box 7690, San Francisco, CA 94120-7690, or visit www.cmanet.org.

4. Partnership for Caring. Call 1-800-989-WILL, or visit www.partnershipforcaring.org.

The Advance Health Care Directive, (also called a "durable power of attorney for health care" or a "medical power of attorney") names someone, a relative or friend, to make medical decisions for you when you are not able. Depending on the state where you live, the person you designate is called an agent, attorney-in-fact, proxy, or surrogate (California uses the first two terms). Now is a good time to think about appointing a trusted person to speak for you in case you become unable to do so later. It is important to select a health care agent who knows you well and whom you trust. You should also name a backup agent in case the first person is unavailable. A relative or friend can serve this role, but an attending physician or hospital staff person usually cannot.

The agent will be able to make all decisions regarding your health care, from flu shots to the need for surgery. For example, your agent will have access to your medical records unless you limit this right. And your agent or proxy can decide whether to withdraw or withhold life-sustaining procedures. While you can be as specific as you wish in the guidelines you give in the document, remember that your agent must also have the flexibility to make decisions in changing circumstances. (See Things to Think About When Writing an Advance Directive on page 363.) You do not need a lawyer to complete an Advance Health Care Directive. However, to be valid, the document must be signed, and some states require a witness. It's a good idea to note the location of the original form on each of the copies you give to your agent, your family, your doctor's office, and your hospital.

It is important to know that you cannot be forced to sign an advance directive as a requirement of admission to a hospital or nursing home or membership in a health plan. However, these organizations may encourage you to consider this so they can better provide for your wishes.

Another form that may be useful to know about is the Do Not Resuscitate order, or DNR. Written by a physician as part of the medical chart, it instructs medical personnel, including emergency medical personnel, not to use resuscitative measures, such as CPR or chest compressions. For older people living at home, there is an Out of Hospital DNR form. This form is free from the California Medical Association. To be effective, this form must be accessible to emergency medical personnel entering the home. The refrigerator door is a good place to keep a clearly labeled copy.

If your wishes for treatment change, complete new advance directive forms. Do not just cross out a line or add new information unless it is simply a change of address or phone number. Make sure that everyone is aware that you have changed the forms.

Keep all your important papers—your Advance Health Care Directive and your medical, long-term care, and life insurance policies—in an accessible place. Do not put them in a safety deposit box unless others have access to it. Tell a trusted person where these documents are located. You should also think about, and write out, instructions for your funeral, burial, or cremation preferences. Include instructions on how they will be paid for.

Hospice Care and the Medicare Hospice Benefit

Suprisingly, many people do not realize that there is an all-inclusive hospice care benefit available to Americans through the Medicare program. Since 1983, the Medicare Hospice Benefit has enabled millions of terminally ill Americans and their families to receive quality end-of-life care that provides comfort, compassion, and dignity.

What is hospice care?

Considered to be the model for high-quality, compassionate care at the end of life, hospice care takes a team-oriented approach to providing expert medical care, pain management, and emotional and spiritual support expressly tailored to the patient's needs and wishes.

Support is extended to the patient's loved ones as well. At the center of hospice is the belief that each of us has the right to die symptom-free and pain-free, with dignity. The focus is on caring, not curing, and in most cases care is provided in the patient's home. Hospice care is also provided in freestanding hospice facilities, hospitals, and nursing homes and other long-term care facilities.

How does hospice work?

Typically, a loved one serves as the primary caregiver and, when appropriate, helps make decisions for the terminally ill individual. Members of the hospice staff make regular visits to assess the patient and provide additional care or other services. Hospice staff are on call 24 hours a day, 7 days a week.

The hospice team develops a care plan that focuses on the patient's need for pain management and symptom control, as well as emotional and spiritual needs. The plan outlines the medical and support services required, such as nursing care, personal care (dressing, bathing, etc.), social services, physician visits, counseling, and homemaker services. It also identifies the medical equipment, tests, procedures, medications, and treatments necessary to provide high-quality comfort care.

The hospice team usually consists of:

- The patient's family and caregivers.
- The patient's personal physician.
- A hospice physician (or medical director).

- Nurses.

- Home health aides.

- Social workers.

- Clergy or other counselors.

- Trained volunteers.

- Speech, physical, and occupational therapists, if needed.

What is included under the Medicare Hospice Benefit?

Hospice care is available as a benefit under Medicare. The Medicare Hospice Benefit is designed to meet the unique needs of those who have a terminal illness, providing them and their loved ones with special support and services not otherwise covered by Medicare.

Under the Medicare Hospice Benefit, beneficiaries elect to receive non-curative treatment, which consists primarily of services to keep them comfortable and out of pain during their terminal illness by waiving the standard Medicare benefits for treatment of a terminal illness. However, the beneficiary is still able to use Medicare benefits for treatment of conditions unrelated to the terminal illness. For more information about Medicare or to receive a Medicare handbook, call 1-800-MEDICARE (1-800-633-4227).

Summing Up

As you have read in this chapter, a variety of tools and techniques are available to keep you independent and in control. Following the guides for taking care of yourself in this chapter and throughout the book can increase your chances of aging well. If you do need some extra assistance, services may be available through SCAN or in your community. Taking steps to begin advance care planning with some of the tools and strategies presented here will go a long way toward ensuring that your care at the end of your life is as you envision it. But the responsibility is yours! The important thing is to begin the planning process and open the conversation.

Selected material from *Fact Sheet: End-of-Life Decision Making* has been used with permission of Family Caregiver Alliance/National Center on Caregiving. For more information, visit www.caregiver.org or 1-800-445-8106.

One of the deep secrets of life is that all that is really worth the doing is what we do for others.
Lewis Carroll

25

Caregiver Secrets

Many people are caring for a chronically ill or disabled spouse, parent, or other family member. Caregiving can be a rewarding experience, especially when you know that your care makes a positive difference. However, caregiving can be difficult. There are three secrets to being a good caregiver:

• Take care of yourself first.

• Don't help too much.

• Don't do it alone.

This chapter will tell you more about these secrets and how they can help you and the person you are caring for.

Caregiver Secret No. 1: Take Care of Yourself First

If you want to give good care, you have to take care of yourself first. Caregivers tend to deny their own needs. This

strategy may work fine for short-term caregiving. For long-term caregiving, however, it is sure to lead to problems.

Several things happen when care-givers don't take good care of themselves:

• They become ill.

• They become depressed.

• They "burn out" and stop providing care altogether.

These things are bad for both the care-giver and the person receiving the care.

On the other hand, when caregivers take time to care for themselves, good things happen:

• They avoid health problems.

• They feel better about themselves.

• They have more energy and enthusiasm for helping others and can continue giving care.

Planning for Caregiving

- Learn as much as you can about the person's illness. Talk to his or her health care providers and find out how the illness may progress, how it is being treated, and what the expected results of treatment are. Know what medications the person is taking, what side effects to expect, and whether he or she has any drug allergies. Find out what kind of problems might come up and what additional health care services might be needed (for example, home nursing, hospitalization, or nursing home care).

- Work with the person's case manager or a social worker to review his or her financial situation. If financial assistance (such as Medicaid) may be needed to pay for long-term care expenses, find out how and when to apply for such assistance. Find out if your state requires you to become a legal guardian before you can manage your loved one's finances.

- Talk to your loved one about his or her after-death wishes. Does he or she want a funeral or memorial service; to be buried or cremated? Does he or she own a burial plot? Has money been set aside for these expenses? If not, it may be possible for you to establish a fund for these needs. Discuss this matter with a funeral director.

When you take on the task of caregiving, time becomes your most important resource. Caregiving requires a large time commitment, perhaps all of the extra time you have for yourself. If that happens, problems can develop.

The best way to prevent the depression, frustration, and resentment that cause caregiver burnout is to hold back some time out of every day for yourself. If you wait until all of your chores and caregiving tasks are done before doing things for yourself, you will wait a very long time. Instead, decide on the minimum amount of time you need each day to meet your basic personal needs. Carve that time out of your schedule. Then figure out how the chores will get done.

Here are some important things that you need to find time to do—just for yourself:

1. Get regular exercise, even just a few minutes several times a day. Exercise can be a good energizer for both physical and emotional health.

2. Maintain a healthy diet. When you are busy giving care, it may seem easier to eat fast food than to prepare healthy, low-fat meals.

However, healthy meals are easy to prepare, and a good diet will give you more energy to carry you through each day.

3. Make time for an activity you enjoy—reading, listening to music, painting or doing crafts, playing an instrument—even if you can only do it for a few minutes each day. If you like to participate in

church activities or take classes, ask a friend or family member to stay with your loved one for an hour or two once or twice a week so you can do those things.

4. Recognize stress and take steps to manage it. Your need for relaxation increases during periods of caregiving. For more information about recognizing and managing stress, see Stress on page 342.

Recognize and deal with signs of depression. Depression is common in caregivers. Maintaining a positive self-image is the most important thing you can do for yourself. Use self-care and ask for extra support when the earliest signs of depression appear. If that doesn't work, seek professional help. Also be on the lookout for signs of depression in the person you are caring for. Depression is common in older adults, especially those who have chronic diseases or who are disabled. Encouraging the person to seek treatment for depression will make your job easier in the long run. See Depression on page 325.

5. Deal with important issues in your life and maintain supportive relationships. Being a caregiver adds another dimension to your life, but it does not mean you have to put the rest of your life on hold. Issues involving your family and other relationships, your finances, your job, and other responsibilities still need to be addressed. Taking time to deal with issues as they arise and planning for the future are an important part of taking care of yourself. Make a conscious effort every day to stay connected with family, friends, and others in your support system.

6. Let go of guilt. The best way to let go of guilt is to accept the fact that you just can't be everything to everyone all of the time. Acknowledge your limitations, and do only what is most important. Tell yourself that you are doing a good job at a very difficult task, and ask for help. Feeling guilty is often a sign that you need a break from your caregiving schedule. Ask your friends and family to pitch in.

Caregiver Secret No. 2: Don't Help Too Much

The biggest mistake most caregivers make is providing too much care. Even if they don't admit it, people like to help themselves. Every time you do something for a person that the person could have done alone, there is a double loss. First, your effort may have been wasted. Second, the person has missed an opportunity to help him- or herself.

As a caregiver, your highest goal is to give the person you are caring for the power and the permission to be in control of his or her own life (as much as possible). Every act your loved one makes to maintain independence is a victory for you as a caregiver.

Long-Term Care Insurance

Medicare and private health insurance do not usually cover nursing home services or extended periods of home health care. (However, if the need is related to an acute medical problem, short-term services may be covered.)

Long-term care insurance is designed to protect families from the high costs of custodial care. When shopping for a policy of this kind, look for:

• Allowance of benefits without requiring a prior hospital stay.

• Premiums that do not increase because of age or health status.

• Benefits for in-home care.

• Guaranteed lifetime renewability.

• Comprehensive coverage for all levels of long-term care.

• Specific coverage for Parkinson's disease, Alzheimer's disease, and any other illness involving dementia.

• A waiver of premiums while receiving benefits in a long-term care facility.

• No waiting period for coverage of preexisting conditions.

For more information about Medicare and long-term care, call the U.S. Health Care Financing Administration at 1-800-638-6833, or contact your state office on aging.

Here are some things you can do to empower the person you are caring for to do things independently:

1. Expect more. People respond to expectations. If you expect the person to get dressed, care for houseplants, or prepare simple meals, the person often will.

2. Limit your availability to help. If you are not always there to help, the person will be forced to do more on his or her own.

3. Simplify. If you are caring for a person who has mild dementia, divide complex tasks into simpler parts for him or her: first, get out the cereal box; next get out the milk and the bowl, etc.

4. Make it easy. One of the most productive things a caregiver can do is to make modifications to the person's home and provide tools that will allow the person to do things without help.

5. Allow for mistakes and less-than-perfect results. The hardest thing about letting someone do something alone is knowing that you could do it better or faster. Mistakes are okay.

6. Reward both the effort and the result. Help the person feel good about doing things independently.

7. Let the person make as many decisions as possible, such as what to wear, what to eat, or when to go to bed. Help the person retain as much control as possible.

8. Give the person responsibility to care for something. Studies show that nursing home residents who are asked to care for pets or plants live longer and become more independent.

9. Match tasks with abilities. Identify the person's skills, and try to match them with tasks that the person can do independently.

10. Take acceptable risks. A few broken dishes or a few bruises are a small price to pay for letting someone explore what he or she can do. You can't eliminate all risks without eliminating all opportunities. See pages 26 and 47 for tips on how to create a safe environment and reduce the risk of accidents.

Elder Abuse

Abuse of an older adult may include any or all of the following:

- Physical or sexual abuse. This may include hitting, shaking, shoving, pinching, or burning a person, or performing sexual acts with the person without his or her consent.

- Psychological abuse. This may include verbal assault, threats, intimidation, humiliation, harassment, or isolating the person from his or her family, friends, or usual activities.

- Financial exploitation. This may include the improper or illegal use of a person's funds, assets, or properties without the person's consent.

- Neglect. This may include abandonment of an older adult by his or her caregivers or self-neglect, in which an older person's behavior threatens his or her own health and safety.

The reasons why elder abuse occurs are complex. The overwhelming amount of stress that comes with taking care of an older person—especially one who has severe health problems—is often a factor. Elder abuse is committed most often by family members, although abuse does occur at the hands of hired caregivers and employees of nursing homes, foster care, and board-and-care homes.

If you suspect elder abuse, contact the local Adult Protective Services agency, your state's office on aging or Area Agency on Aging, or the county Department of Social Services. Your state may have an Elder Abuse Hot Line; you may also call the Eldercare Locator at 1-800-677-1116.

Caregiver Secret No. 3: Don't Do It Alone

Some caregivers live under the impression that they are the only available source of help. However, there are often other sources of assistance available that can make your caregiving easier. If you want to be a good caregiver, know where to find help when you need it. The more support you have, the more successful you are likely to be.

See page 359 for a descriptive list of services that can help with a variety of needs, from shopping to personal care. Other types of services that may be useful to caregivers are discussed in this section.

Respite care may be the most important service for caregivers. Respite services provide someone who will stay with the person while you get out of the house for a few hours. If the person you are caring for needs routine medical care, you may be able to arrange to have the person stay in a nursing home for a few days while you get away for a break.

Ten Ways to Make Extra Time for Yourself

Five Ways That Don't Cost Money

- Trade one morning or afternoon "off" each week with another caregiver.

- Ask several relatives, friends, church members, or neighbors if each would relieve you for a few hours per week on a regular schedule.

- Sign up for respite services. Some are available for no cost or for a voluntary donation. For more information about respite care services, see page 372.

- Barter for services: offer a loaf of bread, a casserole, or errands in exchange for an hour of care.

- Plan some time each day to be alone, perhaps during a time when the person you care for doesn't need your attention.

Five Ways That Can Cost Money

- Hire a teenager or older adult to stay with the person for a few hours each day.

- Sign up for homemaker or chore services. By saving a few hours of housekeeping, you might have more time and energy for more important caregiving tasks.

- Sign up for a home-delivered meal service.

- Enroll the person in an adult day center. Even a part-time placement for several hours per week can be helpful to both you and the person you are caring for.

- Hire a home health aide or personal care assistant.

Adult day centers are "drop-off" sites where a person who does not need individual supervision can stay during the day. This service is usually offered during working hours and may or may not be available on weekends. Meals, personal care services, and social activities are provided.

Adult foster care or **board-and-care homes** are private homes where older adults receive around-the-clock personal care, supervision, and meals. Some states require board-and-care homes to be licensed.

Nursing homes generally have two levels of care. Intermediate care includes assistance with using the toilet, dressing, and personal care for people who do not have serious medical conditions. Skilled nursing care is usually for people who have just come from the hospital or for others who have medical conditions that require more intensive nursing care. Some facilities have special units for people with dementia.

Hospice programs provide social, personal, and medical services for terminally ill patients who wish to spend their remaining time at home or in a less formal environment than that of a hospital or nursing home.

Support groups give you an opportunity to discuss problems or concerns about caregiving with other caregivers.

To learn whether these services are available in your community, look under "Senior Citizen Services" in your Yellow Pages.

Your Rights as a Caregiver

As a caregiver you have the right:

- To take care of yourself. This is not an act of selfishness. It will allow you to take better care of your relative.
- To seek help from others even though your relative may object. Recognize the limits of your endurance and strength.
- To maintain parts of your life that do not include the person you care for, just as you would if he or she were healthy.
- To get angry, be depressed, and express other difficult feelings occasionally.
- To reject any person's attempt (either conscious or unconscious) to manipulate you through guilt, anger, or depression.
- To receive consideration, affection, forgiveness, and acceptance from your loved one as long as you offer these qualities in return.
- To take pride in what you are accomplishing and to applaud your courage in the sometimes difficult task of caregiving.
- To protect your individuality and make a life for yourself that will sustain you when your relative no longer needs your full-time help.
- To expect and demand that as new strides are made in finding resources to aid physically and mentally impaired older persons, similar strides will be made toward aiding and supporting caregivers.

Adapted from the AARP's "Caregiver's Bill of Rights."

Take Pride

Now that you know the three secrets of caregiving, you can see that they really aren't secrets at all. There is nothing magical or mysterious about being a good caregiver.

- Care for your own needs first. Your physical and mental health depend on it. Give yourself as much special attention as you give the person you are caring for.

- Help the person you care for to be independent. This is a gift to both of you.

- Recognize when you need extra help, and know where you can get it. A helping hand at the right time can make all the difference.

Take pride in being a caregiver. It is not easy, and those who do it are special people. The three secrets of caregiving can help you feel good about yourself and the care you give.

Caregiver Needs for Respite

If you can answer yes to any of the following questions, it's time to get more help.

- Do I feel overworked and exhausted?

- Do I feel dissatisfied with myself?

- Do I feel isolated?

- Do I feel depressed, resentful, angry, or worried?

- Do I feel that I have no time for myself?

- Do I lack time for exercise and rest?

- Do I lack time for fun with people outside of my family?

A merry heart doeth good like a medicine.
Proverbs 17:22

26

Your Home Health Center

Your health care takes place in your home more often than anywhere else. Having the right tools, medicines, supplies, and information on hand will improve the quality of your self-care.

Store all of your self-care tools and supplies in a central location. Use the Self-Care Supplies chart on page 376 as a checklist for keeping your home health center well stocked.

Note: If small children live in or visit your house, keep your supplies out of reach or stored in containers or cabinets with childproof safety latches.

Be familiar with the disaster preparation and response plan for your area. Keep the appropriate supplies on hand.

Home Medical Tests

Many common medical tests are now available in home kits. Combined with regular visits to your health professional, home tests can help you monitor your health and, in some cases, detect problems early.

Home medical tests must be very accurate to be approved by the Food and Drug Administration (FDA). However, they must be used correctly to give such accurate results. Follow the package directions exactly. If you have questions, ask your pharmacist or call the toll-free phone number on the product label.

Home medical tests are especially helpful if you have a chronic condition that requires frequent monitoring, such as diabetes, asthma, or high blood pressure. Ask your doctor which home medical tests would be appropriate for you. Some common tests are described next.

Self-Care Supplies

Item	Use	Comments
Bandages (Band-Aids, butterfly bandages, sterile gauze pads, adhesive tape, gauze)	Closing and protecting cuts and scratches.	See p. 43.
Blood pressure cuff and stethoscope	Measuring your blood pressure at home.	Your pharmacist can help you pick a blood pressure kit and show you how to use it.
Cold pack (keep in freezer)	Helping the healing of bumps, bruises, sprains, sore joints, or any other health problem that calls for ice.	Make your own: Put 1 pint of rubbing alcohol and 3 pints of water in a 1-gallon plastic freezer bag. Place inside another freezer bag and freeze.
Dental supplies (dental mirror, disclosing tablets, floss)	Removing plaque from teeth.	See p. 228.
Elastic "Ace" bandages	Supporting a strained or sprained joint.	See p. 60.
Eyedropper	Putting liquid medication in eyes or ears.	See p. 208.
Heating pad	Applying heat to sore joints or bruises after a day or so of cold packs. Do not use on a newly swollen joint.	Do not fall asleep with a heating pad on. Be careful if you have a condition such as diabetes that may make it hard for you to notice if the pad is too hot.
Humidifier or vaporizer	Adding water to the air to soothe coughs and make it easier to breathe. Humidifiers produce a cool mist. Vaporizers produce hot or cool mist.	Humidifiers should be cleaned and disinfected regularly, or mold may grow in them. Steam or hot water from vaporizers can cause burns.
Thermometer	Taking temperatures.	Temperature strips are easy to use, but not as accurate as other thermometers.
Tweezers	Removing splinters or ticks.	See p. 35.

Blood Pressure Monitoring

If you have heart disease or high blood pressure, it's a good idea to have a home blood pressure monitor so you can check your blood pressure regularly. By checking your blood pressure at home, when you are relaxed, you will be able to track changes resulting from your home treatment and medications.

The two general types of blood pressure monitors commonly available are manual and automatic. Automatic types may also be called electronic or digital.

A manual blood pressure monitor is similar to the one that your doctor or nurse might use to take your blood pressure. Called a sphygmomanometer, this device usually includes an arm cuff, a squeeze bulb for inflating the cuff, a stethoscope to detect blood pulsing through the artery, and a mechanical gauge or column of mercury to measure the blood pressure. Manual blood pressure monitors require good eyesight and hearing for correct use. Some models have a stethoscope head permanently attached to the cuff. With models that don't, you need to use a separate stethoscope with the monitor.

Automatic blood pressure monitors use a microphone to detect blood pulsing in the artery, so you don't need a stethoscope. The cuff, which is attached to your wrist or upper arm, is connected to an electronic monitor. Some models automatically inflate and deflate the cuff when you press a button. First you place your wrist or upper arm inside the cuff. Then you press a button to start the monitor and wait for a reading to appear on the display. The monitor records your pulse as well as your blood pressure. Automatic monitors are by far the easiest to use, but they are also the most expensive. Generally, the electronic models that use an arm cuff are more accurate than those that use a wrist cuff.

A pharmacist can help you select a home blood pressure monitor and make sure you get the right size cuff for your arm. Ask your doctor or another health professional to teach you how to use your blood pressure monitor. It's a good idea to take your monitor to your health professional's office once a year to have it calibrated against the monitor in the office.

Check your blood pressure at different times of day to see how rest and activities affect it. For regular readings, check it at the same time every day. Blood pressure is usually lowest in the morning and rises during the day. For the most accurate reading, sit still for 5 minutes before taking your blood pressure.

Do not make any changes to your medications based on your home blood pressure readings without consulting your doctor first.

Tests for Blood in Stool

The fecal occult blood test can detect hidden blood in your stools, which may indicate colon cancer or other problems. This test is inexpensive and easy to do, and it has been proven to save lives. It does not detect colon cancer as well as other screening tests can. Your doctor may recommend a more accurate screening test for colon cancer, such as flexible sigmoidoscopy or colonoscopy. See page 71.

Blood Glucose Monitoring

If you have diabetes, you may already monitor your blood glucose levels using a finger prick and a test strip. Some test strips can be read visually, but putting the strip into an electronic monitor is more accurate.

This test should always be used under a doctor's supervision. Never adjust your insulin dose based on a single abnormal test, unless your doctor has specifically instructed you to do so.

Check with your doctor if you have symptoms of abnormal blood glucose levels, even if the test is normal. See page 178.

Managing Your Medications

Medications have special importance for older adults. People over age 50 receive more prescriptions than do people of other ages. Because of changes in many body processes, your body absorbs and uses medications differently as you age. So managing your medications becomes increasingly important as you get older.

- You may weigh less than you did when you were younger, and your body composition may have changed in ways that affect the amount of medication you may need.

- Your circulatory system, liver, and kidneys may work more slowly than they did before. These changes affect how quickly your body uses and disposes of medications.

- You may need to take several different medications, which increases the risk of drug interactions.

Be Smart About Medications

Good medication management begins in your doctor's office when a prescription is written, but it doesn't stop there. Here are some tips on how to organize and take medications as well as some guidelines for recognizing and avoiding problems caused by medications.

- Keep a medication record that lists:
  - The name of each medication you are taking.
  - The dosage you are taking.
  - Why you are taking each medication.
  - Who prescribed the medications.

- Include prescription and nonprescription medications, eyedrops, vitamins, skin ointments, and herbal supplements in your medication record.

- Discuss all medication decisions with your doctor. See page 13 for a list of questions to ask when medications are prescribed. Periodically ask your doctor if there are any medications you can safely stop taking.

- Ask about other treatment options besides medication. For some problems, exercise, diet changes, and stress management can provide many of the same benefits as medications do.

- Start low; go slow. Ask your doctor if you can start taking new medications at a low dose and increase the dose only as needed. Many drugs are tested on young adults. Older adults may need a lower dose.

- Learn about each medication you take. Talk to your doctor or pharmacist about the side effects of each of your medications and possible drug interactions.

- Go over your list of medications regularly. Check for outdated prescriptions and possible interactions. Clinics, hospitals, and senior centers often offer "brown-bag" medication days. So, if you prefer, you can put all of your medications in a brown bag and have a doctor or pharmacist review them with you to check for outdated prescriptions and other problems.

- Don't make any change in the number, kind, or dosage of medications you take without consulting your doctor first.

- Remember that your pharmacist is part of your health care team. Pharmacists can answer your questions about prescription and nonprescription medications as well as herbal, vitamin, and mineral supplements.

Organize Your Pills

Good medication management also means organizing your bottles and pills. Taking several different drugs at different times each day can be confusing, but taking your medications exactly as prescribed helps them work better. Develop a system to keep track of when and how you take each medication.

- Show your doctor a complete list of the drugs you take and when you take them. Ask if other medications or doses can be used to reduce the number of times you take pills each day.

- List your medication schedule on a daily planner that has spaces for hourly notations. Post it in a prominent place near your medicine cabinet. Take it with you when you travel.

- Post reminders near clocks or on the bathroom mirror to help keep you on schedule. Set an alarm clock or kitchen timer to remind you to take your medication.

- Use a pillbox designed to hold a week's worth of pills. You can also label empty egg cartons and use them to organize a day's or week's worth of medications.

- Ask if your pharmacist can provide color-coded containers, easy-open caps, and large-print labels.

- Keep medications in a cool, dry place. Heat and steam cause medications to lose their strength. Some drugs need refrigeration. Ask your pharmacist.

- Store drugs in their original containers, or clearly label any drugs that you put in different bottles.

- Inspect your medications at least once a year. Dispose of expired, unused, unlabeled, or discolored drugs by flushing them down the toilet.

Home Medical Records

You can keep medical records at home for your family. A 3-ring binder with dividers works just fine. Each person's section should start with a page that lists:

- Any diagnosed chronic conditions (for example, diabetes or asthma).

- Any known allergies to drugs, foods, or insects (list the allergy and the type of reaction).

- Information that would be useful in an emergency. For example, make a note if someone has a pacemaker, wears a hearing aid, has epilepsy, or has impaired vision.

- Medications the person is currently taking. Include the name of the drug, the reason why it was prescribed, the dosage, any special instructions, the doctor who prescribed it, and the date it was first prescribed.

- The name and phone number of the person's primary care doctor.

In addition, for each person's record you may want to include:

- An immunization record with date of last tetanus booster, flu shot, and pneumococcal vaccine.

- The most recent screening results for blood pressure, cholesterol, vision, and hearing.

- The results from recent cancer screenings, such as Pap tests, mammograms, colonoscopy, and PSA (prostate-specific antigen) tests.

- A list of major illnesses or injuries with dates when they occurred (for example, pneumonia or a broken bone).

- A record of all major surgeries or hospitalizations with the dates and the diagnoses.

- A list of conditions (such as heart disease, stroke, cancer, or diabetes) that have occurred in the person's family (parents, siblings, children).

- A copy of the person's advance directives, living will, and medical power of attorney.

Spend Less Money on Medications

Medications are expensive and the costs of several prescriptions add up quickly. Successful medication management will not only prevent adverse health effects but may help you save money as well. Besides avoiding unneeded drugs, you can cut your medication costs in these ways:

- Ask your doctor if generic forms of your medications are available and appropriate for you. Generics work just as well as brand-name drugs in most instances, and they cost less.

- Compare prices between several pharmacies. It may be worth paying a little more if you are comfortable with the pharmacist, but do shop around. Prices can vary.

- Ask your doctor for samples of newly prescribed medications, or ask your pharmacist to fill only the first week's worth of pills. If the medication has to be changed later, you won't have wasted the price of the full prescription.

- If you can choose where to buy your pills, consider buying regularly used, expensive medications from mail-order pharmacies (see Mail Order or the Local Pharmacy? on page 381). If your medication has a long shelf life, you may be able to buy larger quantities at a lower price.

Mail Order or the Local Pharmacy?

If you regularly take the same medications, buying them through a mail-order pharmacy (including on the Internet) may save you money. However, before you place your order, talk with your local pharmacist. Most pharmacies offer a senior citizen discount, and many compete well with mail-order prices. Your local pharmacy also offers a number of valuable services:

- Convenience and immediate availability

- The pharmacist's professional advice and personal service

- The ability to monitor all of your prescriptions for possible interactions

Before you switch to a mail-order drug company, be sure that the savings are worth the other services that you may be giving up. Your insurance coverage may also limit your choices of where to buy medications.

Nonprescription Medications and Products

A nonprescription medication (sometimes called an over-the-counter or OTC medication) is any drug that you can buy without a doctor's prescription. Don't assume that all nonprescription drugs are safe for you. These drugs can interact with other medications and can sometimes cause serious health problems.

Carefully read the label of any nonprescription drug you use, especially if you also take prescription medications for other health problems. Ask your pharmacist for help in finding a nonprescription drug best suited to your needs.

Common nonprescription medications include the following:

• Antacids and acid reducers

• Bulking agents and laxatives

• Antidiarrheals

• Cold and allergy remedies

• Pain relievers

These drugs can be very helpful when used properly but can cause serious problems if used incorrectly. The following tips will help you use common nonprescription drugs wisely and safely. In some cases, you may find that you don't need to take them at all.

Antacids and Acid Reducers

Antacids relieve heartburn or indigestion caused by excess stomach acid. While they are safe if used occasionally, antacids may cause problems if taken regularly. There are several kinds of antacids. Learn what ingredients are in each type so you can avoid any adverse effects.

• Sodium bicarbonate antacids (such as Alka-Seltzer and Bromo Seltzer) contain baking soda. Avoid these antacids if you have high blood pressure or are on a salt-restricted diet. If used too often, these antacids may interfere with heart and kidney function.

• Calcium carbonate antacids (such as Tums and Alka-Mints) are sometimes used as calcium supplements (see page 310). These products may cause constipation, so drink plenty of water when taking them.

• Aluminum-based antacids (such as Amphojel) are less potent and work more slowly than other products do. They may also cause constipation. Some may cause calcium loss and should not be taken by postmenopausal women. If you have kidney problems, check with your doctor before using aluminum-based antacids.

• Magnesium compounds (such as Phillips' Milk of Magnesia) may cause diarrhea. Diarrhea increases the risk of becoming dehydrated.

• Aluminum-magnesium antacids (such as Maalox, Di-Gel, Mylanta, and Riopan) are less likely to cause constipation or diarrhea than are aluminum-only or magnesium-only antacids.

Acid reducers reduce the amount of acid produced by the stomach. There are several types of nonprescription acid reducers on the market. Each has slightly different cautions for use. Read and carefully follow the instructions included with the package.

Antacid and Acid Reducer Precautions

• Try to eliminate the cause of frequent heartburn instead of taking antacids or acid reducers regularly. See Heartburn on page 78.

• Consult your doctor or pharmacist before taking an antacid if you take other medications. Antacids may interfere with the absorption and action of some prescription medications. Also consult your doctor if you have ulcers or kidney problems.

• If you have a problem with the function of your kidneys or liver, you should be careful in using acid reducers. All drugs are broken down and removed from the body by the combined action of the liver and kidneys. If your liver or kidneys are not working correctly, it is possible that too high a dose of the acid-reducing drug will build up in your body.

Bulking Agents and Laxatives

Two types of products are used to prevent or treat constipation: bulking agents and laxatives.

Bulking agents, such as bran or psyllium (found in Metamucil, for example) ease constipation by increasing the volume of stool and making it easier to pass. Regular use of bulking agents is safe and helps make them more effective.

Laxatives (such as Correctol, Ex-Lax, Senokot, and Dulcolax) speed up the passage of stool by irritating the lining of the intestines. Regular laxative use is not recommended.

There are many other ways to treat constipation, such as drinking more water. See page 72.

Precautions

• Drink plenty of water and other liquids when taking a laxative or bulking agent.

• Do not take laxatives regularly. Overuse of laxatives decreases muscle tone and sensation in the large intestine, causing laxative dependence. If you need help keeping your bowels regular, use a bulking agent.

• Regular use of some laxatives (such as Correctol, Ex-Lax, and Feen-a-Mint) may interfere with your body's ability to absorb vitamin D and calcium; this can lead to weakened bones.

Antidiarrheals

There are two types of antidiarrheal drugs: those that thicken the stool and those that slow intestinal spasms.

The **thickening** mixtures (such as Kaopectate) contain clay or fruit pectin and absorb bacteria and toxins in the intestine. They are safe because they do not go into the blood, but these products also absorb the bacteria needed for digestion. Long-term use is not advised.

Antispasmodic antidiarrheal products slow the spasms of the intestine. Loperamide (the active ingredient in products such as Imodium A-D and Pepto Diarrhea Control) is an example of this type of preparation. Some products (such as Donnagel and Parepectolin) contain both thickening and antispasmodic ingredients.

Antidiarrheal Precautions

- Do not use an antidiarrheal if you have glaucoma, kidney or liver disease, or prostate problems.

- Diarrhea helps rid your body of infection, so try to avoid using antidiarrheal medications for the first 6 hours after the onset of symptoms. After that, if cramping and pain continue, use antidiarrheal medication only if there are no other signs of illness, such as fever.

- Be sure to take a large enough dose. Take an antidiarrheal preparation until your stools thicken; then stop taking it immediately to avoid becoming constipated.

- Replace lost body fluids. Diarrhea increases your risk of becoming dehydrated. See Rehydration Drinks on page 74 for a recipe for a rehydration drink you can make at home.

Cold and Allergy Remedies

In general, whether you take medications for your cold or not, you'll get better in about a week. Rest and liquids are the best treatment for a cold (see page 142). Antibiotics will not help. However, other medications help relieve some cold symptoms, such as nasal congestion and cough.

Allergy symptoms, especially runny nose, often respond to antihistamines. Antihistamines are also found in many cold medications, often together with a decongestant. However, the value of antihistamines in treating cold symptoms is under debate.

Saline Nose Drops

Nonprescription saline nasal sprays (such as NaSal and Ocean) are convenient, inexpensive, and sterile. They will keep nasal tissues moist so the tissues can filter the air. Saline nasal sprays will not cause mucous membranes in the nose to swell.

Saline nose drops can also be easily made at home. Mix ¼ teaspoon salt in 1 cup of water warmed to body temperature (too much salt will dry nasal membranes). Place the solution in a clean bottle with a dropper (available at drugstores). Use as necessary. Make a fresh solution every 3 days.

Insert the drops while lying on your back on a bed, with your head hanging over the side. This will help the drops get farther back. Try to keep the dropper from touching your nose.

Decongestants

Decongestants make breathing easier by shrinking swollen mucous membranes in the nose so that air can pass through.

They also help relieve runny nose and postnasal drip, which can cause a sore throat.

Decongestants can be taken orally or used as nose drops or sprays. Oral decongestants are probably more effective and provide longer relief, but they cause more side effects. Pseudoephedrine, the active ingredient in products such as Sudafed, is an oral decongestant.

Sprays and drops provide rapid but temporary relief. Nasal sprays containing phenylephrine (such as Neo-Synephrine) are effective. Decongestant sprays and drops are less likely to interact with other drugs than oral decongestants are.

Decongestant Precautions

- Do not use medicated nasal sprays or drops more than 3 times a day or for more than 3 days in a row. Continued use will cause a "rebound effect": your mucous membranes swell up more than they had swollen before you used the spray.

- Drink extra fluids when taking cold medications.

- Decongestants can cause problems for people who have heart disease, high blood pressure, glaucoma, diabetes, or an overactive thyroid. Decongestants may also interact with some drugs, such as certain antidepressants and high blood pressure medications. Read the package carefully or ask your pharmacist or doctor to help you choose a decongestant.

- Decongestants can cause drowsiness or increased activity in some people. Some brands also interfere with sleep.

- Taking too much of a decongestant can cause hallucinations and convulsions in older people. Use long-acting formulas only as directed.

Cough Preparations

Coughing is your body's way of getting foreign substances and mucus out of your respiratory tract. Coughs are often useful, and you shouldn't try to eliminate them. However, if a cough is severe enough that it interferes with your ability to breathe or rest, you may want to relieve it.

Water and other liquids, such as fruit juices, are probably the best cough syrups. They help soothe the throat and also moisten and thin mucus so it can be coughed up more easily.

You can make a simple and soothing cough syrup at home by mixing 1 part lemon juice with 2 parts honey. Use as often as needed.

There are two kinds of cough medicines: expectorants and suppressants.

Expectorants help thin the mucus, making it easier to bring up when you have a productive cough. Look for expectorants containing guaifenesin, such as Robitussin and Vicks 44E.

Suppressants control or suppress the cough reflex and work best for a dry, hacking cough that keeps you awake. Look for suppressant products that contain dextromethorphan, such as Robitussin-DM or Vicks Dry Hacking Cough.

Don't suppress a productive cough too much (unless it is keeping you from getting enough rest).

Cough Preparation Precautions

- Cough preparations can cause problems for people with certain health conditions, such as asthma, heart disease, high blood pressure, or an enlarged prostate. Cough preparations may also interact with sedatives, certain antidepressants, and other medications. Read the package carefully or ask your pharmacist or doctor to help you choose a cough preparation.

- Cough suppressants can stifle breathing. Use caution when giving a cough suppressant to a person who is very old or frail or who has a chronic respiratory problem.

- Read the label so you know what the ingredients are. Some cough preparations contain a high percentage of alcohol; others contain codeine. There are many choices. Ask your pharmacist to advise you.

Antihistamines

Antihistamines dry up nasal secretions and are commonly used to treat allergy symptoms and itching.

If your runny nose is caused by allergies, an antihistamine will help. For cold symptoms, home treatment and perhaps a decongestant will probably be more helpful. It is usually best to take a single-ingredient allergy or cold preparation, instead of one that contains several active ingredients. Products such as Chlor-Trimeton (chlorpheniramine) and Benadryl (diphenhydramine) are single-ingredient antihistamines. Products such as Dristan, Coricidin, and Triaminic contain both a decongestant and an antihistamine.

Antihistamine Precautions

- Using antihistamines to treat the stuffiness caused by a cold will often thicken the mucus, making it harder to get rid of.

- Drink extra fluids when taking antihistamines.

- Antihistamines can cause problems for some people who have health conditions such as asthma, glaucoma, epilepsy, or an enlarged prostate. Antihistamines may also interact with certain antidepressants, sedatives, tranquilizers, and other medications. Read the package carefully or ask your pharmacist or doctor to help you choose an antihistamine that will not cause problems.

- Antihistamines may cause drowsiness, dizziness, and abnormally low blood pressure in older adults. They may cause increased activity in some people. Do not drive or operate machinery when taking antihistamines.

- Antihistamines that don't cause drowsiness are available by prescription. Ask your doctor if these are appropriate for you.

Pain Relievers

There are dozens of pain reliever products. Most contain either aspirin, ibuprofen, or acetaminophen. These three drugs, as well as ketoprofen and naproxen sodium, relieve pain and reduce fever. Aspirin, ibuprofen, ketoprofen, and naproxen sodium also relieve inflammation. They belong to a class of drugs called nonsteroidal anti-inflammatory drugs (NSAIDs).

When purchasing pain relievers, keep in mind that generic and brand-name products are chemically equivalent. Generic products work just as well as brand-name products, and they cost less.

The product's package label will tell you how much medicine is in each pill (in milligrams or mg), how much you should take, and how often you should take it. Do not exceed the dosage limits, and if you have health problems that may make it unsafe for you to take the usual dosage of a product, follow the special instructions on the package with extra care.

Aspirin

Aspirin is widely used for relieving pain and reducing fever in adults. It also relieves minor itching and reduces swelling and inflammation. Most tablets contain 325 mg of aspirin. Although it seems familiar and safe, aspirin is a very powerful drug.

Aspirin Precautions

- Aspirin can irritate the stomach lining, causing bleeding or ulcers. If aspirin upsets your stomach, try a coated brand, such as Ecotrin. Talk with your doctor or pharmacist to determine what will work best for you.

- Some people are allergic to aspirin. They may also be allergic to ibuprofen.

- Throw aspirin away if it starts to smell like vinegar.

- Do not take aspirin if you have gout or if you take blood thinners (anticoagulants).

- Do not take aspirin for a hangover. Aspirin used with alcohol increases your risk for stomach irritation.

- High doses may result in aspirin poisoning. Stop taking aspirin and call a health professional if any one of these symptoms occurs:
  - Ringing in the ears.
  - Visual disturbances.
  - Nausea.
  - Dizziness.
  - Rapid, deep breathing.

Other Aspirin Uses

In addition to relieving pain and inflammation, aspirin is effective against many other ailments. Because of the danger of side effects and the interactions aspirin may have with other medications, do not try these uses of aspirin without a doctor's supervision.

- **Heart attacks and strokes:** In low but regular doses, aspirin helps prevent heart attacks and strokes in certain people. Aspirin may also help as a first aid measure for heart attacks. See page 53.

- **Stomach and colon cancer**: Some studies have shown that taking 1 aspirin tablet per day can reduce the risk of cancer in the digestive system.

- **Migraines**: Regular, low-dose aspirin use may reduce the frequency of migraines.

Other Pain Relievers

Ibuprofen (the active ingredient in products such as Advil and Nuprin), **ketoprofen** (in products such as Orudis KT and Actron), and **naproxen sodium** (in products such as Aleve) are other nonsteroidal anti-inflammatory drugs (NSAIDs). Like aspirin, these drugs relieve pain and reduce fever and inflammation. Also like aspirin, they can cause nausea, stomach irritation, and heartburn. People who take blood thinners (anticoagulants) should use these pain relievers with caution.

Do not take more than one type of anti-inflammatory medication at a time. Do not take these medications while you are taking a prescription anti-inflammatory medication unless your doctor advises you to do so. Taking these medications together increases the risk of severe irritation to the stomach lining.

Acetaminophen (the active ingredient in products such as Tylenol) reduces fever and relieves pain. It does not have the anti-inflammatory effect of NSAIDs, such as aspirin and ibuprofen, but it also does not cause stomach upset and other NSAID side effects. Acetaminophen is commonly recommended to treat osteoarthritis pain. Acetaminophen is also useful in relieving cold and flu symptoms, such as muscle aches and fever.

Prescription Medications

There are thousands of different prescription medications used to treat hundreds of different medical conditions. Your doctor and your pharmacist are your best sources of information about your prescription medications.

Guidelines for proper use of every kind of prescription medication could fill several books. Common types covered here include antibiotics, minor tranquilizers, and sleeping pills.

Antibiotics

Antibiotics are drugs that kill bacteria. They are effective against bacteria only and have no effect on viruses. Therefore, antibiotics will not cure the common cold, flu, or any other viral illness. Unless you have a bacterial infection, it's best to avoid the possible adverse effects of antibiotics, which may include:

• **Side effects**, including **allergic reactions**. Common side effects of antibiotics include nausea, diarrhea, and increased sensitivity to sunlight. Most side effects are mild, but some, especially allergic reactions, can be severe. A severe allergic reaction usually causes shortness of breath and can be life-threatening. If you have any unexpected reaction to an antibiotic, tell your health professional before another antibiotic is prescribed.

• **Secondary infections**. Antibiotics kill most of the bacteria in your body that are sensitive to them, including the bacteria that help your body. Antibiotics can destroy the bacterial balance in your body, leading to stomach upset, diarrhea, vaginal infections, or other problems.

• **Bacterial resistance**. When antibiotics are used too often, bacteria change so that the antibiotics are no longer effective against them. This increases the difficulty of treating bacterial infections.

When you and your doctor have decided that an antibiotic is necessary, carefully follow the instructions that come with the prescription.

• Take the whole dose for as many days as prescribed, unless you have unexpected side effects (in which case, call your health professional). Antibiotics kill off many bacteria quite quickly, so you may feel better in a few days. However, if you stop taking the antibiotic too soon, the weaker bacteria will have been killed, but the stronger ones may survive and multiply.

• Be sure you understand any special instructions for taking the medication. The instructions should be printed on the label, but double-check with your doctor and pharmacist.

• Store antibiotics in a dry, cool place. Check the label carefully to see if they need refrigeration.

• Never give an antibiotic prescribed for one person to someone else.

• Do not save leftover antibiotics, and do not take an antibiotic prescribed for another illness without a health professional's approval.

Minor Tranquilizers and Sleeping Pills

Minor tranquilizers (such as Valium, Librium, Xanax, and Tranxene) and sleeping pills (such as Dalmane, Restoril, and Ambien) are widely prescribed.

Minor tranquilizers can be effective for short periods of time. However, long-term use is often of limited value and introduces the risk of memory loss, confusion, injuries from falls caused by drug-induced unsteadiness, and addiction.

Sleeping pills may help for a few days or weeks, but using them for more than a month generally causes more sleep problems than it solves. For other approaches, see Sleep Problems on page 333.

If you have been taking minor tranquilizers or sleeping pills for a while, talk with your doctor about whether you can stop taking the medication or reduce your dosage. If you have experienced any unsteadiness, dizziness, or memory loss, tell your doctor. These adverse effects of medications are often mistaken for "normal" signs of aging.

Adverse Drug Reactions

Side effects, drug-drug and food-drug interactions, overmedication, or addiction may cause the following symptoms:

- Nausea, indigestion, and vomiting
- Constipation, diarrhea, or problems with urination
- Dry mouth
- Headache, dizziness, ringing in the ears, or blurred vision
- Confusion, forgetfulness, disorientation, drowsiness, or depression
- Difficulty sleeping, irritability, or nervousness
- Difficulty breathing
- Rashes, bruising, or bleeding problems

Don't assume any symptom is a normal side effect that you have to suffer with. Call your doctor or pharmacist anytime you suspect that your medicines are making you sick.

Medication Problems

As the body ages, it becomes more susceptible to medication-related problems. One in five older adults has experienced an adverse drug reaction to a prescription medication.

Aging brings on changes in the stomach, circulatory system, and kidneys, and in body composition. These changes affect the body's absorption, use, and excretion of medications.

Several different kinds of adverse medication reactions can occur, including:

- **Side effects.** Side effects are predictable but unpleasant reactions to a drug. They are usually mild, but they can be inconvenient. In some cases, side effects can be severe.

- **Allergies.** Drug allergies can cause symptoms such as rashes and nausea. Some people have severe, life-threatening allergic reactions (called anaphylaxis) to certain medications. See Allergies on page 131 for symptoms of an allergic reaction.

- **Drug-drug interactions:** These occur when two or more prescription or nonprescription drugs or herbal medicines mix in a person's body and cause an adverse reaction. The symptoms can be severe and may be improperly diagnosed as a new illness.

- **Drug-food interactions:** These occur when medications react with certain foods. Some drugs work best when taken with food, but others should be taken on an empty stomach. Some drug-food reactions can cause serious symptoms.

- **Overmedication:** Sometimes the full adult dose of a medication is too much for people over age 60. Taking too large a dose may cause severe reactions soon after a drug is taken or after the drug has been taken for a while and has built up in the body.

- **Addiction:** Long-term use of some medications can lead to dependency, and severe reactions may occur if the medications are withdrawn suddenly. To prevent addiction to prescribed narcotics, tranquilizers, and barbiturates, these drugs must be taken very carefully. See page 320.

Prevention

- Take a list of every medication you are taking (prescription and nonprescription, including herbs) to every doctor visit. Don't forget eyedrops, skin ointments or patches, and vitamins.

- When a new medication is prescribed, ask your doctor whether it may interact with other medications you are already taking, including nonprescription medications and herbal supplements.

- Tell your doctor and pharmacist if you have any medication allergies.

- Never take a prescription that was written for another person. Don't share your medications with anyone. A drug that works wonders for you might harm someone else.

- Do not ignore symptoms that you suspect are related to a medication. Even mild symptoms can sometimes cause serious problems. If any symptom is bothersome, your doctor should know about it. Sometimes the dose can be adjusted or a different medication can be recommended to reduce side effects.

- Keep a record of any symptom or side effect you have, even if it is minor. Show it to your doctor.

When to Call a Health Professional

- If any symptom, such as vomiting, difficulty breathing, headache, confusion, or drowsiness, is severe or persistent.

- If symptoms develop soon after you have started taking a new medication, changed the dose of a medication, or eaten a certain food.

- If symptoms such as forgetfulness, depression, confusion, or fatigue develop slowly over a period of weeks or months. Some adverse drug effects take a while to show up.

- If you suspect that a symptom you are having is related to a medication you are taking.

- If any side effect, such as dry mouth or constipation, interferes with your enjoyment of life or makes it hard for you to keep taking the medication as directed.

Health Information at Home

Getting the right health information at the right time is the key to making good health decisions. If the information you need is not in this book, keep looking. Here's how:

On the Internet. Follow the instructions on the back cover of this book to get to the Healthwise® Knowledgebase. With over 100 times the information in the book, the Healthwise Knowledgebase has accurate, unbiased, and regularly updated information on almost all health problems. It is written in language that is easy to understand. And, it is free. If you have Internet access, go to this site first.

If you don't find everything you need in the Healthwise Knowledgebase, don't give up. There is plenty of reliable information out there if you know where and how to look for it. See Five Tips for Finding Good Web Sites on page 392.

On the phone. Many hospitals and health plans have nurse call centers that can respond to your health questions. Local offices of national organizations like the American Cancer Society, American Heart Association, Arthritis Foundation, or American Diabetes Association can help connect you with information resources in your area. Check your phone book.

At your library or bookstore. Research librarians at public libraries spend a good part of their time helping people find information. Ask for their help if you are trying to learn more about a health problem. Libraries can also be a good place to use the Internet if you don't have a computer at home. Be aware that the information found in books and magazines is not guaranteed to be any more accurate than that found on the Internet. Use some of the tips for finding good Web sites as a guide for finding helpful books.

Health information you find on the Internet or in books or magazines should never replace the medical expertise and experience of a health professional. Discuss what you find with your doctor to learn if and how it relates to your particular situation.

Five Tips for Finding Good Web Sites

As a source of health information, the Internet has two major drawbacks. First, there is little to no regulation of what gets published. Misleading, contradictory, inaccurate, and even fraudulent health information is all over the Internet. Second, the amount of information available on the Internet can make your search overwhelming and time-consuming.

With so much information out there, how do you separate the good from the bad? We hope these guidelines will help you find information you can trust.

1. Don't rely on search engines. Instead, go to trusted sources recommended by your health professional, hospital, or health plan. If you have to use a search engine, be sure to follow the other four tips closely.

2. Don't trust the information on a health Web site unless the site clearly indicates:

- Who wrote and reviewed the information.

- When the information was last updated.

- What sources and references the information is based on. (Look for a bibliography or reference list.)

If information is missing, be skeptical of the site's reliability.

3. Check the site's privacy policy. It should tell you that your personal information will not be given to any third party without your explicit permission. Web sites displaying the URAC Health Web Site Accreditation seal should be safe.

4. Check the site ownership or sponsorship. Web sites displaying the URAC Health Web Site Accreditation seal should indicate any influence that the owner or sponsor has on the site's content.

5. Watch out for these clues that a Web site is of questionable quality:

- Heavy use of personal testimonies without references to good research.

- Unsupported claims of a "secret" or "revolutionary" cure.

- Promotion of a specific drug, dietary supplement, medical device, or other product.

- Requirement of a financial investment.

Your final test should be the common sense test. If information doesn't make sense to you, don't trust it without first talking with your health professional. Never make a health care decision based solely on what you read on the Internet.

Index

Notes

Notes

Notes

Notes

Notes

Notes